Legal, Ethical, and Issues in Nursing

Second Edition

Tonia Dandry Aiken, RN, BSN, JD

President and Co-founder of Nurse Attorney Resource Group, Inc.
Louisiana State University Health Sciences Center School of Nursing—
Adjunct Faculty
New Orleans, LA
A Past President
The American Association of Nurse Attorneys and the Foundation

F. A. DAVIS COMPANY • Philadelphia

F. A. Davis Company
1915 Arch Street
Philadelphia, PA 19103
www.fadavis.com

Printed in the United States of America

Last digit indicates print number: 10 9 8 7 6

Acquisitions Editor: Joanne Patzek DaCunha, RN, MSN
Developmental Editor: Caryn Abramowitz
Cover Designer: Louis Forgione

As new scientific information becomes available through basic and clinical research, recommended treatments and drug therapies undergo changes. The author(s) and publisher have done everything possible to make this book accurate, up to date, and in accord with accepted standards at the time of publication. The author(s), editors, and publisher are not responsible for errors or omissions or for consequences from application of the book, and make no warranty, expressed or implied, in regard to the contents of the book. Any practice described in this book should be applied by the reader in accordance with professional standards of care used in regard to the unique circumstances that may apply in each situation. The reader is advised always to check product information (package inserts) for changes and new information regarding dose and contraindications before administering any drug. Caution is especially urged when using new or infrequently ordered drugs.

Library of Congress Cataloging-in-Publication Data

Aiken, Tonia D.
    Legal, ethical, and political issues in nursing / Tonia Dandry Aiken.—2nd ed.
      p. cm.
    Includes bibliographical references and index.
    ISBN 13: 978-0-8036-0571-8 (alk. paper)
    ISBN 10: 0-8036-0571-4 (alk. paper)
      1. Nursing—Polical aspects—United States. 2. Nursing—Law and legislation—United States. 3. Nursing ethics—United States. I. Title.

RT86.5.A37 2003
362.1-73—dc21
                                  2003046061

Preface

The success of the first edition of *Legal, Ethical, and Political Issues in Nursing* made it clear that its user-friendly, practical approach was just what student and clinical nurses needed to understand the often complex legal aspects of providing health care. The second edition continues to use this foundation for the content, and improvements have been made to ensure that content is relevant to all levels and specialty practices, is easier to locate, and is applicable to today's clinical practice.

The second edition has been reorganized into five parts.

Part 1: *Nursing Practice* introduces the legal and ethical issues that lay the foundation for one's ability to practice. It focuses on both the legal right to practice and the responsibility to practice using the highest standards of care.

Part 2: *Nursing and the Law* explains the underlying concepts on which the principles that underlie health care laws are based and illustrates the political processes leading up to developing or changing laws. Understanding this process and the nurse's role in it can empower nurses to be positive change agents and patient advocates.

Part 3: *Nursing Ethics* explains the fundamental principles on which ethical decision making is based. It helps the nurse distinguish between what is often legal but not necessarily ethical.

Part 4: *Liability in Professional Practice* focuses on the doctrines, such as intentional and quasi-intentional torts, risk management, and informed consent, that form the basis of determining right from wrong actions, in turn helping determine how to justly compensate the injured party. It covers how to identify potentially harmful actions and procedures to assist in setting up procedures to reduce or eliminate avoidable negative patient outcomes and to protect the nurse and institution from being held wrongfully liable. It provides practical, useful advice for nurses who may find themselves involved in a malpractice suit, including what to do when being deposed and how to be an expert witness. It helps the student understand the importance of choosing and maintaining professional liability insurance.

Part 5: *Professional Issues* helps the nurse entering into a contract understand the rights a contract provides and, should disputes arise, some positive ways to deal with conflicts. For those nurses with entrepreneurial aspirations, Carolyn Zagury provides details on starting one's own business and empowers the nurse to creatively design his or her own professional career.

We added several new features in this edition.

Each chapter opens with a discussion of the ethical considerations and the underlying ethical principles for the topic that the nurse may encounter in clinical practice.

Numerous *A Case in Point* boxes within the chapters clearly illustrate what happens in real court cases when laws and procedures are challenged or when care provided is alleged to be negligent.

The *What Would You Do?* boxes challenge the reader to consider all the legal and ethical ramifications of real-life cases.

In a Nutshell and *Keep in Mind* sections at the end of each chapter capture the most essential information of the chapter. *Afterthoughts* and *Ethics in Practice* help the reader to think critically about the information and see how it applies to clinical practice.

A list of useful resources at the end of each chapter directs the reader interested in finding out more detail where to find the information.

For the Instructor, a CD is available with an instructor's guide that includes practical tips for teaching legal content, legal issues specific to nurse educators, additional cases, and an electronic test bank.

The textbook is a wonderful resource, but it is not intended to be used as a substitute for legal advice. If legal advice is warranted, the nurse should find an attorney that is qualified and competent in the appropriate area of law.

TONIA D. AIKEN

Acknowledgments

I want to thank my wonderful friend and editor, Joanne DaCunha, the talented contributors, and my colleagues, who were all instrumental in creating the second edition.

Thanks to the following individuals who were instrumental in helping me obtain and organize the most relevant and current legal information:

Sharon L. Alborn
Legal Assistant/Medical Researcher
American Hospital Association
Chicago, IL

David Quidd
Paralegal/Researcher
New Orleans, LA

Theresa Nicholson
Research/Secretarial Services
New Orleans, LA

Ruth A. Takeda
Administrative Program Specialist
State of Colorado Board of Nursing
Denver, CO

I would also like to acknowledge contributors to the first edition, without whose expertise and input this edition would not have been possible.

Mary Powers Antoine, RN, JD
Linda M. E. Auton, RN, BS, JD
Patricia Gauntlett Beare, RN, PhD
Sandra Lee Berkowitz, BSN, JD
D. M. Boulay, RN, JD
Joseph Catalano, RN, CCRN, PhD
Tamara Todd Cotton, BSN, JD
Mical De Brow, RN, MSN, CCRN
Michele L. Deck, RN, BSN, Med, ACCE-R

Thania Savole Elliott, RN, MSH, JD
Anne Goldman, RN, BSN
Nancy S. Jecker, PD
Elizabeth Bowyer Malacoff, RN, BSN, JD
Melinda Mercer, RN, CS, MSN
Katherine J. Pohlman, RN, MSN, JD
Felice Quigley, RN, JD
June Smith Tyler, RN, JD
Ann Verderber, BSN, RPN

TONIA D. AIKEN

Dedication

To my loving husband and soul mate, Jim, and our wonderful children, Brett, Alexes, and Candace, for their support.

To my parents, Shirley and Anthony Dandry, who taught me perseverance.
To my sister, Tina Dandry-Mayes, who has shared so much with me.
To my circle of family and friends, who are always there for me:
Larry, Klye, and Matthew Mayes
Sally, Jack, Lynn, and Larry Aiken
Julie and Courtney Bounds
Kathy Moisiewicz
Jean Farquharson
Rita, Ragus, Andrea, and Ali Legendre

Contributors

James B. Aiken, MD, MHA, FACEP
Assistant Clinical Professor of Emergency Medicine
Louisiana State University School of Medicine
New Orleans, LA
Past President
Orleans Parish Medical Society
Medical Director for Emergency Preparedness at the
Medical Center of Louisiana
New Orleans, LA

Tonia Dandry Aiken, RN, BSN, JD
President and Co-founder of Nurse Attorney Resource Group, Inc.
Louisiana State University Health Sciences Center School of Nursing—
Adjunct Faculty
New Orleans, LA
A Past President
The American Association of Nurse Attorneys and the Foundation

Julia W. Aucoin, DNS, RN, BC
Assistant Professor
University of North Carolina School of Nursing
Greensboro, NC

Julia A. Bounds, CRNA, APRN, BSN
President and CEO
Julia A. Bounds CRNA and Associates
Metairie, Baton Rouge, and Alexandria, LA

Tamela B. Esham, RN, JD
Associate Attorney
Ambrecht Jackson, LLP
Mobile, AL

Jean M. Farquharson, RN, JD
Administrator
Interlink Home Health Services of Southeast Louisiana
New Orleans, LA

Nancy M. Matulich, RN,C, MSN
Legal Nurse Consultant
New Orleans, LA

Carolyn S. Zagury, RN, PhD
President and Founder
Vista Publishing, Inc.
Long Branch, NJ
Director of Clinical Project Development
Monmouth Medical Center
Long Branch, NJ

Consultants

Lynn C. Aiken, RN, BSN, BA
New Orleans, LA

Patricia Ann Bemis, RN, CEN
President
National Nurses in Business Association
Rockledge, FL

Janis M. Campbell, PhD, RN
Chair, Division of Nursing
Walsh University
North Canton, OH

Winifred Carson, JD
Practice Counsel
American Nurses Association
Washington, DC

Dolores J. Eitel, RN, MA, ANP, FNP, CAN, CSN
HealthCare Consultant
Union, NJ

Thania Elliott, RN, MSH, JD
Regional Manager for Disciplinary
Louisiana State Board of Nursing
Metairie, LA

Beth Furlong, RN, PhD, JD
Associate Professor, School of Nursing
Faculty Associate, Center for Health Policy and Ethics
Creighton University
Omaha, NE

Paula Dimeo Grant, RN, BSN, MA, JD
Of Counsel
McGuire Woods, LLP
Washington, DC

Gina Henning, RN, PHN
Project Coordinator
California Department of Health Sciences

Patricia Kimball, RN, MN
Assistant Professor of Nursing
Louisiana State University Health Sciences Center School of Nursing
New Orleans, LA

Kathleen A. Moisiewicz, PhD, RN
Assistant Professor of Clinical Nursing
Louisiana State University Health Sciences Center School of Nursing
New Orleans, LA

Barbara Morvant, RN, MN
Executive Director
Louisiana State Board of Nursing
Metairie, LA

Debbie Fischer Petersen, RN, MSN
Adjunct Assistant Professor
Montana State University—Bozeman College of Nursing
Billings, MT

Winifred J. Ellenchild Pinch, RN, EdD
Professor, School of Nursing
Creighton University
Omaha, NE

Tawna J. Pounders, RN, MNSc
Executive Director
Louisiana State Board of Nursing
Metairie, LA

Frances G. Snodgrass, RN, MA, MS, JD
Chair, Department of Nursing
West Virginia University Institute of Technology
Montgomery, WV

Carolyn R. Tuella, RN, EdD
Chairperson, Presbyterian Division of Nursing
Bloomfield College
Bloomfield, NJ

Diane Trace Warlick, RW, BSN, JD
Co-owner and Founder
Nurse Attorney Resources Group, Inc.

Contents

12 Facility Liability: Employment Issues 277

13 Liability of the Nurse Manager 311

Jean M. Farquharson, RN, JD

To the Student:

Two bonus chapters are available on the F.A. Davis web site:

Licensed Practical Nurse Areas of Liability
Julia W. Aucoin, DNS, RN, BC

Enterepreneur: The Nursing Cycle of Success
Carolyn S. Zagury, RN, PhD

You can download each chapter to read on your computer or to print out. To access these bonus chapters, point your web browser to this address: *http://www.fadavis.com/online_store/catalog/catalogdetail.cfm?section=online_ store&publication_id=1554&subsection-catalog*

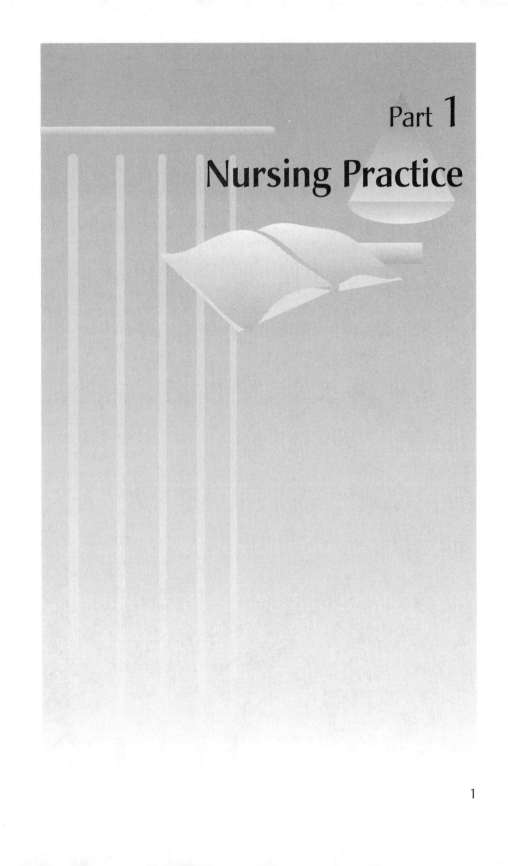

Part 1

Nursing Practice

Nursing Practice   1

Key Chapter Concepts

Licensure

Permissive licensing legislature

Mandatory licensure

Credentialing

Parens patriae power

Nurse practice acts

Boards of nursing

Certification

Board-level certification

Advanced practice certification

Nursing administration certification

Scope of nursing practice

Alternative dispute resolution

Advanced nursing practice

Prescriptive authority

Facility privileges

Third-party reimbursement

Traditional disciplinary system

Disciplinary diversion acts

Disciplinary defense insurance

National Practitioner Data Bank

National Nurses Claims Database

Chapter Thoughts

Today's elaborate and complicated system for licensing and credentialing nurses is a recent development of the health care system. Prior to the early 1900s, a willingness to care, a strong back, and a rudimentary understanding of the treatments used by Florence Nightingale were all that were required to be called a nurse. As nursing became more independent and began to be recognized by the public as a separate occupation, if not profession, some type of safeguard was needed to protect the public from unqualified practitioners. The processes of licensure and credentialing were developed to address the public concern.

Although licensure laws have been in place in one form or another since 1903, it was not until the 1950s that the various nursing organizations began initiating standards to regulate the profession. The first step in developing standards of care for nurses was the American Nurses Association's (ANA) *Code of Ethics for Nurses*. Although this code presents only general guidelines, it forms the basis for most of the standards of care that are used today.

One of the primary functions of state boards of nursing is to protect the public from unqualified persons who attempt to practice the profession of nursing or who pose potential harm to a patient through unsafe practices. Through such mechanisms as the nurse practice act, standards of care, and the code of ethics, the state boards of nursing are able to ensure a degree of public safety where nursing care is involved. The nurse practice act is a legal code, and although stated in very general terms, it does have the force of law and mechanisms for enforcement. Standards of care and codes of ethics are not laws, but they have their own means of enforcement. When a nurse violates either the standards of care or the code of ethics (or both) frequently and with disregard, that person is not acting in a professional manner. Most state boards of nursing have the authority to discipline nurses who are not acting in a professional manner. This discipline can range from a reprimand to licensure suspension or even revocation.

OBJECTIVES

Upon completing this chapter, the reader will be able to:
1. Discuss the relationship between the state nurse practice act and the requirements for entry into practice.
2. Describe how state nurse practice acts define the scope of nursing practice.
3. Describe the role of state boards of nursing.
4. Discuss licensure issues.
5. Discuss what should be done if you find evidence of an impaired colleague.
6. Discuss disciplinary actions and grounds for licensure revocation, suspension, or probation.
7. Discuss the disciplinary process.
8. Discuss common areas for discipline.
9. Define the sanctions that can be imposed on the nurse.
10. Describe components of diversionary programs.

Introduction

Nursing practice has changed considerably over time and will continue to change as health care delivery evolves. As technology advances and the profession responds to societal needs, the regulatory agencies and professional associations continue to redefine the roles, functions, and responsibilities of nurses.

This chapter discusses nursing practice—specifically, the relationship between the state nurse practice act and entry into practice requirements and the scope of practice. The chapter also outlines the role of state boards of nursing and discusses licensure and disciplinary issues.

Licensure

Licensure is the process by which an agency of a state government grants permission to an individual to engage in a given occupation. There must be evidence that the applicant has attained a minimal degree of competency to ensure that public health, safety, and welfare are reasonably protected.[1] Licensing can be described as either permissive or mandatory.

Permissive v. Mandatory Licensing

Permissive licensing legislation regulates the use of a title and requires compliance with the licensing statute only if an individual intends to use the title granted by the licensing authority.

Mandatory licensure regulates the practice of a profession such as nursing and requires compliance with the licensing statute if an individual engages in the activities defined within the scope of that profession.

Prior to the early 1900s, anyone could provide care to those in need. The first nursing licensure laws regulated the use of the title *nurse,* allowing any unlicensed individual to practice provided he or she did not use that title. North Carolina was the first state to adopt a nurse practice act. Eventually, licensure laws regulated not only the use of the title *nurse,* but also the practice of nursing. The laws defined the scope of practice and created requirements for entry into practice, as well as penalties for proscribed actions and penalties for practicing without the requisite license.

Licensure v. Credentialing

Licensure can be contrasted with **credentialing,** or certification, which is a voluntary form of self-regulation seen in many health care disciplines. Whereas *licensure* implies that an individual has met the minimum competency levels set by the state for the public's protection, *credentialing* implies that the individual has met even higher standards. Usually, the profession sets credentialing standards that serve the purpose not only of protecting the public, but also of advancing the profession. In many health care professions, credentialing standards exist for the various subspecialties within that profession. The professional association that represents the subspecialty often contributes to or sponsors the development of the standards for the certification programs for practitioners.[2]

Educational programs and institutions also often seek some type of credentialing certification, such as the accreditation granted to hospitals by the Joint Commission for the Accreditation of Healthcare Organizations (JCAHO) or the accreditation granted to nursing programs by the National League for Nursing (NLN). As in professional subspecialties, educational or institutional accreditation implies that the program or facility has met standards that exceed those of the licensing agency.

Source of the State's Authority

In areas unregulated by the federal government, each state remains free to exercise control over its citizens, provided that state decisions do not conflict with federal laws.

Each state possesses **parens patriae power** (literally translated as "parent of the country" power), which allows it to create laws designed to protect the public's health, safety, and welfare.[3] In creating laws necessary to carry out its responsibility for public protection, a state can reasonably limit individual rights by virtue of its police power.[4]

Licensure laws represent an example of a state's exercise of its police power. States also have **nurse practice acts,** which regulate nursing practice, including requirements to enter into practice and obtain and maintain a license to practice. Requirements for entry into practice typically include graduation from an accredited nursing education program, successful completion of an examination, and payment of a fee to the state (Box 1–1).

Most state nurse practice acts define the scope of practice, establish the requirements for licensure and enter into practice, create and empower a board of nursing to oversee licensees, and identify grounds for disciplinary action.[5] Requirements for entry into practice typically include graduation from an accredited nursing education program, successful completion of an examination, and payment of a fee to the state.

Boards of Nursing

To enforce its nurse practice act, each state creates a board of nursing. Most boards function in a manner typical of a governmental or administrative body, exercising only powers conferred by statute or reasonably implied as necessary to carry out their authority.[6] The board usually exercises rule-making power over regulatory and disciplinary matters involving licensees. The authority of boards varies among states from fully autonomous to advisory power only.[7] Similarly, the composition of boards varies from all-professional boards to those composed of registered nurses (RNs), licensed practical nurses (LPNs) or licensed or vocational nurses (LVNs), and representatives of the public.

Legal representation of the boards also varies. Some boards share legal counsel with other administrative agencies, whereas boards in densely populated states may enjoy counsel dedicated solely to representing health care boards. The increased attention paid to impaired professionals has led to more administrative activity for many boards and a reason to have competent legal counsel. An attorney dedicated

---

BOX 1–1

Nurse Practice Acts

Nurse practice acts perform the following functions:
1. Define the scope of practice
2. Establish the requirements for licensure and entry into practice
3. Create and empower a Board of Nursing to oversee licensee
4. Identify grounds for disciplinary actions

solely to a health care board offers better representation of the board, more efficient and fairer proceedings, and hopefully fewer successful challenges to board decisions and actions.

Regulation of Educational Institutions

Most state boards of nursing also regulate nursing education programs. Many require those programs to obtain accreditation, often from the National League for Nursing (NLN) or the American Association of Colleges of Nursing (AACN). Accreditation by any objective organization is usually granted only after that organization conducts a thorough evaluation to determine whether the applicant program meets the standards established by the accrediting body. Accreditation may affect a program's ability to obtain funding or an individual graduate's chances of later admission for advanced study or the armed services.

In addition to the NLN accreditation required by a state Board of Nursing, other state agencies (such as the Department of Education) may require that the nursing education program obtain accreditation from its official body. To the extent that accrediting bodies publish criteria that must be met before accreditation status is granted, those criteria represent standards for nursing education.

Regulation of Practice

State boards of nursing regulate the requirements to enter the profession and maintain licensure, and the disciplinary actions taken for those who do not comply.

ENTRY-INTO-PRACTICE REQUIREMENTS

Long a source of controversy within the profession, entry-into-practice requirements may differ from state to state. Historically, most state licensure laws created two categories of nurses—licensed practical nurses (LPNs) or LVNs and RNs. LPN licensure requirements usually include successful completion of a 1-year education program and the LPN examination.

RN licensure requirements usually include completion of either a 2-year community college program (associate degree), 3-year hospital-based program (diploma), or 4- or 5-year university program (baccalaureate degree) and successful completion of the RN examination. Despite the variability of the RN educational preparation, most state laws require RN applicants to complete the same examination and grant all successful candidates an identical RN license. Many within the nursing profession have lobbied for standardization of entry requirements. Citing other health care professions as an example, some nursing leaders have proposed the baccalaureate degree as a requirement for entry into practice for professional nurses and the associate degree as a requirement for entry into practice for associate or technical nurses. The struggle to accomplish that objective has been long and complicated.

In 1964 the ANA passed a resolution that specified that all states require a bachelor of science degree in nursing (BSN) for entry into professional practice by 1985.[8] In 1984 the ANA adopted a more realistic timetable, calling for all states to achieve the goal by 1995.[9] In 1985 the ANA urged the state nurses' associations to establish a BSN as the minimum entry level for professional nurses and the associate degree (ADN) as the minimum entry level for associate (technical) nurses.[10]

Although opinions differ within the profession, many who support the BSN for entry into professional nursing practice also support abolishment of the traditional LPN role. They propose expanding LPN educational and licensure requirements to equal associate degree requirements for entry into practice as an associate or technical nurse. Others advocate the elimination of LPN programs but support the licensing of ADN graduates as associate or technical nurses. Still others advocate a single category of licensure as a professional nurse with a BSN as the entry requirement. Supporters of the latter position advocate elimination of all LPN, ADN, and diploma nursing programs. Despite the fact that all states plan to grandfather currently licensed RNs into the professional category, those prepared at the ADN level often speak out against the BSN as the entry requirement, citing the lack of data in support of that position.[11]

Factors cited as responsible for the delay include division among nurses, lack of the necessary commitment from organized nursing, failure to mobilize nursing's natural allies, and the legislature's desire to maintain the security of the status quo.[12]

CERTIFICATION

In 1973 the ANA established the ANA Certification Program to provide tangible recognition of professional achievement in a defined functional or clinical area of nursing. In 1991 this group became the American Nurses Credentialing Center (ANCC), a distinct corporation dedicated to certifying RN and advanced practice nurses in specialty roles. ANCC's Open Door 2000 program has resulted in the Commission on Certification approving the implementation of two major levels of credentialing:

1. Certified (RN,C)
2. Board certified (RN,BC)

Certification is based on several factors:

1. Formal educational preparation
2. Recognition of knowledge
3. Skills
4. Competence developed through experience in a specialty area of practice

Both formal educational preparation and competence in practice are key criteria for *all* certification programs regardless of discipline.

Certification, designated by the RN,C credential, is awarded by the Committee on Certification for Diploma and Associate Degree Nursing Practice and the Committee on Modular Certification. RN,C credential examples include RNs with a bachelor's or higher degree taking the modular exams and RNs with a diploma or associate degree taking the pediatric, perinatal, gerontology, medical-surgical, and psychiatric and mental health nurse exams.

Board-level certification, designated by the RN,BC credential, is awarded by the Board on Certification for Baccalaureate Nursing Practice and the Board on Certification for Advanced Nursing Practice.

Advanced practice certification, designated by the APRN,BC credential, is the new credential approved for advanced practice nurses (nurse practitioners and clinical nurse specialists). The credential BC can be attached to the designation required by the state in which the nurse practices.

Nursing administration certification is designated by the CNA,BC and CNAA,BC credentials.[13]

Certification can also be obtained through nursing specialty organizations such as the American Association of Legal Nurse Consultants, the National Certification Board for School Nursing, the American Association of Nurse Anesthetists, and the American Association of Nurse Practitioners.

MANDATORY CONTINUING EDUCATION

The last decade has seen a trend toward mandatory continuing education for nurses. Most states that have adopted such legislation require nurses to have a specific number of continuing education units (CEUs) or contact hours as a condition for license renewal. See Table 1–1 for individual states' requirements. Renewal of certification status is also usually dependent on completing specific continuing education requirements that are dictated by the specialty certifying organization. See Table 1–2 for some organizations' requirements.

Scope of Nursing Practice

Many social factors, including limited resources and the increasing complexity of health care delivery, have affected the evolution of nursing practice and other health care disciplines. In its Nursing Social Policy Statement, the ANA describes the **scope of nursing practice** as multidimensional and characterized by four major elements.[14] The elements include a core of professional practice common to all members of nursing, dimensions or characteristics of nursing practice, intraprofessional and interprofessional relationships between nursing and other disciplines, and boundaries of nursing practice (Box 1–2).

TABLE 1-1

Continuing Education Requirements for Licensure Renewal and Reentry

State	Renewal	Reentry	Continuing Education Approval/Accreditation Organization		
			SBN	SNA	Other
Alabama	24 hours every 2 years	24 hours in preceding 2 years	*	PN	
Alaska	30 hours	30 hours	PN	PN	
American Samoa	None	Refresher course or retake of licensure examination within 5 years	*		
Arizona	None	30 hours in last 5 years or refresher course		*	
Arkansas	None	None			
California (RN)	30 hours in 2 years	30 hours in 2 years; after 8 years of inactive status, NCLEX-RN required	*		
California (LVN)	30 hours in 2 years	After 4 years of nonrenewal, NCLEX-PN required	PN		Psychiatric technicians
Colorado	None	None			
Connecticut	None	When license has lapsed for more than 3 years, Board may review application and require continuing education			*
Delaware	RN: 30 hours in 2 years PN: 24 hours in 2 years	30 hours for RN, 24 hours for PN, regardless of the number of years	*		*
District of Columbia	Only for inactive license	12 hours per year	*		

PN = Practical nurse; RN = Registered nurse; SBN = State Board of Nurses ; SNA = State Nurses Association.

TABLE 1–1

Continuing Education Requirements for Licensure Renewal and Reentry

| State | Renewal | Reentry | Continuing Education Approval/Accreditation Organization | | |
			SBN	SNA	Other
Florida	25 hours in 2 years, which includes 1 hour of human immuno-deficiency virus/aquired immuno-deficiency syndrome (HIV/AIDS) and 1 hour of domestic violence education	1 hour per month (1 hour of total for HIV/AIDS educa-tion) plus 1 hour of domestic violence educa-tion	*		
Georgia	None	None			
Guam	None	160 hours of clinical learning	*	*	
Hawaii	None	None			
Idaho	None	Varies in 5-year increments up to 20 years		*	
Illinois	None	If absent 5 years: RN, 48 hours theory and 96 hours clinical; PN, 32 hours theory and 64 hours clini-cal	*		
Indiana	None	Varies			*
Iowa	45 hours in 3 years	15 hours in 12 months prior to reinstatement	*		
Kansas	30 hours in 2 years with 15 hours inde-pendent study	10 hours didactic and 180 hours clinical	*		

(continued)

TABLE 1–1

Continuing Education Requirements for Licensure Renewal and Reentry *(continued)*

State	Renewal	Reentry	Continuing Education Approval/Accreditation Organization		
			SBN	SNA	Other
Kentucky	30 hours in 2 years, including 2 hours of AIDS education; must have a one-time 3-hour course on domestic violence within first 3 years of initial licensure	15 hours per year up to a maximum of 150 hours	*	*	
Louisiana (RN)	5, 10, or 15 hours depending on full-time, part-time, or nonpracticing status	60 hours within the past 4 years or refresher course or retake the NCLEX-RN	*	*	*
Louisiana (LPN)	None	Refresher course if out of practice 4 or more years	*		
Maine	None	None			
Maryland	None	Successful completion of (1) Board-approved refresher course; (2) Board-approved reorientation program; (3) minimum of 3 semester hours of nursing credit (after 5 years out of practice)			
Massachusetts	15 hours in 2 years	15 hours in 2 years immediately preceding license reactivation			

TABLE 1–1

Continuing Education Requirements for Licensure Renewal and Reentry

State	Renewal	Reentry	Continuing Education Approval/Accreditation Organization		
			SBN	SNA	Other
Michigan	25 hours in 2 years	25 hours in 2 years	*	*	*
Minnesota	RN: 24 hours in 2 years PN: 12 hours in 2 years	RN: 1 hour for every month out of practice, with a maximum of 150 hours PN: 1 hour for every 2 hours out of practice, with a maximum of 75 hours			
Mississippi	Only if nurse has not practiced within previous 3 years	20 hours every 2 years prior to application for reinstatement, or successful completion of Board-approved reorientation program, or successful completion of minimum of 3 semester credit hours of nursing (after 5 years out of practice)	*	*	*
Missouri	None	None			
Montana	None	If unlicensed anywhere for 3 years, must retest			
Nebraska	20 hours in 2 years plus 500 hours of clinical practice in 5 years	20 hours in last 2 years and 500 hours of clinical practice in last 5 years or Board-approved refresher course		*	

(continued)

TABLE 1–1

Continuing Education Requirements for Licensure Renewal and Reentry *(continued)*

| State | Renewal | Reentry | Continuing Education Approval/Accreditation Organization | | |
			SBN	SNA	Other
New Hampshire	30 hours in 2 years	900 hours active practice within 4 years immediately prior to application; 30 hours in 2 years			
New Jersey	None	None			
New Mexico	30 hours in 2 years or national certification	Meet 30 hours requirement in reentry activity; after 5 years must retake the NCLEX, take refresher course, or complete preceptorship of 75 hours each of didactic and clinical		PN	*
New York	None	None			
North Carolina	None	Board-approved refresher course if licensed is lapsed for 5 years or more	*		
North Dakota	None	Required refresher course if nonpracticing for 5 years or more			
Ohio	24 hours in 2 years	24 hours in preceding 2 years			
Oklahoma	None	None			
Oregon	None	Formal program required if not practiced 900 hours in last 5 years		*	

TABLE 1–1

Continuing Education Requirements for Licensure Renewal and Reentry

| State | Renewal | Reentry | Continuing Education Approval/Accreditation Organization | | |
			SBN	SNA	Other
Pennsylvania	None	None			
Puerto Rico	RN: 36 hours in 3 years PN: 24 hours in 3 years	12 hours per year	*	*	*
Rhode Island	None	None	*		
South Carolina	None	60 hours theory, 80 hours clinical if practiced less than 960 hours in past 5 years	*		
Tennessee	None	None			
Texas (RN)	20 hours in 2 years	20 hours in 2 years		*	*
Texas (LVN)	20 hours in 2 years	20 hours in 2 years; refresher course or supervised employment if inactive more than 2 years	*	*	*
U.S. Virgin Islands	18 hours in 2 years	After 5 years, refresher course of 90 hours didactic and 70 hours clinical	*		
Utah	30 hours in 2 years plus practice	30 hours up to 3 years		*	*
Vermont	None	RN: 120 hours each of theory and clinical after 5 years PN: 60 hours each of theory and clinical after 5 years			
Virginia	None	None			

(continued)

TABLE 1–1

Continuing Education Requirements for Licensure Renewal and Reentry *(continued)*

State	Renewal	Reentry	Continuing Education Approval/Accreditation Organization		
			SBN	SNA	Other
Washington	None	RN: 160 hours clinical and 80 hours theory if absent for 3 years PN: 120 hours clinical and 60 hours theory if absent for 3 years	*		
West Virginia (RN)	30 hours in 2 years	12 hours in 1 year	*	*	
West Virginia (LVN)	24 hours plus 400 hours practice in 2 years	24 hours plus 400 hours practice in 2 years; or, within 90 days of limited license, 12 hours and 200 clinical hours; or refresher course of 80 hours each of theory and clinical	*	*	*
Wisconsin	None	At the discretion of the Board			
Wyoming	20 hours in 2 years	20 hours in 2 years	*	PN	

TABLE 1–2

Web Site Contact Information for the National Certification Boards

Organization	Web Site
American Academy of Nurse Practitioners	http://www.aanp.org/5
American Association of Critical-Care Nurses Certification Corporation	http://www.certcorp.org/
American Association of Diabetes Educators	http://www.nursingworld.org/ancc/ http://www.aadenet.org
American Board for Occupational Health Nurses, Inc.	http://www.abohn.org/certif.htm

TABLE 1–2

Web Site Contact Information for the National Certification Boards

Organization	Web Site
American Board of Neuroscience Nursing	http://www.aann.org/credential/
American Board of Perianesthesia Nursing Certification, Inc.	http://www.cpancapa.org/
American College of Nurse Midwives Certification Council	http://www.accmidwife.org/
American Holistic Nurse Certification Corporation	http://ahna.org/edu/certification.html
American Legal Nurse Consultant Certification Board	http://www.aalnc.org/certification/ http://www.nursingworld.org/ancc/
American Nurses Credentialing Center	http://www.aone.org/
American Organization of Nurse Executives	http://www.apna.org/
American Psychiatric Nurses Association	
American Society of Plastic and Reconstructive Surgical Nurses	http://asprsn.inurse.com/
Association of Pediatric Oncology Nurses	http://www.oncc.org/
Board of Certification for Emergency Nursing	http://www.ena.org/BCEN/
Certification Board Perioperative Nursing	http://www.certboard.org/
Certifying Board of Gastroenterology Nurses and Associates	http://www.cbgna.org/
Council on Certification of Nurse Anesthetists	http://www.aana.com/
Dermatology Nursing Certification Board	http://www.dna.inurse.com/ Certification/
Intravenous Nurses Certification Corporation	http://www.ins1.org/certify2.htm
National Certification Board of Pediatric Nurse Practitioners/Nurses	http://www.pnpcert.org/
Society of Urologic Nurses and Associates	http://www.suna.org/cert/
National Board for Certification of School Nurses	http://www.nbcsn.com/
National Board for Nutrition Support Certification	http://www.nutritioncertify.org/
National Certifying Board for Ophthalmic Registered Nurse	http://webeye.ophth.uiowa.edu/ asorn/certif.htm
Nephrology Nursing Certification Commission	http://anna.inurse.com/
Oncology Nurses Certification Corporation	http://www.oncc.org/
Orthopedic Nurses Certification Board	http://www.orthopaedicnurse.org/ Certification/default.htm
Rehabilitation Nursing Certification Board	http://www.rehabnurse.org/ index5.htm
Wound, Ostomy and Continence Nursing Certification Board	http://www.wocncb.org/

BOX 1–2

ANA's Social Policy Statement: Elements of Scope of Nursing Practice

The ANA's scope of nursing practice includes the following:
1. Core of professional practice common to all members of nursing
2. Dimensions or characteristics of practice
3. Intraprofessional and interprofessional relationships
4. Boundaries

TRADITIONAL NURSING ROLES

ROLE OF THE RN AND LPN: In the beginning of the century, registered nurses provided health-related service, care, and treatment to patients and families. Nurses also were instrumental in organizing hospitalized patients' nursing care and working in the communities to improve health. The emphasis was on the RN's improving the health of patients whether in the hospital or community.[15]

Four factors have stimulated the redesign of the health care roles:

1. The supply of nurses
2. The cost of nursing salaries
3. Redefinition of the role of nursing
4. Changes in other health care professions that impact the role of nurses[16]

Through the years, the registered nurse's role changed to become part of not only the hospital and community, but also of long-term care facilities, home care, and public health services, caring for the sick in all arenas.

Because of the changing demands, nurses must be prepared and clinically competent to handle the vast areas of health care needs. Nurses now can be very mobile in providing health care, and work schedules and sites can vary—a day, a week, an 8-hour shift, or a 12-hour shift. Roles and facilities can vary—hospital, risk manager, or nurse executive. The nurse must have the clinical competence to handle the specialized needs of the patients, along with leadership and managerial skills. The nurse's role has changed through the years to one that is not just a bedside caregiver working in a hospital. Today's nurse must have the clinical competence, leadership skills, and critical thinking skills to work in the highly competitive health care arena in different settings, such as ambulatory, preventive, long-term care, home, and hospital. The nurse must also be computer literate and have effective communication skills and effective skills in negotiation and conflict resolution.

NONTRADITIONAL NURSING ROLES DEFINED

As the health care delivery system continually evolves to meet society's changing needs and financial limitations, more nontraditional roles may emerge.

Nurse attorneys, nurse paralegals, and legal nurse consultants are nontraditional roles that use both professions for a career in the legal world. Nurse attorneys commonly practice in the fields of medical negligence, medical products liability, personal injury, worker's compensation, guardianship, social security, and toxic torts. They also serve as counsel for insurance companies, governmental bodies, or other health care organizations.

Nurse paralegals and legal nurse consultants work with attorneys in an assistant or advisory capacity, are employees of firms or companies, own their own consulting businesses, or serve as independent contractors.

Other nontraditional nursing roles include public speaking and writing books. Many nurses also enjoy teaching, including educating patients, family members, other health care providers, and the public.

AUTHOR TIP: *If you want to be a public speaker, educator, or author, it is important to perform in-depth background research relevant to your audience. Here are some preliminary questions to ask yourself:*

1. Do you know your topic?
2. Is there a need for your type of information?
3. Who is your target market?
4. Who would be interested in buying your book or materials or listening to what you have to say?
5. Who are your competitors?
6. How can you make your book or presentation different or better?
7. What do competitors charge for the book, materials, or seminar?
8. Can you get a sponsor to pay for the seminar or publication costs?

As many nurses strike out on their own these days, other nontraditional roles include nurse entrepreneur or business owner. In addition to the expanded roles discussed earlier, many nurses have become involved in professional activities that require nursing expertise but do not clearly fall within the scope of practice as defined by most nurse practice acts. Health promotion and managed health care represent two of these nontraditional areas.

ALTERNATIVE DISPUTE RESOLUTION AND NURSING

A wave of the future for nurses involves their learning, teaching, and applying mediation and negotiation skills. This area of expertise is called **alternative dispute resolution** (ADR) and is discussed more fully in later chapters (Box 1–3). Nurses who are trained mediators and negotiators become invaluable in the following ways:

1. Negotiating contracts (with employers, vendors, physicians, and others in the health care arena)
2. Mediating and facilitating disputes among employees, independent contractors, patients and their families, or coworkers
3. Acting as consultants in cases involving personal injuries or medical negligence and assisting in the actual mediation

---

BOX 1–3

Alternative Dispute Resolution

Features of alternative dispute resolution include some of the following:

Mediator: Neutral third party who facilitates agreements by helping both sides to identify their needs and underlying interests.

Mediation: The process in which both sides agree on a third party who facilitates an analysis and, step by step, a mutually beneficial resolution to the issues.

Arbitration: A process during which both sides select a neutral third-party arbitrator usually with technical knowledge in the area of contention. The arbitrator hears the case and renders a decision and award. The arbitration decision can be binding or nonbinding, depending on what the parties agreed on prior to beginning the arbitration.[17]

ADVANCED NURSING PRACTICE AND THE EXPANDING ROLE OF NURSING

Historically, nursing has struggled with boundaries, particularly with respect to the overlap between nursing and medical practice. Physicians' assistants, certified medical assistants, unlicensed assistive personnel, wound care technicians, and registered care technicians represent several types of "physicians' extenders" that further cloud the boundaries between the various medical practitioners. The historical overlap has led to the development of **advanced nursing practice** or expanded nursing roles. As health care delivery has changed, many of the functions once defined as expanded practice now have been legally absorbed into the scope of professional nursing practice of the RN. Expanded nursing roles usually include nurse midwives, nurse anesthetists, nurse practitioners, and clinical nurse specialists. The latter category often includes nurse administrators, as well as nurses practicing in subspecialties (such as pediatrics and mental health).

Nurse midwifery and nurse anesthesia actually developed prior to the regulation of nursing.[18] As early as 1912, the literature proposed training nurse midwives, and by the 1920s nurse anesthetists were relatively common. Clinical specialization dates back to 1936, and history can trace the nurse practitioners' movement back to 1965. After a report by the United States Department of Health, Education, and Welfare in 1971, Congress made available federal funding to train nurse practitioners as primary care providers.[19]

Not all states have adopted the same approach to regulation of the expanded role. Some states control advanced nursing practices through specific statutes separate from the state's nurse practice act. In some states, the nurse practice act authorizes advanced nursing practice, but the Board of Nursing has established regulations that define and control that practice. Such expanded role regulations usually require that a nurse demonstrate evidence of additional education or experience and, in some cases, the existence of a supervisory relationship with a physician. Many state boards require that the nurse obtain certification through the ANCC or another specialty organization.

LEGAL CHALLENGE TO SCOPE OF ADVANCED NURSING PRACTICE

In some states, nursing has met with success in legal challenges related to the control of practice. In a landmark case, *Sermchief v. Gonzales*,[20] the Missouri court recognized the actions of certified nurse practitioners as the legal practice of nursing rather than the illegal practice of medicine. The nurse practitioners were providing routine gynecologic care (including such things as Papanicolaou [Pap] smears and pregnancy testing) pursuant to protocols developed jointly by the nurses and supervising physicians. The Missouri Nurse Practice Act did not require direct physician supervision or identify nurse practitioners separately, but instead defined professional nursing as "The performance of any act which requires substantial specialized education, judgment and skill...including, but not limited to: ...teaching health care and the prevention of illness...assessment, nursing diagnosis, nursing care and counsel...the administration of medications and treatments as prescribed by a person licensed in this state to prescribe."[21]

Sermchief represented a significant victory in the struggle for nursing autonomy. That struggle continues in many states, supported by the ANA and its strong belief that nurse practice acts should broadly define nursing.[22] A broad definition allows flexible boundaries and minimizes the need for frequent legislative amendments to respond to changes in health care delivery.

PRESCRIPTIVE AUTHORITY

Prescriptive authority is the limited authority to prescribe or dispense certain medications or devices incidental to routine health or family planning, according to established protocols.

Two issues emerge when discussing prescriptive authority for nurses: (1) Does the state recognize the prescriptive authority of nurses? (2) Does the state regulate that authority within the context of professional nursing practice? As with scope of practice and other professional nursing issues, the Board of Nursing rather than state agencies should retain control.

California was the first state to grant prescriptive authority to nurses. Since 1991 nurse practitioners (as distinguished from registered nurses) in several states have had limited authority to prescribe certain medications pursuant to protocols, often developed jointly by a nurse and physician. Most states permit advanced practice nurses to prescribe to some degree. Restrictions to prescribing are constantly being revised or challenged. The latest regulations are compiled by the ANA and are available on their Web site at *http://www.nursingworld.org/gova/charts/dea.htm.*

Many of the prescriptive authority provisions also allow nurses to dispense certain medications, although comments accompanying the ANA-suggested legislation on prescriptive authority urge caution in the area of dispensing,[23] recommending that legislation limit dispensing authority to no more than the doses of medication necessary until a patient can obtain a full prescription from a pharmacist.[24] Presumably, such limited authority represents a balance among such variables as the additional liability associated with dispensing and the overlapping boundaries between nursing and pharmacy.

FACILITY PRIVILEGES

As more and more nurses enter independent practice in their expanded roles, hospital and other **facility privileges** become an increasingly controversial issue. In many subspecialties, such as mental health, a nurse cannot practice to the fullest scope of the profession without first obtaining privileges.

For the most part, privileges are handled by the granting facility rather than the state legislature. The extent of nursing privileges varies widely among facilities. At some facilities, privileges merely include the opportunity to visit the patient outside regular visiting hours. At other hospitals, privileges allow nurses to make entries in the medical record. Few facilities consider privileges to include the right to admit a patient without a supervising physician. Nurses have received some assistance from the courts in their efforts to secure privileges.[25]

THIRD-PARTY REIMBURSEMENT

Many of the issues discussed earlier, including the expanded role, prescriptive authority, and facility privileges, have had an indirect effect on the nursing profession's efforts to obtain **third-party reimbursement** (e.g., payment from the patient's insurance carrier for services rendered). As nurses legally assume increased responsibility for the primary care of patients, third-party reimbursers have been forced to provide benefits for services. In some states, the legislature has forced the issue by adopting laws that require reimbursement of nurses to the extent that they provide services identical to those for which other providers receive reimbursement. Nurse psychotherapists have benefited most often from such legislation.

Unfortunately, certification and third-party reimbursement requirements sometimes limit direct reimbursement to nurses practicing in expanded roles, such as nurse practitioner.[26] When such requirements rely on broadly worded language, a nurse may successfully challenge the provisions through administrative channels. In some states that have not passed legislation, third-party reimbursers have voluntarily offered coverage for such services, realizing that reimbursement for the less costly nursing services minimizes the need for the more costly services of a physician.

Disciplinary Proceedings

TRADITIONAL DISCIPLINARY PROVISIONS

All nurse practice acts provide a **traditional disciplinary system.** Such systems empower the state board to take action against a nurse's license for certain violations that are specifically outlined by the board or defined by regulations. In addition to granting the power to take action against a license, the nurse practice act also empowers the board to reinstate licenses.

Traditionally, boards can deny, revoke, suspend, probate, limit, or otherwise condition a license for violations in areas such as substance abuse, negligence, endangerment, patient safety, incompetence, criminal activity, or other violations of the nurse practice act.

In fact, some acts include broad language that allows the board to discipline for *unprofessional conduct,* a term interpreted differently in various states (Box 1–4). Often regulation or case law interprets broad language such as this.

Although each state's administrative procedures act (or its equivalent) specifically defines the manner in which the board must proceed when disciplining a licensee, most involve a similar process. The board usually must investigate a complaint prior to taking any action, unless the law provides for summary suspension, a rare action reserved for situations involving extreme danger to the public. Even where the law permits summary suspension, the licensee has the right to exercise due process rights similar to those available to all licensees subjected to disciplinary charges (Box 1–5).

Unless waived, a nurse is entitled to notice of the time and place of the investigatory hearing.[27] The nurse also has the right to an attorney, to a clear statement of the charges, to confront and produce witnesses, to a record of the proceedings, and to a fair determination by the presiding body based on the evidence presented. Finally, the nurse is entitled to some type of appeal or judicial review, whether by the full board or the state court.

BOX 1–4

Disciplinary Actions

Disciplinary actions by a Board of Nursing can include:
a. Denial of the license
b. Revocation
c. Suspension
d. Probation
e. Placement of conditions such as educational requirements, fines, drug screens, psychological/psychiatric evaluations, evaluation by an addictionologist, supervisory requirement, periodic evaluations, or restrictions on the type of nursing you can perform (e.g., home health)

BOX 1–5

Nurses' Rights Before, During, and After Administrative Disciplinary Proceedings

Nurses have the rights to the following:
1. Notice of the time and place of the investigatory hearing
2. An attorney
3. A clear statement of the charges
4. Confront and produce witnesses
5. A record of the proceedings
6. A fair determination by the presiding body, based on the evidence
7. An appeal or judicial review

Despite the variability among states, the rules of evidence applied by most administrative proceedings are less formal than those used in civil or criminal cases. The burden of proof, or amount of evidence required to support a particular board decision, also varies from state to state. Many states apply a variation of the substantial evidence test, a burden defined by Arkansas as "evidence that is valid, legal and persuasive and such relevant evidence as a reasonable mind might accept as adequate to support a conclusion."[28] The most common reasons for disciplinary actions are listed in Box 1–6.

BOX 1–6

Common Grounds for Disciplinary Actions

1. Committing Medicare/Medicaid fraud
2. Patient abuse
3. Diverting or stealing narcotics
4. Failure to use good nursing judgment
5. Documentation errors
6. Aiding and abetting a criminal
7. Falsifying information on your renewal or application;
8. Failure to report previous criminal actions (e.g., driving while intoxicated)
9. Practicing outside the scope of the nurse practice act
10. Practicing without a valid license
11. Substance abuse
12. Negligence
13. Incompetence
14. Criminal activity
15. Violation of the Nurse Practice Act
16. Unprofessional conduct

The development of a defense against disciplinary charges involves the same principles applicable in any administrative, civil, or criminal case. Perhaps the most critical variable is retaining a knowledgeable attorney who can assist with preparation of the defense. Although many attorneys offer such assistance, nurse attorneys often serve as particularly well-qualified advocates, based on their understanding of the profession and its regulations. Regardless of the nurse's choice of advocate, thorough investigation forms the foundation of any defense.

Although the nurse practice act may empower a state Board of Nursing to discipline a licensee for negligence, that administrative action remains separate from a civil action. Any individual who believes that he or she has suffered an injury as a result of a nurse's professional negligence can file a lawsuit against that nurse for damages. Unlike a criminal conviction, a finding of negligence in a civil action (i.e., a medical malpractice claim) does not necessarily serve as the basis for disciplinary action. The board can conduct an investigation at the same time as the civil lawsuit or after the suit has ended. If the board is empowered by the nurse practice act, the board can take action against the licensee.

If a nurse signs a consent order or the board renders a decision, the following disciplinary actions may be part of the final document:

1. Fines
2. Requirement of a certain number of continuing education hours
3. Additional skill training
4. Reports from supervisors
5. Drug testing (if drugs or alcohol are at issue)
6. Consultation reports from a psychiatrist, psychologist, or addictionologist if drugs, alcohol, or mental illness are at issue
7. Notification if the nurse is prescribed medication by a physician (if drugs or alcohol are at issue)
8. Notification of a change in employment
9. Notification of a change in address
10. Monitoring fees

The most common results of disciplinary actions are the following:

1. The allegation or claim is dismissed.
2. A formal or informal letter of reprimand is placed in the nurse's file and will remain there as long as the nurse practices.
3. Probation, which allows the nurse to practice, but he or she may be required to perform certain tasks, such as the following:
   a. Have supervisory reports sent to the board
   b. Be monitored by another RN
   c. Attend educational classes
   d. Pay a fine
   e. Pay a monitoring fee
   f. Take random drug tests (blood or urine)

    g. Be evaluated by a psychologist, psychiatrist, or addictionologist

    h. Receive approved treatment for substance abuse

    i. May be prohibited from practicing in certain areas that are unsupervised (e.g., homes, long-term care facilities)

4. Suspension of the license will prohibit the nurse from practicing for a period designated by the board. The nurse may have to do several of the tasks indicated in number 3 before the board allows the nurse to request to be reinstated. (The nurse may also receive a suspension with stay, meaning he or she will be allowed to practice.)

5. Revocation means that the nurse is not allowed to practice. The period of revocation may be indicated.

DISCIPLINARY DIVERSION ACTS

Over the last decade, the nursing profession has demonstrated a commitment to the rehabilitation of nurses impaired by psychological dysfunction or substance abuse, particularly drugs and alcohol, supporting legislative initiatives known as **disciplinary diversion acts,** such as rehabilitative programs under the state Board of Nursing, to divert impaired nurses from traditional disciplinary procedures (Box 1–7).

When determining whether to reinstate a nurse's license, the criteria judged most significant among board members include active treatment and an ability to function safely in the workplace, as certified by a psychiatrist, psychologist, or addictionologist. Whether these two criteria are met is determined by the results of a board evaluation, letters of recommendation, evaluations of the nurse, and the persuasiveness of a physician's statement of support. These same criteria represent the conditions required by many nursing disciplinary diversion acts. In some circumstances, as long as a nurse is able to meet these two conditions, the nurse is allowed to retain a limited nursing

---

BOX 1–7

Diversionary Programs

Diversionary programs are effective alternatives to the disciplinary process. Confidentiality is a key factor in the program. Other features can include the following:

1. Confidential consultation with the employer, coworkers, family, and friends
2. Ongoing monitoring
3. Mandatory drug and alcohol screening
4. Education
5. Group sessions with other health care providers
6. Assistance with employers
7. Referrals to local support groups
8. Immediate intervention to protect the public

license, which permits the nurse to rehabilitate, enjoy the rehabilitative benefits of employment, and earn money.

Failure to comply with the voluntary rehabilitation program, sometimes called the Recovery Nurse Program, can result in reversion to the traditional disciplinary procedures. The model diversion program allows a nurse to avoid traditional disciplinary actions such as license revocation, provided that the nurse complies with the rehabilitative program overseen by the committee. Records of rehabilitation and board action remain confidential and, unless a relapse occurs, may be destroyed after 5 years. Immunity provisions exist for those providing information related to a nurse's functioning or rehabilitation.

If a nurse suspects that a colleague is impaired, he or she must act to protect patients and prevent potential for liability and legal actions against the facility. Warning signs of impairment may include but are not limiting to the following:

Physical signs

- Slurred speech
- Alcohol odor
- Irrational or irritable behavior
- Mood swings
- Blackouts (temporary amnesia)

Job-related signs

- Numerous narcotics or documentation errors
- Frequent sleeping on the job
- Only a minimum amount of work performed
- Isolation from the social group
- Untidy appearance
- Excessive tardiness and absenteeism
- Increased somatic complaints
- Elaborate excuses for behavior[29]

The nurse should contact his or her supervisor, who should counsel the colleague suspected of substance abuse. Some facilities have assistance programs. Other facilities may send the information to the state Board of Nursing's Recovering Nurse Program. Such programs may be coordinated and monitored internally by the board. Some boards refer nurses to approved facilities and health care providers.

DISCIPLINARY DEFENSE INSURANCE

Many facilities provide professional liability insurance policies for nurses that will cover legal fees and expenses incident to a civil suit or malpractice case. But if a nurse is faced with disciplinary proceedings and must defend his or her nursing license, **disciplinary defense insurance** can provide for such things as the following:

1. Legal fee reimbursement or payment to the attorney
2. Wage loss reimbursement
3. Travel, food, and lodging reimbursement
4. Qualified attorneys for representation

AUTHOR TIP: *Check with your insurance company to see if disciplinary defense insurance is offered. The cost may be included in the premium for your professional liability policy or may be an additional rider or separate policy cost.*

National Practitioner Data Bank

The **National Practitioner Data Bank** (NPDB) is a central repository of information on physicians, dentists, and, at times, other health care practitioners. The NPDB became operational on September 1, 1990.[30] Congress enacted the Health Care Quality Improvement Act (HCQIA) based on a belief that the need to improve the quality of care and slow down the increasing malpractice litigation could no longer rest solely with the licensing bodies in the states.[31] The intent of the HCQIA is to provide "positive incentives" for participation in peer review, predominantly in the form of good faith immunity for those providing information to the NPDB.[32]

The NPDB contains information on the following:

1. Medical malpractice payments
2. Adverse licensure actions
3. Adverse clinical privilege actions
4. Adverse professional society membership actions

The NPDB was created in an effort to improve the quality of health care by encouraging facilities, state licensing boards, and others to report those health care professionals who were unprofessional. The NPDB also restricts the incompetent providers from moving from state to state without disclosure of previous medical malpractice payment or adverse action history (Box 1–8).

Some features of the NPDB include the following:

1. The NPDB is intended to facilitate a comprehensive review of practitioner's professional credentials.
2. The NPDB should not replace a credential's review.
3. The Data Bank reports information confidentially at the risk of civil money penalties imposed by the Office of Inspector General. For each violation of confidentiality, a civil money penalty of up to $11,000 can be levied. If more than one party (individual, entity, or organization) has improperly disclosed information, each can be assessed up to $11,000.

The NPDB is available to state licensing boards, hospitals and other health care entities, professional societies, federal agencies, and others according to law.

BOX 1–8

National Practitioner Data Bank

1. NPDB addresses the following types of data:
   a. Information relating to medical malpractice payments made on behalf of health care practitioners
   b. Information relating to adverse actions taken against clinical privileges of physicians, osteopaths, or dentists
   c. Information concerning actions by professional societies that adversely affect membership
   d. Information relating to adverse licensure actions
2. Types of information reported:
   a. Required reporting—adverse professional review actions against physicians, osteopaths, and dentists
   b. Optional reporting—adverse professional review actions against other health care providers (including nurses)
   c. Required reporting—medical malpractice payments made on behalf of all health care providers

---

Keep in mind the NPDB is legally prohibited from disclosing information on a specific practitioner provider or supplier to a member of the general public.

Although public attention has focused predominantly on its effect on the practice of medicine, the NPDB does impact the nursing profession. NPDB information is available on request to hospitals and health care entities engaged in credentialing. The Web site is *www.npdb-hipdb.com*.

Reports to the NPDB

Reporting of information relating to adverse professional review actions against physicians, osteopaths, and dentists is required. Reporting regarding other health care providers (including nurses) is optional. On the other hand, reporting medical malpractice payments is required on behalf of all health care providers. Optional reporting most likely will affect nurse midwives, nurse anesthetists, and nurse practitioners, because those professionals often are subject to credentialing procedures similar to those associated with clinical privileges.

Although health care providers receive notice of reports filed, they can request copies of any report filed against them. Procedures for appeal exist for those hoping to challenge the validity or accuracy of reported information.

The ANA runs the **National Nurses Claims Database,** which attempts to collect data on nursing malpractice claims. However, the database relies on voluntary reporting by the nurse involved in the malpractice litigation.

▒ Financial Responsibility for Practice

The financial burden of defending against an administrative or civil proceeding can be significant. As a result, many nurses arrange for professional liability insurance and disciplinary action insurance as protection against such burdens. Many do so regardless of the coverage available through an employer. The American Association of Nurse Attorneys maintains that financial responsibility for practice is a fundamental component of professional accountability.[33] Given the increasing incidence of litigation against health care professionals and the costs to the health care system and society, many states have undertaken tort reform. In an attempt to reverse the litigious trend, some states have explored state compensation pools for individuals injured by a professional with inadequate insurance or financial resources to compensate the injured party otherwise. A nurse should be familiar with the various sources of financial relief for injured patients and should consider those when making a decision regarding insurance and accountability for professional practice.

KEEP IN MIND

▶ Licensure is the process by which an agency of a state government grants permission to an individual to engage in a given occupation.

▶ Credentialing implies that the professional has met higher standards than licensure.

▶ Nurse practice acts define the scope of practice, establish licensure requirements and entry into practice, empower a board to oversee licensees, and identify grounds for disciplinary actions.

▶ Prescriptive authority allows limited authority for nurses to prescribe medications.

▶ Third-party reimbursement requirements may limit direct reimbursement to nurses.

▶ Mandatory continuing education for nurses is a trend that is increasing throughout the United States.

▶ Several grounds for state Board of Nursing disciplinary actions include substance abuse, negligence, endangerment of patient safety, incompetence, criminal activity, unprofessional conduct, or violation of the nurse practice act.

▶ Disciplinary defense insurance can pay for such costs as attorney fees, lost wages, travel, and lodging.

▶ The National Practitioner Data Bank was created by the Health Care Quality Improvement Act of 1986.

▶ The ANA's National Nurses Claims Database collects data on nursing malpractice claims, but the database only contains information contributed voluntarily.

In a Nutshell

Understanding state nurse practice acts and licensure issues are essential to safe, legal nursing practice. Because disciplinary process and grounds for such actions vary among the states, it is essential for every nurse to obtain, read, and understand the laws and standards governing nursing practice. A copy of the nurse practice act and standards of care can be obtained from the state Board of Nursing and may often be found on their Web site. Additionally, the National Council of State Boards of Nursing has a wealth of information to help nurses understand their rights and the responsibilities of professional nursing practice.

Afterthoughts

1. Discuss the source of the state's authority for licensure and its purpose in exercising that authority.
2. Discuss the source of the board's disciplinary authority.
3. Discuss at least three grounds for disciplinary action, the potential defenses to each, and the actions available to the board of registration for each.
4. Discuss the differences between entry requirements for practice as a professional nurse and as an associate nurse and the history of the development of the different requirements.
5. Discuss the implications of separate expanded role licensure for nurse practitioners.
6. Discuss the functions of the state Board of Nursing.
7. What is licensure, and what are the differences between licensure and credentialing?
8. Discuss third-party reimbursement and how it can affect the nursing profession.
9. Discuss the purpose of the National Practitioner Data Bank. How does it differ from the ANA's National Nurses Claims Database?
10. Discuss what can happen if a disciplinary action is filed against you.
11. What is the nurse's role today with regard to prescriptive authority in your state?
12. How has the nurse's role expanded over the last 10 years in the health care arena?
13. Discuss the disciplinary defense insurance policy.
14. Discuss two types of nontraditional nursing roles. Talk to individuals practicing in these roles and report to the class.
15. How can the nurse use Alternative Dispute Resolutions in the health care setting?

16. Does your state require mandatory continuing education for licensure and license renewal? What are the specific requirements?

ETHICS IN PRACTICE

After her initial 6-week orientation period, Patty N., a new graduate RN, was beginning her first job on the 11 to 7 shift in a busy surgical unit of a city hospital. Patty enjoyed the busy pace of the unit, the development of new skills in the care of complicated post-operative patients, and the spirit of cooperation and camaraderie with the other nurses on the shift. She particularly liked to see the patients recover and resume a normal life.

Because of the nature of the surgical unit and the fact that most of the patients were in pain to some degree, large quantities of narcotics and other pain medications were used. Occasionally the narcotic count was off at the end of the shift, but the nurses were usually able to track down who forgot to sign out a medication. After several weeks of working on the unit, Patty began to notice that the narcotic count was always wrong when Vickie L., an older RN who had worked on the unit for 5 years, was on duty. Patty also noticed that Vickie signed out pain medications for her patients at the minimal intervals ordered all through the shift, even if the patient had not received any medication for the previous 24 hours.

Patty asked one of the other nurses about Vickie. The nurse told Patty that Vickie was an excellent nurse, a hard worker, and would be virtually impossible to replace if she were to leave or be fired. Patty was also reminded that she was the newcomer to the unit and that she really should not make waves. If Patty really wanted to help, she was informed that she could cover for Vickie, as the other nurses did, when she was "sick," which was often.

After observing Vickie more closely, Patty recognized the symptoms of drug abuse that she had been taught in school, including moody and erratic behavior, frequent absences because of "illness," forgetting to give scheduled medications on time, and frequent and prolonged bathroom breaks throughout the shift. Patty felt that Vickie's behavior and problem were dangerous to the patients she was caring for at the hospital.

What should Patty do? What are the key elements in this ethical dilemma? What does the Code of Ethics for Nurses say about incompetent practitioners? Are there any legal or ethical obligations that apply to Patty's actions?

References

1. Shimberg, B: Occupational Licensing: A Public Perspective. Center for Occupational and Professional Assessment, Educational Testing Service, Princeton, 1982.
2. Driscoll, VM: Legitimizing the Profession of Nursing: The Distinct Mission of the New York Nurses' Association. Foundation of the New York Nurses' Association, New York, 1976.
3. Parens patriae, literally "parent of the country," refers traditionally to the role of the state as sovereign and guardian of persons under legal disability. State of W. Va. v. Chas. Pfizer & Co., C.A.N.Y., 440 F.2d 1079, 1089. Parens patriae originates from English Common Law, in which the king had a royal prerogative to act as guardian to persons with legal disabilities, such as infants, idiots, and lunatics. In the United States, the parens patriae function belongs with the states. See Black's Law Dictionary, ed 5. West Publishing, St. Paul, Minn, 1979, p 1041.

4. Police power is the power of the state to place restraints on the personal freedom and property rights of a person for the protection of the public safety, health, and morals or the promotion of the public convenience and general prosperity and is an essential attribute of government. Police power is subject to the limitations of the federal and state constitutions and especially to the requirements of due process. See Black's Law Dictionary, ed 5. West Publishing, St. Paul, Minn, 1979, p 1041.
5. Velsor-Friedrich, B, and Hackbarth, DP: A house divided. Nursing Outlook 38(3):129–133, 1990.
6. Northrop, CE: Licensure revocation. In Northrop, CE, and Kelly, ME (eds): Legal Issues in Nursing. Mosby, St. Louis, 1987, pp 405–422.
7. Ibid.
8. Pohlman, KJ, et al: Should nursing implement the 1985 resolution? In McCloskey, J, and Grace, HK (eds): Current Issues in Nursing. Blackwell Scientific Publications, Boston, 1981, pp 149–159.
9. Hood, G: At issue: titling and licensure. American Journal of Nursing 85(5):592–594, 1985.
10. Lewis, E: Taking care of business: the AMA house of delegates. Nursing Outlook 33(5):239–243, 1985.
11. Ibid.
12. Velsor-Friedrich, B, and Hackbarth, DP: A house divided. Nursing Outlook 38(3):129–133, 1990.
13. http//www.nursingworld.org/ancc/index.htm (2002).
14. American Nurses' Association: Nursing Social Policy Statement (Publ. No. NP-68A). American Nurses' Association, Kansas City, MO, 1980, pp 3–4.
15. The Evolving Role of the Registered Nurse. American Oragonization of Nurse Executives, 1999.
16. Kerfoot, K: Role redesign: what has it accomplished? Online Journal of Issues in Nursing, Dec. 22, 1997.
17. Aiken, J, Aiken, T, Grant, P, and Warlick, D: The basics of alternative dispute resolution. In Legal and Ethical Issues in Health Occupations. WB Saunders, Philadelphia, 2002.
18. Kelly, ME: Control of the practice of nurse practitioners, nurse midwives, nurse anesthetists and clinical nurse specialists. In Northrop CE, and Kelly, ME (eds): Legal Issues in Nursing. Mosby, St. Louis, 1987, pp 469–485.
19. Ibid, p 469.
20. Sermchief v. Gonzales, 660 S.W.2d 683 (Mo., banc., 1983).
21. Mo. Rev. Stat. Sec. 335.016.8(A)-(E), 1975.
22. Mechanic, HF: Redefining the expanded role. Nursing Outlook 36(6):280–284, 1988.
23. American Nurses' Association: Suggested State Legislation: Nursing Practice Act, Nursing Disciplinary Diversion Act, Prescriptive Authority Act (Publ. No. NP-78). American Nurses Association, Kansas City, MO, 1990, pp 1–46.
24. Ibid.
25. Wrable v. Community Memorial Hospital, 205 N.J. Super. 428 (1985), aff'd, 517A.2d 470 (10/22/86), cert. denied, 526 A.2d 210 (4/28/82).
26. Mechanic, HF: Redefining the expanded role. Nursing Outlook 36(6):280–284, 1988.
27. Northrop, CE: Licensure revocation. In Northrop, CE, and Kelly, ME (eds): Legal Issues in Nursing. Mosby, St. Louis, 1987, pp 405–422.
28. Arkansas State Board or Nursing v. Long, 651 S.W.2d 109 (Ark .1983).
29. Louisiana State Board of Nursing, Recovering Nurse Program Brochure, January 6, 1998.
30. Health Care Quality Improvement Act of l986 (Title IV of P.L. 99–660) (11/14/86), 42 U.S.C. 11101 et, seq., as amended by Sec. 402 of P.L. 100–177, Public Health Service Amendments of 1987 (12/1/87) and Sec. 6103(e)(6) of P.L. 101–239 Omnibus Budget Reconciliation Act of 1989 (12/19/89) amending Sec. 402 of P.L. 100–177.
31. Ibid.
32. Ibid.
33. American Association of Nurse Attorneys: Demonstrating Financial Responsibility for Nursing Practice. American Association of Nurse Attorneys, Baltimore, 1989.

Resource

American Nurses Credentializing Center
600 Maryland Ave.
SW Suite 100
West Washington, D.C., 20024–2571.
800–284–2378

Part 2

Nursing and the Law

Standards of Care 2

Key Chapter Concepts

ANA Code of Ethics for Nurses with Interpretive Statements
Standards of care
Comprehensive Accreditation Manual for Hospitals
Statutes
Regulations
Standards of professional performance
Standard

Guideline
Bylaws
Policy
Procedures
Expert
Relevant
Hearsay evidence
Error-in-judgment rule
Two-schools-of-thought doctrine

Chapter Thoughts

Standards of care are used daily in all aspects of nursing care. Standards of care form the basis for competent, high-quality nursing care. The basic purpose of these standards is to protect and safeguard the public. Standards of care are the "yardsticks" by which the legal system measures the actions of a nurse in a malpractice suit.

In the **ANA Code of Ethics for Nurses with Interpretive Statements**, nine provisions are listed that state the ethical obligations and duties of nurses. The provisions describe such things as (1) the nurse's fundamental commitment and values, (2) boundaries of duty and loyalty, (3) aspects of duties related to advancing the profession, and (4) collaborative efforts with other health care professions to shape policy and meet the health needs of society. The ANA Code of Ethics for Nurses provides a framework to aid nurses in resolving ethical dilemmas and in analysis and decision making in day-to-day work settings.[1]

Nurses can best maintain the patient's optimal well-being by providing nursing care that reflects and incorporates the latest techniques, knowledge, and practices. The only way a nurse can maintain this high level of competency is by knowing the standards of care and seeking the knowledge required to meet these standards. Quite apart from the legal demands, the ethical principle of fidelity to the profession underlies this obligation on the part of nurses.

The profession of nursing is based on understanding and using a body of knowledge, some of which is borrowed from other disciplines, some of which is unique to nursing. This body of knowledge is reflected in the various standards of care that have been adopted by professional organizations representing nurses. To be most effective, standards of care need to change as technology progresses, society changes, and the demands of the profession are altered. Nurses have a responsibility to monitor these standards on an ongoing basis and to improve and update their techniques and service accordingly. This responsibility translates to mean that nurses must be active, participating members on the many committees that deal with standards of care. These committees range from local institutional committees on standards of care to state, national, and international level committees. They may meet and make decisions with or without the participation of nurses. If nurses are not active in this process, then others who do not necessarily have nurses' and the patients' best interests in mind will decide the standards of care to which nurses will be held in the future.

OBJECTIVES

Upon completing this chapter, the reader will be able to:
1. Define the term *standard of care*.
2. Describe how sources of standards of care are used in a disciplinary proceeding and in a malpractice case.
3. Describe the role of an expert in establishing the standard of care in a malpractice case.
4. Distinguish between standards and guidelines.
5. Understand the process used to develop standards.
6. Understand the importance of defining the scope and purpose of documents that may be used as evidence of standards of care.
7. Distinguish between a national and local standard of care.
8. Describe how the error-in-judgment rule and the two-schools-of-thought doctrine relate to standard of care.

Introduction

This chapter provides an overview of the concept of standard of care. It reviews sources of standards of care and discusses the points to remember in developing standards of care. It also focuses on the legal implications of standards in a disciplinary proceeding and a nursing malpractice case, including the crucial role of expert testimony in establishing deviations in the standard of care.

Standards of Care

Standards of care exist to provide guidance and to define appropriate levels of quality patient care that patients should receive from health professionals. The standards of care came about to protect patients from inferior care. In the context of a malpractice case, the standard of care is a scale against which the judge or jury measures the care provided, to determine whether or not the care was negligent. The **standard of care**

A CASE IN POINT

Postoperative Chemical Burns

The Facts

A patient who had surgery on an infected finger suffered chemical burns post-operatively from the irrigation solution used on the wound dressing. The patient complained of burning in his hand but his complaints were ignored by the nurses. Six additional surgeries, including skin grafts and a finger amputation, were required.

It was discovered that the hospital pharmacist was talking on the telephone while the student extern mixed the irrigation solution and therefore was unable to see and effectively supervise the student extern who mixed the solution improperly.

Violations of the nursing standards of care included the following:

1. Failure to check the dressing
2. Failure to call the physician
3. Failure to use good judgment and recognize a problem when the numerous pain shots were ineffective

The Jury Decides

The jury found that the nurses, pharmacist, and hospital were 100% liable. The student extern and the university were found 0% liable. The jury found the nurses, pharmacist, and extern were negligent.[2] However, the jury found that the extern's negligence was not a legal cause of the injury.

is the average degree of skill, care, and diligence exercised by members of the same profession under the same or similar circumstances. If a practitioner's care does not meet this level, it is negligent care. In the context of a disciplinary proceeding, by contrast, the standard of care is assessed in terms of incompetence or gross negligence, rather than ordinary negligence.

Sources of Standards

Joint Commission on Accreditation of Healthcare Organizations

The Joint Commission on Accreditation of Healthcare Organizations (JCAHO) publishes numerous manuals, books, periodicals, and newsletters, such as the **Comprehensive Accreditation Manual for Hospitals,** the official handbook that is designed to support health care providers' efforts in continuous improvement of performance.

The *Hospital Accreditation Standards* are published annually and contain all the intent statements, accreditation policies and procedures, and hospital standards such as staffing effectiveness standards, restraint and seclusion standards, and patient safety standards. The standards are drafted in a general way so as to apply to nursing care in a variety of settings. (JCAHO's Web site is http://www.jcaho.org; telephone 630-792-5006; fax 630-792-5005.)

State Statutes and Regulations

Nursing licensure is regulated by states. As discussed earlier, the scope of practice, entry to practice requirements, criteria for credentialing, and grounds for disciplinary action are contained in state statutes and regulations. **Statutes** are laws passed by the state legislature. Lobbying by groups such as the state nurses' association, special interest groups, or specialty nursing organizations can impact legislation. Nurse practice acts also take the form of statutes. **Regulations,** on the other hand, are rules or orders issued by various regulatory agencies, such as state boards of nursing. From a practical perspective, regulations have the force and effect of law because their intent is to carry out the law. They tend to be more detailed and specific and offer guidelines and methods to comply with the law.

Although statutes and regulations do not always directly pertain to patients, they dictate standards of practice for nurses and affect the delivery of health care. Generally, nurses are required to demonstrate competent practice; however, there may be different levels of standards, in addition to competency, in licensing legislation. For example, in certain states, licenses can be revoked for criminal actions (e.g., murder) or repeated acts of negligence.

American Nurses Association

The American Nurses Association published its first standards of practice in 1973. Since then, the ANA, in collaboration with specialty nursing organizations, has adopted standards that apply to many different fields of nursing. (See Box 2–1 for a list of standards available from the ANA.) The ANA's standards contain both standards of care and standards of professional performance.

In many states, disciplinary action is taken when the nurse negligently and willfully acts in a manner inconsistent with the health or safety of the patient or negligently and willfully practices nursing in a manner that fails to meet generally accepted standards of such nursing practice. The incorporation of the term *willful* means that disciplinary action should not be based on ordinary negligence alone, but rather on gross negligence; in other words, the subjective component of willfulness is required. The difference between these two terms is significant. *Ordinary negligence* implies carelessness or omission of care; it can be seen as a failure to take the precautions that any ordinary person would have taken in a similar situation. *Gross negligence,* on the other hand, involves an intentional, reckless disregard of the consequences to a person or property.

Because licensing laws differ from state to state, nurses must be familiar with those statutes and regulations that apply to their nursing practice. In fact, some states' nursing regulations require knowledge of statutes and regulations governing nursing and

---

BOX 2–1

ANA Nursing Standards Available from the American Nurses Association

ANA Nursing Standards Package
Scope and Standards for Nurse Administrators
Scope and Standards of Advanced Practice Registered Nurses
Scope and Standards of College Health Nursing Practice
Scope and Standards of Diabetes Nursing
Scope and Standards of Forensic Nursing Practice
Scope and Standards of Home Health Nursing Practice
Scope and Standards of Nursing Practice in Correctional Facilities
Scope and Standards of Parish Nursing Practice
Scope and Standards of Pediatric Oncology Nursing
Scope and Standards of Practice for Nursing Professional Development
Scope and Standards of Psychiatric-Mental Health Nursing Practice
Scope and Standards of Public Health Nursing Practice
Scope of Cardiac Rehabilitation Nursing Practice
Scope of Practice for Nursing Informatics Practice
Standards and Scope of Gerontological Nursing Practice (ed 2)
Standards Case
Standards of Addictions Nursing Practice with Selected Diagnoses and Criteria
Standards of Clinical Nursing Practice (ed 2)
Standards of Clinical Practice and Scope of Practice for the Acute Care Nurse
Statement on the Scope and Standards for the Nurse Who Specializes in Developmental, Disabilities and/or Mental Retardation
Statement on the Scope and Standards of Genetics Clinical Nursing Practice
Statement on the Scope and Standards of Oncology Nursing Practice
Statement on the Scope and Standards of Otorhinolaryngology Clinical Nursing Practice
Statement on the Scope and Standards of Pediatric Clinical Nursing Practice
Statement on the Scope and Standards of Respiratory Nursing Practice
The Scope and Standards of Public Health Nursing Practice

other topics related to nursing.[3] Failure to possess such knowledge may result in disciplinary action on the grounds of incompetence.[4]

Standards of professional performance are professional activities such as continuous quality improvement, education, research, ethics, and peer review. Standards of care and standards of performance are both described in terms of competency, rather than in terms of reasonable care or optimal level of performance. According to the ANA, the standards remain stable; however, the criteria used to measure compliance with the standards of practice may change as dictated by technological advances. There is also a distinction between standards and guidelines. A **standard** is an authoritative statement, whereas a guideline is a recommended course of action. This distinction certainly has important legal implications. **Guidelines** suggest or recommend practices by which standards of care can be met; however, the standards do not mandate compliance with the guidelines.[5]

Although the ANA standards are based on competency, they recognize that a nurse's ability to provide care depends on the working environment. It is the employer's responsibility to provide adequate resources and working conditions.

Bylaws, Facility Policies, and Procedures

Bylaws are rules that are adopted to regulate practice and privileges. Bylaws affect the medical, surgical, and nursing staff. Bylaws may incorporate standards for credentialing and other aspects of professional conduct, such as staff privileges and patient care.

Health care facilities may have rules and regulations relating to specialty practice areas, such as obstetrics and gynecology. Although their primary purpose is to regulate the care provided by physicians, rules and regulations can also set standards of care for nursing.

Nurses must be familiar with all rules and regulations pertinent to their area of practice because these may be used as sources of evidence regarding standards of care.

Nurses must also have a good working knowledge of the facility's policy and procedure manual. A **policy** is an overall plan to accomplish general goals. **Procedures** are the tools used to implement the policies.

Policies, which are broader than procedures, may deal with many different services within the health care facility. For example, a policy on fire safety includes all individuals within the facility regardless of their job or profession. In addition to the policy on fire prevention, a facility will likely have procedures that specifically outline particular responsibilities, such as evacuation plans and safety equipment maintenance.

Health care facilities must have policies and procedures covering all aspects of patient care. They must address everything from how to deal with staffing shortages to how to change intravenous tubing. The manuals that contain these policies and procedures are an important source of standards and are often introduced as evidence in legal proceedings.

A CASE IN POINT

Fractured Hip from a Fall

The Facts

A 92-year-old disoriented patient fractured her hip while trying to get out of bed. A nurse was assigned exclusively to this patient.

The Court Decides

The court held that the nurse was 35% liable for failure to notify the physician that the patient was disoriented earlier that morning. She had left the patient unattended to respond to an emergency code pursuant to the hospital's policy. The hospital was held 55% liable for failure to properly staff and requiring a nurse to be in two places at one time. The physician was held 10% liable for failing to order restraints, although expert testimony was to the contrary.[6]

AUTHOR TIP: *A word of caution—policy and procedure manuals should not be thrown away when new policies are created. Policy and procedure manuals should be maintained for a time based on the statute of limitations and state or federal laws.*

If a facility has created standards that are based on the highest standards available, rather than reasonable standards, the facility may be held to the higher level. For example, if your national specialty nursing organization requires "level one" standards, which are reasonable standards, but your institution guarantees the "highest level of nursing care in the world," the facility has created a higher standard to which the nurse may be held in a court of law.

The sophistication of rules, regulations, policies, procedures, and standards of care may depend on the level of the health care facility. Major university teaching institutions tend to be more progressive; their standards may be higher than those reflected in the policies or rules of a small community facility. If procedures and rules have not been properly updated and maintained, the nurses working in the facility could be practicing under parameters that do not meet acceptable standards of care. Following facility policy does not automatically excuse a nurse from liability.[7] In other words, if the conduct at issue is not consistent with an appropriate standard of care, adherence to an outdated facility procedure will not excuse a nurse and may be grounds for holding a nurse negligent. The nursing profession must also take an active part in developing standards and in reviewing, evaluating, and updating policies and procedures.

Other Sources of Standards

Standards of care are also found within nursing texts and articles. To be a competent source of standards, the text or publication must be recognized as an authoritative work in the field.[8] Instruction manuals, job descriptions, and expert witnesses can also be use to define a standard.

Developing Standards of Care

When in a situation where standards must be developed for an institution, nurses should take advantage of the lobbying efforts and expertise demonstrated by associations drafting standards of care. Nurses should obtain these documents by writing to associations such as the ANA, state nursing associations, boards of nursing, and national specialty nursing organizations. Nursing administration or staff development offices should have these standards available, as well as copies of state statutes, nurse practice acts, and regulations pertinent to the nursing profession.

How Standards Vary

Standards vary according to the level of care being measured and according to whether they dictate general or more specific aspects of patient care.

A standard of care that is framed broadly enough to address general aspects of patient care affects a large segment of health care providers. For example, a standard of care on disaster safety (e.g., a hurricane or flood) involves every person who is responsible for patient care—administrators, medical staff, nurses, and biomedical engineers. Achieving that standard depends on compliance with procedures, guidelines, or criteria by many individuals, all of whom may have different positions within the health care setting.

Standards that dictate specific aspects of patient care are restricted to a particular segment of health care providers or to a subspecialty within that segment. They should be drafted keeping in mind the practitioner's education, training, and experience. Standards that measure a particular clinical aspect of patient care and have significance for a smaller segment of practitioners are referred to as profession specific because they are tailored only to those whose conduct they are dictating. For example, a standard assessing intravenous placement may only apply to perivascular nurses.

Understanding the Terms

Nurses must have a clear understanding of such terms as *incompetence, gross negligence, negligence,* and *malpractice* and understand the distinction between the actual standards and the criteria used to assess compliance with standards.

Competency is a level of care used to determine whether grounds exist for disciplinary action by a state licensing board. Competency is also used to assess civil liability against a nurse in a malpractice case. Under the theory of corporate liability, a health care facility can be held liable for damages caused by its employees or staff when it has reason to know that a nurse rendering care is incompetent to do so.[9]

Legal Implications of Standards of Care

Standards as Evidence

A nurse can be held liable for damages under a number of different legal theories. Depending on the proceedings, liability can result in civil judgments, criminal penalties, imprisonment, and restrictions on licenses to practice. In a judicial or administrative proceeding, a nurse defendant is almost always faced with the question of whether his or her conduct was consistent with a particular standard of care. State statutes, regulations, ANA standards, criteria, guidelines, state nurse practice acts, JCAHO standards, facility policies and procedures, instruction manuals for medical equipment, job descriptions, specialty organization standards, and authoritative textbooks can all be used as evidence of standards of care. In malpractice litigation, the nurse's attorney argues that the nurse was following a particular standard and that the judge, jury, or hearing board should not hold the nurse liable because (1) the nurse did not breach the standard or (2) even if the nurse breached the standard, it did not cause the patient's injury. The opposing counsel presents evidence of standards and argues that the nurse defendant failed to comply with those practices that caused damages to the patient.

Whether evidence of standards is admissible depends on the legal theories involved, the standard, the type of proceeding, and the jurisdiction.

Standards in Disciplinary Proceedings

A state Board of Nursing administrative proceeding decides issues involving licensing violations. State statutes and regulations indicate the grounds on which the disciplinary action is based, such as drug addiction, criminal conduct, or incompetence. Administrative procedure, along with other statutes or regulations, set parameters for disciplinary action. Both types of provisions affect how standards are used in an administrative proceeding. The statutes and regulations determine whether the alleged conduct constitutes a licensing violation. In addition to serving as evidence of standards, statutes and regulations also determine whether other sources of standards are admissible because they provide procedural guidelines that indicate what evidence is admissible.

A CASE IN POINT

Postoperative Heating Pad Burns

The Facts

The physician verbally ordered a "heating pad to abdomen PRN" for a postoperative patient. He failed to specify under what conditions it was to be applied, which type of pad to use and at what settings, and what periods of use were appropriate. The heating pad was placed on her abdominal surgical incisions for more than 22 hours, and the patient subsequently sustained second- and third-degree heating pad burns.[10]

It was discovered that the nurses breached the standard in the following ways:

1. After removing the pad to check the area, the nurse noted that the abdomen was red but failed to remove the pad entirely or contact the physician.
2. The pad displayed warnings against use on patients who were sedated, had sensitive skin, or were sleeping or disoriented.

Questions that may be asked by an attorney representing a patient who suffers burns may include the following:

1. What is the policy, procedure, rules, or regulations regarding monitoring heating pads and documenting heating pad use and skin integrity?
2. How often should the patient be checked to ensure that the heating pad is not burning the skin and is at the proper temperature?
3. Why did the nurse fail to follow the rules, regulations, policies, and procedures of the facility?
4. Was an incident report written?
5. Are the same heating pads still in use at the time of the deposition? At the time of trial? If the heating pads are no longer in use, why did the facility discontinue their use? Were other types of heating pads available but not used? Why?
6. Did the nurse know of the standard of care that applies to the use of heating pads?
7. How could this injury have been prevented?
8. What could the nurse or physician have done to prevent the injury?

The Court Decides

The hospital (60%) and physician (40%) were held liable.

A nurse's attorney should object to the indiscriminate introduction of standards that dictate levels of care that are more stringent than the grounds for disciplinary action.

The rules of evidence that apply to disciplinary proceedings are not as stringent as those used in a malpractice case.[11] A hearing board is more likely to admit documents that are subject to objections in a trial.

Standards as Evidence in a Malpractice Case

As stated in Chapter 1, to establish malpractice or professional negligence against a nurse, the plaintiff must prove the elements of negligence: (1) duty, (2) breach of duty (which is where standard of care comes into play), (3) proximate cause, and (4) damages. Once a duty to the patient by the health care provider has been established, it is the burden of the plaintiff to prove that the nurse breached the duty, or in other words, did not live up to the standard of care.

The Role of the Expert

The standard of care in a malpractice case is most often brought into evidence through expert testimony. The role of the expert is to describe the "reasonable" care that is required under the circumstances. Expert testimony is needed to educate judges and jurors who do not have the training, education, and experience to make decisions about health care practices. The purpose of the **expert** is to assist the court in determining the applicable standard of care.[12]

The plaintiff and defendant usually present expert testimony on the issues of standard of care, breach of the standard, causation, and damages. In many cases, there is disagreement between the experts concerning what standard of care is required. For example, in a wrongful death and survival action brought by the parents on behalf of their stillborn infant, it is likely that there may be contradictory expert testimony focusing on whether or not the standard of care required the nurse to institute and to continue fetal monitoring.

Standards, facility procedures, treatises, and forms of documentary evidence, along with expert testimony, may be used in a malpractice case to establish the standard of care. However, the effect of those documents and their admissibility as evidence depend on the rules of evidence and case law of the jurisdiction. The judge makes a preliminary determination concerning whether evidence should be admitted in a case. The two main issues the judge must deliberate before admitting documents into evidence are whether they are relevant and whether they are considered hearsay.

Relevance

Evidence is **relevant** when it tends to either prove or disprove a contested matter.[13] Documents containing standards of care must be relevant to the factual issues involved. The documents must relate to both the subject matter and the time at issue in the case. A guideline that simply promotes the best patient care is not relevant and should not be used to decide whether a nurse exercised the skill and judgment that are routinely exercised by nurses under similar circumstances. For a text to be relevant, the party must prove, usually by means of expert testimony, that the text is an authoritative work in the profession and that members of the profession recognize it as containing well-established and accepted principles.

In a case involving a specialty area of practice, documents incorporating standards that generally relate to nursing may be relevant; however, in a case involving general aspects of nursing care, standards relating to a specialized field of nursing may not be relevant.

Hearsay Evidence

In addition to relevancy, a judge must also decide whether documents introduced as evidence of the standard of care should be excluded as hearsay. **Hearsay evidence**[14] is evidence that is derived from sources other than witnesses testifying at the hearing. Documents containing standards are likely to be considered hearsay evidence if the authors of the documents are not in court. The thinking behind the hearsay prohibition is that because the opposing side has no opportunity to cross-examine the author or challenge the credibility of the statements made in the documents, it may be unfair to admit that evidence into trial. Note, however, if the documents contain the type of information on which an expert would rely, then the expert may be allowed to read that information into evidence.[15]

The Effect of Standards as Evidence

Even if documents are admitted as evidence of the standard of care, they are not necessarily conclusive evidence.[16] That is, just because a judge permits a procedure to be introduced as evidence does not necessarily mean that a nurse's failure to follow the procedure automatically amounts to malpractice. The judge will instruct the jury on the law regarding the use of that evidence. Depending on the judge's instructions, the impact of the evidence on the issue of malpractice is decided by the jury.

▓ Legal Theories and Standards of Care

National v. Local Standards

Standards of care can be based on local or national standards. In a medical malpractice case, the standard of care is based on reasonableness and is the average degree of skill, care, and diligence exercised by members of the same profession. With increased specialization, most courts hold health care practitioners to a national, rather than a local, standard of care.[17] In a state following the locality rule, a health care provider's conduct is evaluated based on the care required by other practitioners in the same profession in that geographic area[18] or in a similar community.[19] On the other hand, states following the national standard of care doctrine evaluate a health care provider's conduct based on the care required by that group practicing throughout the country. Applying a national standard holds a nurse or physician in a rural community facility to the same standard of care as a nurse working in a large, well-funded university medical center.

Standard of Care Defenses

Nurses in Training

Some jurisdictions hold licensed physicians and nurses to a higher standard of care than practitioners who are still involved in the training process. The students are held to the standard of care that another student with the same knowledge and experience would have followed.

Error-in-Judgment Rule

Another theory regarding standard of care is the **error-in-judgment rule.** The error-in-judgment rule can be used successfully to defend a claim of malpractice by arguing that the standard of care was met by the nurse even though a mistake was made.[20] An error in judgment, including a mistaken diagnosis, does not necessarily prove malpractice if a nurse follows the standard of care required by using the skill, knowledge, and care routinely exercised by nurses with the same background and experience.

Two-Schools-of-Thought Doctrine

The **two-schools-of-thought doctrine** may also be used to defend a malpractice claim. When there is more than one method of treatment recognized among nurses as being proper, a nurse is not considered negligent for adopting any of these modes of treatment.[21] A nurse may choose to follow a school of thought that differs from the majority—as long as the nurse treats the plaintiff according to a method or school of thought deemed proper by a considerable number of nurses.

KEEP IN MIND _____

▶ Standard of care in a malpractice case is based on negligence and means the average degree of skill, care, and diligence exercised by members of the same profession under the same or similar circumstances.

▶ Depending on the law of each jurisdiction, standard of care in a disciplinary proceeding may be assessed in terms of incompetency, gross negligence, or negligence.

▶ Standard of care in a disciplinary proceeding can be assessed in terms of whether the nurse negligently and willfully acted in a manner inconsistent with the health or safety of the patient or negligently and willfully practiced nursing in a manner that fails to meet generally accepted standards of such nursing practice.

▶ Standards are created by accreditation bodies, state and federal legislatures, professional associations, and health care facilities.

▶ Standards may be used for evidentiary purposes to determine whether the standard of care has been violated in any given case.

▶ The JCAHO's *Comprehensive Accreditation Manual for Hospitals* and the ANA's standards of nursing practice both dictate competency as the level of care required by nurses.

▶ Adherence to an outdated facility procedure that is a standard at a facility may leave a nurse open to liability.

▶ Standards are drafted for different purposes and vary in the level of practice they dictate. In drafting standards, it is important to clearly identify to whom the standard should apply and whether it is meant to dictate optimal, competent, reasonable, or minimally acceptable parameters of care.

▶ A standard is not automatically admissible as evidence in a malpractice case. It must be relevant and must overcome any hearsay objections.

▶ The standard of care in a malpractice case is primarily established by expert testimony. The expert may rely on documents containing standards, such as facility procedures or treatises, if the expert establishes that such documents contain principles that are accepted by the profession.

IN A NUTSHELL

There are many different sources of standards of care. Familiarity with these sources improves patient care and promotes awareness of legal responsibilities. All nurses should have a working knowledge of the state statutes, regulations, and various legal theories in their jurisdiction regarding standards of care. Failure to adhere to standards of care may result in disciplinary action or malpractice liability. Understanding the purpose and concepts of standards of care is an important step in the process of standards development. Because various sources of standards may be used as evidence in a legal proceeding, it is essential that all nurses be familiar with this process.

AFTERTHOUGHTS

1. Discuss where you can find the various sources of standards of care for your area of practice.

2. Develop standards of care for (a) a nursing treatment, (b) a risk management issue, (c) an ethical dilemma, or (d) a case management issue.

3. Why are standards of care developed by nursing facilities and institutions?

4. Discuss two state statutes or regulations that affect nursing practice standards of care in your state.

5. Develop policies and procedures for an area of nursing practice that you see as a problem area.

6. Develop a list of resources for standards available to you in your facility, institution, or nursing school.

7. Discuss various standards of care that your state nurse practice act requires.

8. Identify and discuss the role of standard of care in (a) a malpractice case and (b) a disciplinary proceeding.

9. Discuss the two factors that a judge in a malpractice case must consider in deciding whether standards are admissible evidence in a malpractice case.

10. Discuss common breaches of the standards of care by nurses.

11. Obtain a copy of standards from ANA or a nursing specialty organization and discuss.

12. Analyze and discuss a nursing negligence case and the applicable standards at issue. Cite your sources of standards.

13. Based on your clinical experience, discuss what standards of care you have noticed that have not been followed in facilities. Discuss the consequences.

14. What other sources do you see or know of that could be considered standards?

15. Discuss nursing malpractice cases and the breaches of standards found in the cases.

ETHICS IN PRACTICE

Bill Z., a 6-foot and 3-inch, 135-pound, 76-year-old retired college professor was admitted to a medical unit in a large metropolitan hospital. He had been diagnosed 6 months previously with metastatic cancer that had spread from his lungs to the liver, gastrointestinal (GI) system, and bones. He had received some chemotherapy but with little effect. He was admitted to the hospital because he had become too weak to walk or care for himself at home and because the large doses of oral narcotic medications were having little effect on his generalized pain.

His physician had decided that further chemotherapy would be useless and ordered Mr. Z. to be kept comfortable with medications. A continuous morphine sulfate intravenous (IV) drip was started to help control the pain. Although he was talkative and friendly by nature, as Mr. Z.'s cancer spread, he would cry out and beg the nurses not to move him. Because he was very tall and underweight, his bony prominences quickly became reddened and showed signs of breakdown. The facility standards of care for bedridden patients required that they be turned from side to side every 2 hours. Mr. Z. yelled so loudly when he was turned that the nursing staff wondered if they were helping him or hurting him.

To decide what should be done, a patient care conference was called by the nurses most often involved in providing care for Mr. Z. The head nurse of the unit stated very clearly that the facility standards of care required that he be turned at least every 2 hours to prevent skin breakdown, infections, and perhaps sepsis. In his already weakened condition, an infection or sepsis would most likely be fatal. Melanie F., who had been a registered nurse (RN) for 15 years, disagreed with the head nurse. Her feeling was that causing this obviously terminal patient such extreme pain by turning him was cruel and violated his dignity as a human being. She stated that she could not stand to hear him yell anymore and refused to take care of him until some other decision was made about his nursing care. Susan B., a new graduate nurse, felt that the patient should have some say in his own care and that perhaps some type of compromise could be reached about turning him, even if less frequently. Ellen R., who had worked on the unit for 2 years, felt that the physician should make the decision regarding turning this patient and then all the nurses would have to do was follow the order. This last suggestion was met with strong negative comments by the other nurses present because patient comfort and turning are nursing measures.

What should they decide? Violation of a standard of care can leave a nurse open to a lawsuit. What about the patient's right to make a decision when this violates a standard of care? Are there ever any situations where a nurse might legally and ethically violate a standard of care? What are the consequences?

What are the sources? List the possible alternatives and consider the ethical principles and values.

References

1. Brown v. Southern Baptist Hospital, 96-1990, 96-1991 (La. App. 4th Cir. 3.99, 715 So. 2d 423).
2. American Nurses Association: Code of Ethics. ANA, Washington, DC, 2001.
3. Md. Code Ann. Title 7, Section 313, 20 (1988).
4. Md. Code of Regulations, Title 10, sub-title 27, 5 (1989).
5. The American Heritage Dictionary of the English Language, ed 4. Houghton Mifflin, New York, 2000.
6. Beckham v. St. Paul Fire & Marine Insurance Company, 614 So. 2d 760, (La. App. 2nd Cir. 1993).
7. Vansstrenburg v. Nason Hospital, 535 A.2d 1177.
8. Graham Handbook of Federal Evidence, sec. 702.1, ed 3, 1991.
9. Thompson v. Nason Hospital, 535 A.2d 1177 (Pa. Supp. 1988), aff'd on appeal.
10. Merritt V. Karcioglu, 95-1335 (La. App. 4th Cir. 1/19/96) 668 So.2d 469.
11. Northrup, C, and Kelly, M: Legal Issues in Nursing. CV Mosby, St. Louis, 1987, p 412.
12. Graham, MH: Handbook of Federal Evidence, ed 5. West Group, St. Paul, Minn, 2001, sec. 702.1.
13. Ibid., 401.1.
14. Graham, MH: Handbook of Federal Evidence, ed 5. West Group, St. Paul, Minn, 2001, sec. 801(c).
15. Ibid., at sec. 803.18.1
16. Darling v. Charleston Memorial Hospital, 50 Ill. App 2d 253, 200 N. E. 2d 149 (Ill. App. Dist 4 06/30/1964).
17. O'Keefe, ME: Nursing Practice and the Law: Avoiding Malpractice and Other Legal Risks. FA Davis, Philadelphia, 2001, p 127.
18. Katsetos v. Nolan, 170 Conn. 637, 646, 368 A.2d 172 (1976).

19. Gittens v. Christian, 600 F.Supp. 146 (D.V.I. 1985), aff'd 782 F.2d 1028 (3rd Cir. 1986).
20. Smith v. Yohe, 194 A.2d 167 (1963).
21. Furey v. Thomas Jefferson University, 472 A.2d 1083 (Pa. Supp. 1984).

Recommended Reading

Ardoin v. Hartford Accident & Indemnity Co., 360 So.2d 1331 (La. 1978).
Berens, MJ: Dangerous Care: Nurses "Hidden Role" in Medical Error. Chicago Tribune, Sept 10-12, 2000.
Berens, MJ: Nursing Mistakes Kill, Injure Thousands—Cost-Cutting Toll on Patients, Hospital Staffs. Chicago Tribune, Sept 10, 2000.
Thompson, I, et al: Nursing Ethics. Churchill Livingstone, New York, 2000.

Resources

American Nurses Association
600 Maryland Avenue, SW
Suite 100 West
Washington, D.C. 20024
(202) 651-7000
(202) 651-7001 (FAX)

American Nurses Credentialing Center
600 Maryland Avenue, SW
Suite 100 West
Washington, D.C. 20020
(202) 651-7001 (Fax)

The Law 3

Key Chapter Concepts

Nurse practice acts

Law

Constitutional law

Statutory law

Statutes

Administrative law

Common law

Precedent

Substantive law

Procedural law

Statute of limitations

Civil law

Contract law

Tort law

Unintentional tort

Negligence

Ordinary negligence

Malpractice

Preponderance of evidence

Damages

General damages

Punitive damages

Intentional torts

Criminal law

Misdemeanor

Felony

Indictment

Grand jury

Arraignment

Discovery

Pretrial motion

Trial

Fraud

Jurisdiction

Trial courts

Appellate courts

Supreme courts

Writ of certiorari

Chapter Thoughts

Patient Dandre has a living will and a do not resuscitate (DNR) order in place. She has a terminal illness but is still competent and has stated that she does not want to prolong her life if there is no chance of recovery and no chance for enhancing her quality of life.

Nurse Bonds, a registered nurse (RN), passes by Mrs. Dandre's room and hears her yelling, "I can't breathe, please help me."

Nurse Bonds runs into the room. Mrs. Dandre states, "I can't breathe. Please don't let me die. Do everything you can to save me." Just at that moment the daughter walks in and says, "No, don't do anything."

1. What should the nurse do?
2. Has the patient revoked her living will and DNR order?

3. Should the nurse follow the daughter's orders?
4. If the daughter is the health care agent, can she determine what should be done? What facts must you consider?
5. What are the potential areas of liability for the nurse? For the facility?
6. Who can sue the nurse? Why?
7. What type of law applies to this situation?
8. How can an individual revoke a living will and DNR according to your state laws?
9. Is this an ethical dilemma?

These are just some of the questions we discuss in this chapter.

OBJECTIVES

Upon completing this chapter, the reader will be able to:
1. Define law and explain how society influences the development of law.
2. Identify the four major sources of law.
3. Differentiate between substantive law and procedural law and between criminal law and civil law.
4. Distinguish between contract law and tort law.
5. Describe the judicial system, including the state and federal court systems.
6. Discuss how criminal law violations apply to nursing.
7. Define the criminal procedure process.
8. Discuss how to implement change through the lobbying process.
9. Discuss various ways to handle legal and ethical dilemmas.

Introduction

The expanded scope of nursing practice has brought increased responsibility and, along with it, increased exposure to liability. Nurses practicing in the health care system must stay informed about changing laws, regulations, and public policies and be aware of the ethical dilemmas that may confront them. This chapter introduces the reader to legal concepts vital for understanding the principles and ideas that underlie health care laws.

Legal Status of Nursing

One sure way to invoke high levels of fear and anxiety in most health care providers in general, and nurses in particular, is to utter the word *lawsuit*. To many nurses, the legal system is an incomprehensible monster poised to devour nurses the first time they make a mistake in patient care. Although the legal system is imposing to those who have not been initiated into its complexities, in reality it is just one part of the total health care picture.

The status of nursing has evolved through the years as changing roles and economic forces have affected health care. Nursing has become a profession requiring increased education, competence, technical skills, and business knowledge.

Nurse practice acts, in particular, are specific statutes passed by the state legislatures to define and regulate the practice of nursing within each state. These acts, which define nursing practice and establish the standards for nurses in each state, are the most important legal statutes or legislative acts for regulating nursing practice. Nurse practice acts vary in scope from state to state; they tend to be worded generally and to follow, to some extent, either the American Nurses Association (ANA) model published in 1980 or the model act of the National Council of State Boards of Nursing published in 1982 and revised in 1988. The practice acts are designed to safeguard patients by defining and establishing standards for nursing practice. Most states now regulate the areas of advanced and specialized nursing practice to provide standards for nurses with increased skills. Violation of the nurse practice act can result in criminal prosecution and disciplinary action or medical malpractice litigation and can affect the nurse's license and livelihood.

As professional responsibility has increased, so has legal accountability. Historically, nurses were not routinely named as defendants in malpractice suits because facilities and physicians were considered the primary defendants. Today, however, nurses are being held accountable for their individual actions or omissions and are being named in malpractice cases, primarily in facility settings. Also, nurses are assuming more responsibility in the role as advanced practitioners, clinical specialists, independent contractors, managers, and administrators. With downsizing, roles have also been combined and job descriptions have been changed, adding to the nurse's responsibility and potential liability.

In malpractice cases, laws, statutes, and case law determine such things as when the lawsuit can be filed, the value of the damages suffered, and how and where the claim must be filed.

▨ Definition of Law

Law is the body of rules and regulations that governs people's behavior and their relationships with others in society and with the state. Laws promote order by resolving conflicts and disputes nonviolently, by defining responsibilities, and by protecting the health, safety, and welfare of the citizens.

Although some laws are constant, most are evolving to adapt to society's changing values, customs, and demands. The changing legal rights of minorities and women in the United States over the past century provide a dramatic example of how laws evolve to meet the political, economic, and social values of society.

Both federal and state governments have the constitutional authority to create and enforce laws (Table 3–1). The United States Constitution, as the supreme law of the

TABLE 3–1

Role of Government in Developing Laws

Governmental Source	Role in Lawmaking	Types of Law
Constitution	Establishes supreme law	Constitutional law; Bill of Rights
Legislative branch	Creates law	Statutes
House	Approves executive	
Senate	appointments	
Executive branch	Executes and administrates	Administrative law; rules and
President or governor	laws	regulations
	Vetoes bills	
Judiciary branch	Interprets laws	Common law or judge-made
Supreme Court	Adjudicates disputes	laws
Appellate courts		
Trial courts		

land, grants certain powers to the federal government. Powers not expressly granted to the federal government by the Constitution are reserved for the state governments. The legal basis for federal government involvement in health care is found in Article 1, Section 8, of the Constitution under the provision of general welfare and the regulation of interstate commerce. The federal government has jurisdiction over everything under the broad umbrella of "interstate commerce"; the business of health care, by its nature, falls under the definition of interstate commerce and therefore can be regulated by federal entities.

State and local governments constitutionally possess the most authority to regulate health care through their police power, which allows them to protect the health, safety, and welfare of their citizens. An example of a state exercising its police power is its regulation of the professional practice of nurses, physicians, and other health care providers in the health care industry.

Sources of Law

There are many different sources of law affecting health care providers and their practices. Some laws affect nurses personally, such as the constitutional amendments that guarantee freedom of speech, whereas other laws such as administrative laws regulate the nurse's professional acts. See Table 3–2 for an overview of the role of government in developing laws. Following are the four sources of law in the United States:

1. Constitutional law
2. Statutory law
3. Administrative law
4. Common law

TABLE 3–2

Sources of Law and Examples

Sources of Law	Examples of Federal Law	Examples of State Law
Constitutional	United States Constitution Civil Rights Act	State constitution La. R.S. 40:1299.37
Statutory	Federal Tort Claims Act (FTCA)	Part XX Medical Malpractice Coverage
Administrative	Social Security Act (Medicare/Medicaid)	Nurse Practice Act Workers' compensation laws
Common	*Miranda v. Arizona,* 384 U.S. 436 (1966) Rehearing denied, 385 U.S. 890 (1966)	*Lovelace v. Giddens,* 652 (La. 1999)

Constitutional Law

We the people of the United States, in Order to form a more perfect Union, establish Justice, ensure domestic Tranquillity, provide for the common defense, promote the general Welfare, and secure the Blessings of Liberty to ourselves and our Posterity, do ordain and establish this constitution for the United States of America.

—The Constitution of the United States of America

Constitutional law is a system of fundamental principles on the limitations of the United States' power and organization of the government.

The Constitution, through its articles and amendments, guarantees individuals certain fundamental freedoms. Very little constitutional law affects health care and nursing practice directly, except for the personal rights protected by the Bill of Rights in the constitutional amendments. These amendments guarantee such rights as privacy, equal protection, and freedom of speech and religion. The Constitution does not protect individuals from the private acts of other individuals. For individuals to allege constitutional violations, a state action or statute must be involved. For example, nurses who work in a state or federal facility may have more constitutional protection for employee rights than do nurses who work for private employers. At the same time, these nurses may be exposed to additional legal challenges by patients because the actions of these nurses are considered to be "state actions" and are therefore vulnerable to constitutional attack.

Statutory Law

Statutory law is based on **statutes,** formal written laws enacted by federal, state, and local legislative authorities or bodies. Federal statutes are published in the United States Code (U.S.C.); state statutes are published in various state publications, such as

Revised Statutes or Revised Codes Annotated. The Medicare and Medicaid amendments to the Social Security Act of 1965 are examples of federal laws that have dramatically affected health care in a number of areas, including facility admissions and discharges, available services, and level of care provided.

Specific Statutory Federal Laws Affecting Health Care

EMERGENCY MEDICAL TREATMENT AND ACTIVE LABOR ACT

Congress passed the Emergency Medical Treatment and Active Labor Act (EMTALA) in 1986. EMTALA prohibits Medicare-participating emergency departments from "dumping" patients who cannot pay for services or who do not have insurance. The act requires that each facility provide an appropriate medical screening exam within the capability of the facility emergency department. It also states that a patient can be transferred to another facility only after the following conditions have been met:

1. An appropriate medical screening has been performed by a physician.
2. The patient has been stabilized.
3. The receiving institution has cleared the patient for transfer.

Stabilize in this context means to provide medical treatment to ensure that no material deterioration will occur from or during the transfer to the other institutions.

Institutions that fail to follow EMTALA guidelines can be required to pay civil penalties of up to $50,000 per occurrence for facilities with more than 100 beds and up to $25,000 per occurrence for facilities with fewer than 100 beds. Also, persons injured by EMTALA violations may file civil actions for damages against the facility under state law.

ANTITRUST LAWS AND TRADE RESTRICTIONS

Federal and State antitrust laws prohibit anticompetitive actions (e.g., boycotts, monopolies, or contracts) that restrict commerce or trade. Nurses in expanded roles may be involved in antitrust situations. An example would be if an institution excludes a nurse anesthetist from providing services because of an exclusive tying agreement with the anesthesiologist that restricts competition. The main antitrust laws are The Sherman Antitrust Act, The Clayton Act, and the Federal Trade Commission Act. The Sherman Antitrust Act was passed by Congress in 1890. Under this act, the government was granted authority to initiate criminal prosecution against anyone forming monopolies or perpetuating restrictive agreements in business. The Clayton Act, passed in 1914, and its amendment, The Robinson-Patman Act, declared specific monopolistic practices (e.g., tying arrangements, mergers, or price discrimination) illegal and was adopted as an amendment to the Sherman Antitrust Act. An activity that has an adverse effect on the competition may be declared illegal. The Act also affirmed the rights of unions to picket, boycott, or strike. The act contained provisions related to labor disputes of corporate activities and remedies for reform.

The Federal Trade Commission Act, also passed in 1914, declared "unfair methods of competition" to be illegal. The Commission was created in part to enforce antitrust provisions and could issue cease and desist orders. This act is broader than the Clayton and Sherman Acts. Other illegal actions under the act include price fixing, market allocation, group boycotts, and exclusive agreements. The act also prohibits deceptive practices such as false or misleading advertisements.

On the state level, state legislatures have broad powers to provide for the public's health. State nurse practice acts define and regulate nursing practice. Statutes that deal with AIDS, other communicable diseases, child or elder abuse, consent for medical treatment, health care for the indigent, and Good Samaritan laws are other examples of state health care regulation.

Administrative Law

Administrative laws are created by administrative agencies under the direction of the executive branch. Once the legislature creates a statute or law, it delegates the authority to implement and establish new regulations to meet the intent of the statute. Under the administrative law system, there are reporting duties for the health care professional. For instance, most states have state statutes or laws to elaborate reporting guidelines for the following:

1. Child abuse
2. Elder abuse
3. Communicable diseases (e.g., sexually transmitted diseases, tuberculosis)
4. Impaired peers
5. EMTALA violations

Specific Administrative Departments and Agencies Affecting Health Care

A number of administrative agencies and departments issue rules and regulations that govern health care. See Figures 3–1 and 3–2 for the organizational structure of governments. All nurses should be familiar with and aware of the departments and agencies included in the following list.

DEPARTMENT OF HEALTH AND HUMAN SERVICES

The Department of Health and Human Services (DHHS) is a department of the executive branch of the federal government and is the main source of health care industry regulations. Five operating divisions of the DHHS include the following:

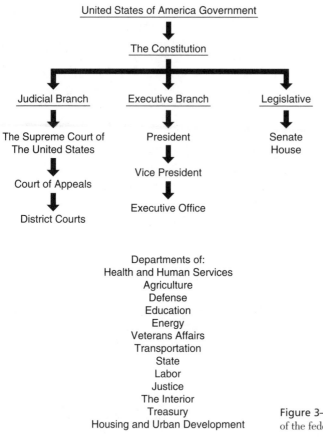

Figure 3–1. Organizational chart of the federal government.

1. *Health Care Financing Administration*
   - ■ Oversees the Medicare and Medicaid programs
   - ■ Is responsible for quality assurance of the programs
   - ■ Develops and implements policies and procedures for Medicare programs
   - ■ Provides grants to states for medical services for the indigent (Medicaid program)
2. *Office of Human Development Services*
3. *Family Support Administration*
4. *Public Health Service*

The Public Health Service (PHS) promotes the protection of the country's mental and physical health through enforcement of laws, policies and agreements, and provision of programs, research and resources, education, and expertise to public and private facilities.

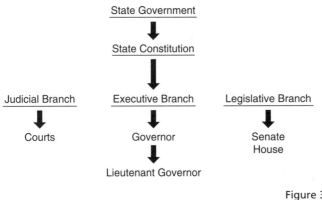

Figure 3–2. Organizational chart of state government.

Two smaller agencies within the PHS are the following:

- Food and Drug Administration (FDA), which controls, regulates, supervises, inspects, approves, and standardizes foods, drugs, cosmetics, and medical devices and issues public warnings when dangerous products have been identified
- The National Institutes of Health (NIH), the principal federal biomedical research agency

5. *Social Security Administration*
   - Supervises the country's social insurance program and provides retirement income to most citizens over 65 years of age (or over 62 years old under certain conditions)
   - Funded by employer and employee contributions
   - Pays benefits to employee or family if earnings are reduced or stopped due to death or disability

DHHS is also responsible for many other programs, including the following:

1. Supplemental Security Income (SSI), a program for needy individuals.
2. Medicaid, a state-administered government program financed by the federal government and some states that provides facility and outpatient medical services to the medically and financially needy. Federal grants are given to those states that have qualifying Medicaid programs.
3. Medicare, a federal program funded through Social Security contributions (e.g., FICA payroll taxes), general revenue, and premiums, that provides health insurance for persons over 65 years of age and some disabled persons. Medicare Part A assists in covering costs of inpatient hospital care and, with qualifying preadmission criteria, up to 100 days in home health or hospice setting or skilled nursing facility. Medicare Part B pays for such things as outpatient hospital services and physician's services.

4. Older Americans Act programs, which provide home-delivered meals, community services, ombudsmen services, and home health services.

FEDERAL COUNCIL ON AGING

The Federal Council on Aging (FCOA) advises and assists the President on issues relating to the needs of older Americans.

NATIONAL INSTITUTE ON AGING

The National Institute on Aging (NIA) is an institute of the NIH that is responsible for conducting and supporting research and training related to the diseases, such as Alzheimer's, that afflict older Americans.

STATE BOARDS OF NURSING

Although state legislators created the nurse practice acts in states, the acts in turn created state boards of nursing as administrative agencies with the authority to develop and enforce regulations concerning nursing practice. Regulations of nursing practice are within the delegated authority of the state boards and are considered administrative laws that are legally binding.

State boards of nursing enforce regulations involving nursing licenses. In most situations, the board receives complaints from a facility's health care providers, patients, or patient families. The board then investigates the allegations to determine if a nurse has breached the nurse practice act and to determine if there is any substance to the allegation. If the nurse is found to be a "danger to the patient's safety" based on the state laws and a board's investigation, the nurse's license may be reprimanded, probated, suspended, or revoked (Box 3–1). Allegations may include the following:

1. Use by the nurse of drugs or alcohol (working under the influence)
2. Failure to properly monitor
3. Endangering patient safety
4. Failure to use good nursing judgment
5. Falsifying documentation
6. Relapse—failure to follow the Recovering Nurse Program or Diversionary Program

The National Council of State Boards of Nursing is a not-for-profit organization whose membership includes the boards of nursing in 50 states, the District of Columbia, the United States Territories, the Virgin Islands, Puerto Rico, Northern Mariana Islands, Guam, and Samoa. The Council is the organization through which all boards of nursing collaborate and work together on common issues and concerns affecting public safety, welfare, and health.

The major functions of the National Council include the following:

> **BOX 3–1**
>
> ## What Can Happen to You and Your License
>
> 1. Dismissed charge
> 2. Investigations agreement
> 3. Letter of reprimand—formal or informal
> 4. Probation with stipulations (e.g., education, fines, monitoring fees, evaluation by psychiatrist, psychologist, or addictionologist)
> 5. Suspension with stipulations
> 6. Revocation
> 7. Diversion program for drug- or alcohol-related charges

1. Developing the NCLEX-PN and NCLEX-RN examinations to test the entry-level nursing competence candidates for licensure as licensed practical/vocational nurses and registered nurses. Exams are computerized and administered through a national test service.
2. Disseminating information related to the licensure of nurses.
3. Conducting pertinent research.
4. Conducting policy analysis.
5. Promoting uniformity in the regulation of nursing practice.
6. Serving as a forum for information exchange.

The Council has also created the NACEM, a nurse aide's competency evaluation program.[1]

Common Law

Common law is one the two ways to classify law according to origin—whether they originated in English common law or written civil code. Common law evolves from the judiciary branch through court decisions. When no written statutes or regulations speak to a given legal issue, the courts are asked to resolve legal disputes through judicial opinions, which take on the force of law. The federal courts and 49 of the state courts in the United States follow common law rules and legal principles developed in England from the days when the king pronounced rules according to his "divine right."[2] After the American Revolution, most states adopted the English common law system and have continued to use it. However, because individual states adopted different statutes and judicial interpretations, variations in common law exist among the states today.

Louisiana is the only state in the United States that has adopted civil code based on the Napoleonic code. The Louisiana Civil Code developed from the civil laws of the Romans, Spanish, and French.[3] The difference between civil code and common law is that in the civil code the law is authorized by the legislature rather than judiciary; the code is a comprehensive written organization of general rules and regulations, rather than a case-by-case analysis of specific legal issues. The other distinguishing feature is that the original basis of civil law is Roman law rather than English law.

Common law is composed of decisions of the court and follows a concept of precedent or stare decisis, which literally means "to stand by things decided." This concept allows courts to refer to previously decided cases and to apply the same rules and principles to current questions. **Precedent,** or prior law, then becomes law, and courts follow their own prior decisions, as well as those of higher courts in their jurisdiction. Common law is the most common source of law for malpractice issues.

Types of Law

There are a number of ways to classify laws. Classifications are based on whether the laws are substantive, procedural, civil, or criminal. All types of law are intermingled in various ways and in different areas of litigation and practice.

Substantive law determines the specific wrong, harm, duty, or obligation that causes an action to be brought to trial. In contrast, **procedural law** determines the form or process that regulates the legal right that is violated. Procedural law includes the various legal procedures required to bring a dispute to trial and determines the rules that parties must follow to litigate a matter before a court.

Both procedural and substantive laws enter the picture when a lawsuit is filed. For example, in a medical malpractice case, substantive laws specify the elements of negligence that must be proved (duty, breach of duty, causation, and damages), whereas procedural laws regulate the statute of limitations and the process for admitting evidence at trial.

The **statute of limitations** is a procedural law that specifies the time during which a plaintiff may bring a lawsuit. This limitation varies with the different types of substantive law. For example, in most instances, malpractice suits must be filed sooner than suits alleging violations of contract or criminal laws. In addition, there are variations among the states regarding the time to file malpractice claims, wrongful death action, and other causes of actions. States also vary regarding the time limit for minors who wish to file suit. If the petition for damages or complaint is not filed within the statutory time limit, the plaintiff is prohibited from filing a lawsuit for that particular injury.

Civil law recognizes and enforces the rights of individuals and organizations. Criminal law defines crimes and punishment.

Civil Law

Two areas of civil law are contract law and tort law.

Contract Law

Contract law is concerned with agreements between two parties that involve an obligation or duty. The elements of a contractual agreement include offer, acceptance, and consideration between two or more competent persons or entities. Consideration is the bargained-for exchange, which one party gives to the other party in exchange for the services offered in the contract (often the consideration is money). Although some contracts must be written in specified forms, others can be oral, and duties can be either overtly expressed or implied. The most common contractual issue that nurses encounter in practice relates to employee/employer agreements. A written contract outlining issues, fees, duties, and other items of interest is better than an oral contract, which is harder to challenge, defend, uphold, or enforce (see Chapter 12).

Tort Law

Tort law is the area of law that nurses are most familiar because it involves negligence and medical malpractice. A tort is a wrongful act committed by one party against another party or against property. The purpose of tort law is to make the injured party "whole again," primarily through monetary compensation.

Torts are divided into two main categories:

1. Negligence, or an "unintentional tort"
2. Intentional tort

UNINTENTIONAL TORTS

Negligence and malpractice, a particular form of negligence, are considered **unintentional torts.** By law, every person is responsible for behaving in a reasonable way. **Negligence** occurs when an unreasonable or careless act or omission of an act causes injury to another. **Ordinary negligence** is the failure to exercise the care that an ordinary prudent party exercises under similar circumstances. For example, if a nursing assistant fails to clean up orange juice on a patient's floor and the patient falls, this would be considered ordinary negligence.

Malpractice is a specific type of professional negligence that occurs when the standard of care that can be reasonably expected from such professionals as nurses, physicians, lawyers, and accountants is not met (Box 3–2); for example, a nurse commits malpractice by improperly administering an injection, causing a sciatic nerve injury. Only a professional can be sued for malpractice; any other misconduct is classified as ordinary negligence. To be liable for malpractice, a professional must fail to act as another reasonable and prudent professional with the same knowledge and education would have acted under similar circumstances.[4] To commit malpractice, the professional must have breached a standard of care. If a nurse infuses intravenous solution into an infant at the rate used for an adult and brain damage results, the malpractice standard applies. If a surgeon improperly performs surgery on a patient and it results in the loss of a limb, professional negligence has occurred and the standard of care applicable to surgeons of that specialty applies.

Although anyone can be sued for almost any reason in today's litigious society, for the nurse or other health professional to be held liable under a malpractice claim, the plaintiff in a court of law must prove each of the elements. The plaintiff must prove the case by a **preponderance of evidence,**[5] which means that the plaintiff must convince the jury that the evidence more likely than not proves the allegations and elements of negligence.

Damages (which are discussed in more detail later in the book) suffered by the plaintiff include "hard" and "soft" damages. Hard damages are damages that are evident through bills, such as past, present, and future medical, facility, or doctor bills; medication costs; funeral expenses; and lost wages. Soft damages are more intangible and include compensation for such things as loss of love and affection, pain and suffering, mental anguish, emotional distress, loss of consortium, loss of nurturance, and loss of chance of survival.

General damages are awards or money given to the plaintiff for pain and suffering caused by the defendant's acts. **Punitive damages** are damages awarded in an amount intended to punish the defendant (or person committing the tort) for the egregious nature of the tort. For a plaintiff to get punitive damages, the defendant's actions must have been willful and wanton. Punitive damages are not based on the plaintiff's actual monetary loss but may be double or triple the amount of the actual monetary loss.

BOX 3–2

Proving Malpractice

To prove liability for malpractice, a plaintiff must prove the elements of negligence:

1. A duty owed to the plaintiff
2. A breach of that duty or a breach of the standard of care by the professional through an act or omission
3. Proximate cause or causal connection between the breach and the harm
4. Actual harm or damages suffered by the plaintiff

Causation can be divided into two parts: cause in fact and proximate cause. Cause in fact means that the damage or injury is actually caused by a breach of duty by the health care professional. A factual connection exists between the act or omission and the harm. Proximate cause means that there is a *legal* connection establishing that within reasonable probability (more likely than not or greater than a 50-percent chance) the breach of the professional's duty to the patient caused the damage or injury.

Punitive damages may be awarded in some states for malpractice actions, depending on state law. Factors considered include the following:

- Concealment of act
- Financial position of the defendant
- Profitability of the actions of defendant
- Extent of harm to plaintiff
- Duration of harm
- Attitude and conduct of defendant

INTENTIONAL TORTS

An **intentional tort** is a willful or intentional act or wrongdoing that violates another person's rights or property (see Chapter 6). The most common intentional torts that affect health care providers include assault and battery, medical battery, false imprisonment, trespass, defamation, and intentional infliction of emotional distress. Intentional torts fall under both the civil (filed as civil suits) and the criminal law (filed as criminal charges) systems.

Criminal Law

Criminal law, as opposed to civil, is a branch of law that defines crimes and punishment. For example, criminal law outlines what act constitutes murder and what punishment should be given to the perpetrator. Criminal law attempts to protect the public from harm by threatening punishment or punishing those who commit crimes. Harm may be physical death, disturbance of the peace, injury to the public health, or loss of or damage to property.

Criminal law is concerned with violations of criminal statutes or laws. Violations of criminal law are offenses against society as spelled out in the written criminal statute or code. The plaintiff in a criminal suit is a governmental body. Depending on the seriousness of the offense, crimes are generally divided into felonies or misdemeanors. A **misdemeanor** is considered a lesser crime, generally punishable by fines or imprisonment. Examples of misdemeanors include driving under the influence or trespassing. A **felony** is a more serious crime with harsher punishments, which may include fines, prison terms, and the death sentence. Murder, kidnapping, and armed robbery are examples of felonies. In many states, felony convictions are grounds for denying, revoking, or suspending a nursing license. In civil proceedings, the injured party receives monetary damages from the defendant. In criminal procedures, the defendant may lose life or liberty if found guilty. At trial, to find the defendant guilty the prosecution must prove beyond a reasonable doubt that the defendant committed the crime.

Although criminal law violations are uncommon in the health care field, nurses may risk being charged with a crime for such actions as withholding life support for terminally ill patients or newborns born with birth defects or for falsifying narcotic records. Nurses also may be called as witnesses in criminal cases when they have cared for a victim or perpetrator of a criminal act, such as in a rape or child abuse case.

Violation of nurse practice acts may also precipitate criminal charges, as reported in a Missouri court involving nurse practitioners. Two nurse practitioners employed by a nonprofit family planning service in Missouri provided services according to specific physician-developed written standing orders and protocols. A complaint was filed with the medical board in Missouri alleging that the nurses were practicing medicine without a license. After investigation, the board recommended criminal prosecution and added that the nurses were practicing beyond the scope of professional nursing as it was defined in the Missouri Nursing Practice Act. The trial court found the nurses' activities constituted the unlawful practice of medicine. However, on appeal, the Missouri Supreme Court overturned the ruling and held that the nurses' practice was authorized by the Nursing Practice Act. The court further noted that when working under medical standing orders, the nurses were making a nursing diagnosis and not a medical diagnosis and that nurses could assume new responsibilities for practice as long as they were consistent with the professional's specialized education and skills.[6]

The Criminal Process

Statutes create the federal system of criminal law, whereas state criminal law is a combination of statutory law and common law. In criminal cases, the right to a jury is a constitutional right for felony cases but not for misdemeanor cases. The following are steps usually followed if a case is brought to federal or state court.

1. **Indictment** or complaint. This is a written document issued to the defendant describing the allegations of wrongdoing.
2. **Grand jury.** If the crime is a federal felony, a grand jury is convened to determine whether evidence is sufficient to indicate probable cause that a crime has been committed by the defendant. Some states also use the grand jury system.
3. **Arraignment.** The person is brought before the judge, pleads guilty or not guilty, and has bail set. If bail is refused or the person cannot make bail, then he or she is taken into custody.
4. **Discovery.** If the defendant pleads not guilty, then the discovery stage is the next step in the process. Evidence is discovered through a variety of means, depending on what is allowed by the court.
5. **Pretrial motions.** These are legal documents filed in court and used to shorten the trial process. For example, motions can be made to suppress or exclude evidence that is improperly seized.
6. **Trial.** At the trial, evidence and witnesses are presented to prove the prosecution's position beyond a reasonable doubt and to defend the accused of the alleged crime.

If the defendant is found innocent, the matter cannot be tried again or appealed by the prosecution. If the defendant is convicted, the defendant receives a sentence or fine for the crime. The defendant may also appeal the ruling of the court, although the prosecution cannot appeal an unfavorable result. Depending on the circumstances, if the person is sent to prison, the person may be eligible for parole after serving part of the sentence.

Health Care Fraud and Abuse

Fraud is intentional misrepresentation that one knows is false and makes anyway, knowing that the deception could result in an unauthorized or illegal benefit to self or others, such as monetary gain.

The most common forms of fraud in health care involve Medicare and include the following:

1. Receiving, offering, or soliciting a kickback
2. Billing for services not rendered
3. Misrepresenting a patient's diagnosis to justify payment
4. Falsification of documents to justify payment, such as certificates of medical necessity, medical records, or plans of treatment
5. Unbundling charges
6. "Upcoding"—billing for a service not provided as billed
7. Waiving patient deductibles and copayments
8. Billing for patient visits not actually done
9. Billing for medically unnecessary testing
10. Inflating bills

If Medicaid fraud is suspected, contact the Office of Inspector General's national fraud hotline for Medicaid and Medicare at 1-800-HHS-TIPS.

Jurisdiction

Jurisdiction is the authority by which courts and judges accept and decide cases. Jurisdictional authority flows from federal and state constitutions and statutes. The federal court jurisdiction extends to cases involving federal questions or disputes between citizens from different states. Certain courts have general jurisdiction, whereas other courts are more specialized, such as the United States customs courts, state juvenile courts, or local traffic courts. If both the state and federal court have jurisdiction over a particular case, then the parties may select which court system will try the case.

Organization of the Court System

Knowledge of the organization of the court system sheds light on how common law decisions are made. There are two separate court systems in the United States: the

A CASE IN POINT

Intentional Torts in Reality

Negligent Homicide

The Facts

In *State of Utah v. Warden,* a pregnant woman's due date was questionable, and she began having cramps and bleeding. Her physician delivered the infant at home. At birth, the infant weighed approximately 4 pounds. Soon after birth, the infant began experiencing respiratory problems (e.g., periodic grunting and purplish-blue skin color). The physician knew the condition was progressive and could end in death; however, he did nothing and gave no instructions to the family. During the night, the infant became worse. At 8:00 AM, the mother attempted to call the physician but was unsuccessful. Her clergyman and a pediatrician then came to the home and rushed the child to the hospital, where the infant died shortly after arrival. The physician lived only five blocks away and was up at 6:00 AM but did not attempt to contact the mother until noon, when he learned of the infant's death.

The Jury Decides

The jury found that the evidence was sufficient to establish beyond a reasonable doubt that his treatment created a substantial and unjustifiable risk that the infant would die. The physician failed to perceive the risk to the infant whom he knew was suffering from prematurity and respiratory distress syndrome. Failure to perceive the risk constituted gross deviation from the standard of care, and thus the physician was found criminally liable for negligent homicide.[7]

Patient Abuse

The Facts

In the *State of Louisiana v. Brenner,* a nurse's aide had physically assaulted three elderly patients by pinching and slapping them. She had also attempted to choke a patient.

The Court Decides

Fifteen nursing home staff members were charged with cruelty, neglect, and mistreatment of the infirm for the following reasons:

1. Failure to adequately feed and care for the patients
2. Failure to properly train the staff
3. Failure to provide adequate medical supplies
4. Failure to supply adequate staff

5. Failure to maintain a sanitary nursing home
6. Failure to maintain patients' records
7. Failure to see that the appropriate and necessary health services were performed

The nurse's aide was sentenced to concurrent prison sentences of 3 years at hard labor, which were suspended for a 9-month imprisonment.[8]

Aggravated Battery

The Facts

In Illinois, a nurse's aide slapped a patient on the head and face and punched him in the chest.

The Court Decides

The nurse's aide was indicted on seven counts of aggravated battery, one count of abuse, and two counts of intimidation and was convicted and sentenced for abuse of a resident of a long-term care facility.[9]

Murder

The Facts

A registered nurse worked on the night shift in the cardiac care and intensive care units. Over a period of three and one-half weeks, 12 patients suffered seizures and respiratory and cardiac arrests during the night shift. Nine of the 12 patients died.

The nurse was hired at another local hospital after the previous hospital closed. Three days later a patient died with the same signs, seizures, and cardiorespiratory arrest. The nurse was arrested shortly after the patient's death.

Evidence showed that the nurse killed the patients by giving them massive doses of lidocaine, a drug that all the patients took routinely, but on a therapeutic basis. Some of the evidence presented consisted of syringes with high concentrations of lidocaine found in the hospital. Lidocaine was also found in the nurse's home.

The Jury Decides

The jury determined that there was sufficient evidence to convict the registered nurse of first-degree murder, and he was sentenced to death in California.[10]

federal system and the state system (Figure 3–3). According to Article III, Section 11, of the United States Constitution, judicial power is vested in the United States Supreme Court and in lesser federal courts as dictated by Congress. Both state and federal courts have trial courts, appellate courts, and a highest appellate-level court,

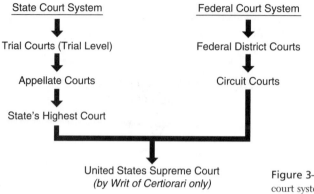

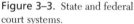

Figure 3–3. State and federal court systems.

which in some states is called the Court of Appeals or Supreme Court. In the state court system, once a case has reached the highest state court, parties can attempt to appeal that case to yet another level—the United States Supreme Court. But the Supreme Court will not necessarily hear any given case. In fact, the Supreme Court does not hear most cases. The party attempting to appeal to the Supreme Court writes a writ of certiorari, which asks the court to hear the case. The Supreme Court either grants or denies the writ.

Similarly, in the federal system, parties can attempt, by writ of certiorari, to appeal cases already heard by the circuit courts to the United States Supreme Court.

Trial Courts

Trial courts are the first courts to hear legal controversies or disputes. The plaintiff, the party alleging harm, files a complaint or petition for damages in either the state, local, or district court or the United States federal district court. In some cases, the plaintiff is the person or entity actually harmed or damaged by the defendant. In other cases, the plaintiffs and their immediate family members (in the case of a wrongful death) are the persons harmed. For example, if the injured party is married, the spouse may be added as a plaintiff because he or she may have suffered losses too. If the injured party dies as a result of malpractice, one of the immediate family members (e.g., the husband or wife) files a lawsuit on behalf of the decedent and that person's estate.

The defendant person or entity sued must answer the complaint within a specified period. Pretrial activities include medical review panels or medical tribunals, and procedures to discover information about the case, such as depositions, interrogatories, admissions of fact, independent medical examinations, and requests for production of documents and specific items (see Chapter 15). If the parties do not settle the dispute, alternative dispute resolutions such as mediation or arbitration may be used (see Chapter 19). Otherwise, the case is set for trial.

The initial trial may be decided by a judge or jury, depending on state or federal laws. In a medical malpractice case, the judge or jury decides whether the facts of the case prove that the defendant breached a standard of care and caused damage or injury to the plaintiff. The judge supervises the court and interprets questions of law. When the jury or judge reaches a verdict, the losing party may seek an appeal of the case to a higher court.

Appellate Courts

The state appellate court and the United States Courts of Appeals have the authority to review and alter the decisions of state or federal trial courts that are under their authority and jurisdiction. In the federal system, 12 circuit courts hear cases from the lower federal courts within their circuit. Each circuit, except for Washington, D.C., consists of three to nine states.

Appellate courts review a case based on the trial record alone. There are no witnesses, no new testimony, and no juries. The appellate court judges review the trial transcripts and the briefs filed by each party's attorney. The opposing attorneys may sometimes present oral arguments to the court; however, because the trial judge has heard the witnesses' testimony, great deference is given to his or her decision. The appellate court renders a decision either to affirm or reverse the trial court's decision or remand the case back to the trial court with special instructions.

The appellate court decisions are written and published in state or regional books called reporters (e.g., *Southern Reporter*), which are distributed to public and private subscribers, including law libraries. Precedent is established through these written appellate decisions.

Supreme Courts

The state **Supreme Court** hears appeals from the state appellate courts. Unless an important federal issue or a constitutional right is involved, the state supreme court is the final authority for state issues. Decisions from the state supreme court are binding on all other courts in that state.

The United States Supreme Court is the court of final decision for both the federal system and the state system in matters involving constitutionally protected rights, such as freedom of speech. Appeals are brought to the Supreme Court under a **writ of certiorari,** which is a written petition by the unsuccessful party requesting that the Supreme Court hear the case. Because the Supreme Court receives requests from thousands of cases annually, only those involving questions of substantial federal importance are selected for review. Once the United States Supreme Court hears a case, the decision becomes binding in all state and federal courts in the nation.

KEEP IN MIND

▶ The state legislature creates the nurse practice act and grants authority for a Board of Nursing to administer and enforce the act.

▶ The nurse practice act creates the legal boundaries for the scope of professional nursing practice.

▶ Both substantive law and procedural law affect the legal process.

▶ Substantive law defines specific rights, duties, obligations, or prohibitions that are imposed by authorities.

▶ Procedural law determines the method or process for legally enforcing these rights and obligations.

▶ *Civil law* refers to the law relating to relationships between private persons.

▶ Criminal law violations are brought by a governmental entity.

▶ The two areas of torts are: (1) unintentional (such as negligence) and (2) intentional (such as battery).

▶ Health care fraud includes: upcoding, unbundling charges, receiving kickbacks, inflating bills, and billing for services not rendered.

IN A NUTSHELL

The legal system in the United States is a complex combination of laws, rules, and regulations that are created at both the federal and state levels. Nurses must stay informed of the legal scope of their nursing practice as society and the profession changes. A basic knowledge of the law and how it works helps nurses avoid litigation while giving them the confidence to practice more competently.

AFTERTHOUGHTS

1. Describe the four major sources of law.
2. What effect do societal values and customs have on the development of laws?
3. How does civil law differ from common law and from criminal law?
4. Discuss the steps in a criminal trial process.
5. Explain the concept of precedent, or stare decisis.
6. Explain the functions of the trial courts, appellate courts, and supreme courts at the state and federal levels.
7. Discuss the differences between a misdemeanor and a felony. Give examples of each.
8. Explain the types of torts.
9. List the elements of negligence that must be present to prove liability for malpractice.

10. Discuss the differences that exist between intentional tort and a tort based on negligence.

11. Explain the difference between ordinary negligence and professional negligence and give examples.

12. List several types of fraud that may have an impact on a nurse's license.

13. Describe the possible ethical conflict with managed care and patient's right to treatment.

14. What is the statute of limitations in your state?

15. Find and discuss a case of patient abuse by a health care provider in your area of practice.

16. Discuss a recent case of Medicare or Medicaid fraud in your area of practice.

17. How has the current economic environment affected patient care and the delivery of care by health care providers?

18. Give an example of professional negligence using the elements of negligence.

19. Obtain a copy of your state's nurse practice act. List the reasons why a nurse's license may be revoked, suspended, or reprimanded.

20. Discuss the two recent cases involving nursing malpractice and negligent homicide.

A CASE IN POINT

Nursing Malpractice

The Facts

Evidence supported the claim that a labor and delivery room nurse failed to observe or recognize signs and symptoms of fetal distress from 8:30 PM to 9:00 PM. The court rejected the defense claim that any negligent conduct of the nurse prior to 8:50 PM was a remote cause of the infant's injuries. The evidence showed that the nurse left the labor room for approximately 10 minutes and should have been in the patient's room doing one-to-one care. The physician testified that the nurse's failure to take action or notify him delayed delivery of the compromised infant and caused and contributed to the infant's damages.[11]

Jury Award

A jury awarded $3.5 million, which was reduced to the applicable statutory cap on damages.

(continued)

Negligent Homicide

The Facts

Over the course of 3.5 weeks, 13 patients in one intensive care unit (ICU) had violent seizures followed by cardiac and respiratory arrest during the night shift. Nine died. In another incident, the same nurse was on duty at a different facility and a patient died with the same symptoms.

The nurse was arrested and charged with murdering a total of 12 patients. He was tried and convicted of killing 12 patients by injecting them with massive doses of lidocaine.

Evidence showed the following:

- The nurse was on the unit and assisted in the patients' care before the seizures.
- He exhibited unusual behavior on the nights the patients had the seizures and died.
- The patients' deaths were consistent with administration of large doses of lidocaine.
- Patients' blood or tissue samples had high concentrations of lidocaine.
- Lidocaine was found at the nurse's home.
- Evidence at trial did not convey that the killings were "mercy killings."

The Court Decides

The nurse was convicted of first-degree murder.[12]

ETHICS IN PRACTICE

Mrs. J., 84 years old, was an active member of a local senior citizens group. One day at a group-sponsored picnic, Mrs. J. experienced an episode of acute chest pain, followed by collapse and cardiac arrest. A member of the group who had taken a cardiopulmonary resuscitation (CPR) course performed CPR on Mrs. J. for approximately 20 minutes, during which time an ambulance was called and the paramedics arrived. Mrs. J. never regained consciousness, although a cardiac rhythm was re-established by the paramedics. She was admitted to the ICU of a local hospital, intubated, and connected to a ventilator. Her two daughters and a son, all of whom lived out of state, were notified of her condition.

Over the several days it took her children to arrive at the hospital, Mrs. J.'s condition gradually deteriorated to the point at which vasoactive medications were required to maintain her blood pressure and urinary output. Although she did not meet all the criteria of brain death, as a result of some reflex reactions that remained, her primary physician believed that because of the extended period of anoxia she had suffered before she was intubated by the paramedics, she had suffered irreversible brain damage.

When the situation was explained to her children, Daughter A and the son agreed that to attempt any further resuscitation on their mother would be futile and cruel. Daughter B, however, disagreed and demanded that "everything" be done to keep her mother alive. After a rather spirited discussion involving the three children, the physician, and the head nurse of the ICU, a compromise was reached. Mrs. J. was to be assigned a "medication-only" code, which meant that antiarrhythmic, vasopressor, and cardiotonic agents would be used to keep the heart beating. The family signed the appropriate form for this procedure, and the physician wrote a medication-only code on the physician order sheet.

The following day, with the family members at the bedside, Mrs. J. went into a sustained episode of ventricular fibrillation. The nurse who was caring for Mrs. J. gave the appropriate medications for the condition. Without chest compressions to circulate the medications, however, there was no change in her cardiac pattern. Approximately 5 minutes into the medication-only code, Daughter B began to yell loudly, "You better do something else, or I'm going to sue you and this hospital for everything you're worth!"

What should the nurse do at this point? Start chest compressions? Tell the family that she cannot do so because of the order? Would Daughter B actually be able to file a lawsuit in this situation?

References

1. National Council of State Board of Nursing: About NCSBN—Overview, Nursing Regulation. http://www.ncsbn.org, accessed December 2002.
2. Creighton, H: Law Every Nurse Should Know, ed 5. WB Saunders, Philadelphia, 1986, p 1.
3. Cazales, MW: Nursing and the Law. Aspen, Germantown, Md, 1978, p 3.
4. Catalano, JT: Ethical and Legal Aspects of Nursing. Springhouse, Springhouse, PA, 1991.
5. Bernzweig, EP: The Nurse's Liability for Malpractice, ed 6. St Louis, Mosby, 1996.
6. Sermchief v. Gonzales, 660 S.W.2d 683 (Mo. 1983).
7. State of Utah v. Warden, 813 P.2d 1146 (Utah 1991).
8. State of Louisiana v. Brenner, 486 So. 2d 101 (La. 1986).
9. People of the State of Illinois v. Johnson, 595 N.E.2d 1381 (Ill. App. 2d 1992).
10. The People v. Diaz, 834 P.2d 117 (Cal. 1992).
11. Fairfax Hospital System, Inc. v. McCurly, 419 S.E. 2d 621 (Va. 1992).
12. People v. Diaz, 11 Cal Rptr. 2d 353 (Cal. 1992).

Resources

National Council of State Boards of Nursing
676 N. St. Clair Street
Suite 550
Chicago, IL 60611-2921
1-312-787-6555
http://www.nscbn.org

Office of the Inspector General
Medicaid and Medicare Fraud Hotline
1-800-HHS-TIPS (1-800-447-8477)

Online Courses

Disciplinary Actions: What Every Nurse Should Know
Tonia A. Aiken, RN, JD, and Julia Aucoin, PhD, RN
Professional Accountability and Legal Liability for Nurses
Laura Mahlmeister, PhD, RN, and Beatrice Yorker, MS, JD, RN
Contact: National Council of State Boards of Nursing

Part 3
Nursing Ethics

Lobbying 4

Julia G. Bounds, CRNA, APRN, BSN

Key Chapter Concepts

Lobbying

Lobbyist

Grass-roots lobbying

Committee

Bill

Law

Veto

Pocket veto

Override

Chapter Thoughts

The health care system in this country is often affected by new legislation and regulations promulgated by the various state and federal governmental bodies. Often lawmakers create these laws in a vacuum, without ever having had hands-on experience in a health care facility. As a result, the laws that they create may not operate as effectively in health care facilities.

For this reason, nurses and other health care practitioners have an obligation to play a role in the future of their own profession. By taking an interest and taking appropriate action to influence the direction of legislation and regulation, nurses will find that the laws and regulations controlling them are founded more, at least in part, on the concepts of beneficence and justice. Nurses have an obligation to patients and to the profession as a whole to take an interest and take part in the formulation of the legal and political infrastructure in which they operate. Also, keep in mind when lobbying for issues affecting nursing practice, any appearance of impropriety must be avoided or it can endanger your license. Payoffs, kickbacks, and gifts of persuasion are illegal, unethical, and certainly unprofessional.

Conflicts of interest may create ethical problems when dealing with lobbyists. For example, the health care industry is lobbying for an issue that is directly opposed by the insurance industry and both are represented by the same lobbyists. An ethical lobbyist should notify both clients and then select one to represent on that particular issue.[1]

The ethical principle of veracity also plays an integral role in the lobbying and legislative processes. Each special interest group views a particular issue in different ways depending on how they see the issue positively or negatively affecting their group's interest. It is easy to see how statements, issues, and things said or discussed are slanted and take on a whole new meaning. Sometimes, it is difficult to determine which group is correctly stating the issues because both positions may sound reasonable. Nurses involved in these processes must do their homework and have the facts available for lobbyists and legislators so it is easier to determine the real truth.

OBJECTIVES

Upon completing this chapter, the reader will be able to:
1. Define lobbying.
2. Learn various ways nurses become involved in the legislative process.
3. Track the process of how a bill becomes a law.
4. Understand the role of committees in the bill process.
5. Learn how to contact legislators effectively.
6. Learn to implement an effective grass-roots campaign.
7. Understand the difference between legislation and regulation.

Introduction

Nurses can take an active role in the legislative and political process to affect change. They may become involved in influencing one specific piece of legislation or regulation, or they can become involved more universally and systematically to influence health care legislation on the whole.

Lobbying: A Primer for Nurses

Lobbying is defined as attempts to influence the passage or defeat of legislation or attempts to create a favorable climate toward legislation affecting goals or sides of various parties, special interest groups, individuals, or organizations. A **lobbyist** is an individual who attempts to influence legislation on behalf of others, such as professional organizations or industries.[2]

There are many ways that nurses can become involved, such as gathering information on issues, visiting or writing to senators and representatives, and lobbying for specific bills. Legislative bills must go through a lengthy process before actually becoming law (Figure 4–1).

When is comes to influencing lawmakers' decisions on health care issues, health care providers have the valuable information needed by both lobbyists and legislators to make rational decisions because for the most part these decision makers do not have a nursing or medical background. Insurance laws, laws involving health maintenance organizations (HMOs), or laws dealing with fraud and abuse in the health care industry can profoundly affect many lives and industries, so decisions should not be made without all the facts. Lawmakers want to be educated and want to know the specifics related to the issues they are dealing with that affect constituents, and as a

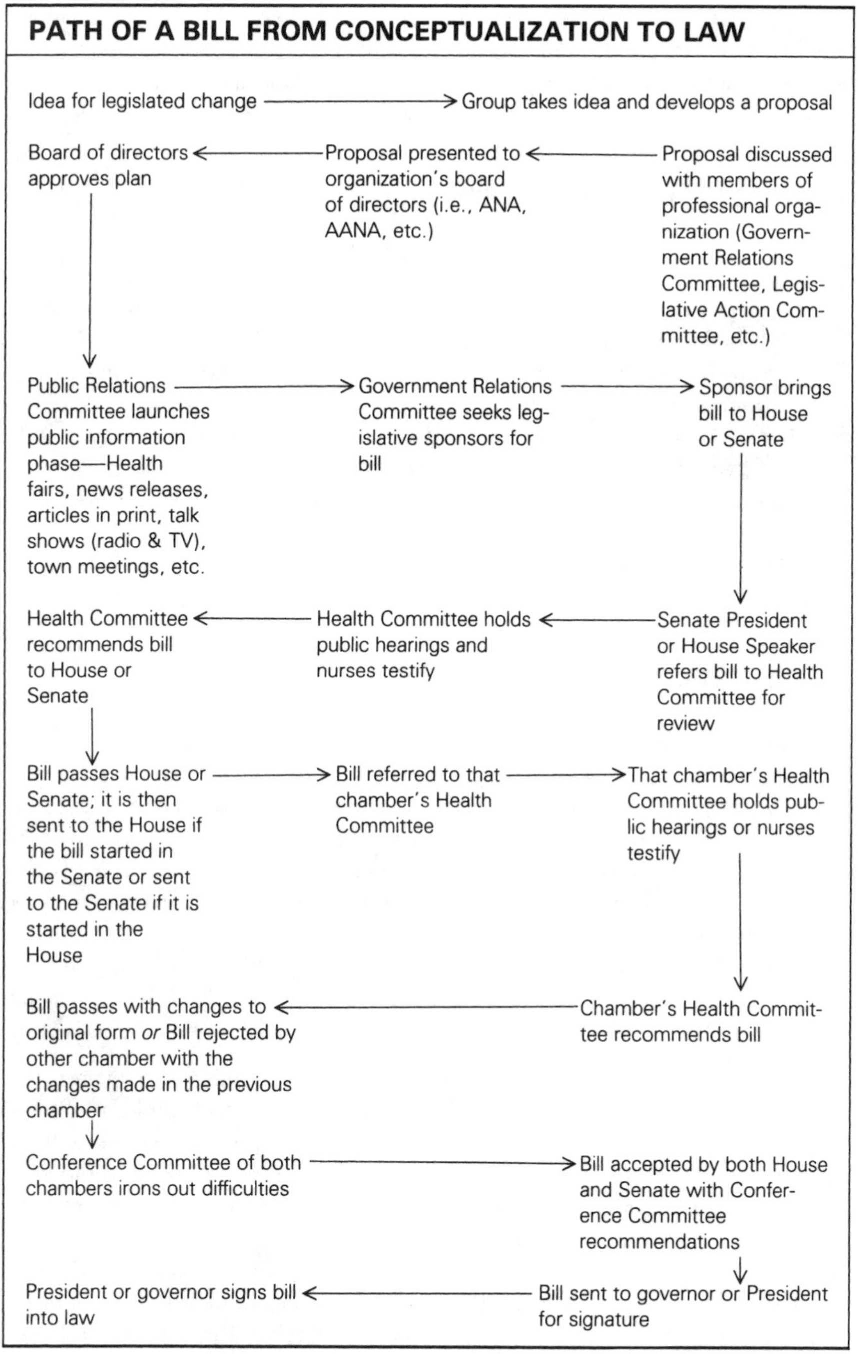

PATH OF A BILL FROM CONCEPTUALIZATION TO LAW

Idea for legislated change ⟶ Group takes idea and develops a proposal

Board of directors ⟵ Proposal presented to ⟵ Proposal discussed
approves plan   organization's board   with members of
                          of directors (i.e., ANA,   professional orga-
                          AANA, etc.)   nization (Govern-
                                                         ment Relations
                                                         Committee, Legis-
                                                         lative Action Com-
                                                         mittee, etc.)

Public Relations ⟶ Government Relations ⟶ Sponsor brings
Committee launches   Committee seeks leg-   bill to House
public information   islative sponsors for   or Senate
phase—Health   bill
fairs, news releases,
articles in print, talk
shows (radio & TV),
town meetings, etc.

Health Committee ⟵ Health Committee holds ⟵ Senate President
recommends bill   public hearings and   or House Speaker
to House or   nurses testify   refers bill to Health
Senate   Committee for
                                                       review

Bill passes House or ⟶ Bill referred to that ⟶ That chamber's Health
Senate; it is then   chamber's Health   Committee holds pub-
sent to the House if   Committee   lic hearings or nurses
the bill started in   testify
the Senate or sent
to the Senate if it is
started in the
House

Bill passes with changes to ⟵ Chamber's Health Commit-
original form or Bill rejected by   tee recommends bill
other chamber with the
changes made in the previous
chamber

Conference Committee of both ⟶ Bill accepted by both House
chambers irons out difficulties   and Senate with Confer-
                                                   ence Committee
                                                   recommendations

President or governor signs bill ⟵ Bill sent to governor or President
into law   for signature

Figure 4–1. Path of a bill from conceptualization to law.

nurse with that knowledge, you are in the best position to provide that information to these lawmakers by giving them statistics, facts, life experiences, and stories that bring the issues before them to life, so that they truly understand the ramifications of their decisions.

Preparing for a Lobbying Campaign

An effective lobbying initiative takes some background work.

1. Develop your plan of action. Consider, rework, revamp, and define your plan in advance of your trip to the legislator's office.
2. Be sure you are fully aware of all similar initiatives on the same topic and the position of those opposing your idea.
3. Check with other nursing organizations to determine their positions and if they have information to help support your position.
4. Fine-tune your presentation to several key points because your time will be limited.
5. Follow up after your meeting with a call or correspondence outlining those points that were discussed.

Getting in Touch with Your Legislators

First, identify the key legislators involved in deciding the issues with which you are concerned. When your legislator is in the home district, invite him or her to your office, hospital, operating room, or business to meet the people who work with you. Invite the legislator to speak to your professional group. You may also invite the members of your state's congressional delegation to lunch or breakfast. This has been done in Washington for several years with success. Remember, legislators need direct contact and exposure to their constituents and their views.

You may also schedule a personal meeting in his or her office either while he or she is in the home district or when you are visiting Washington, D.C., or the state capital.

Regardless of the visit site, be well prepared for the meeting. Follow this advice:

1. Call ahead to make meeting arrangements. Scheduling for senators and representatives is handled by an appointment person in the local office in the major cities in the senator's home state or the representative's district.
2. Send pertinent information to the office ahead of the meeting so the legislator has a chance to consider the issues and prepare questions that he or she may have concerning those issues.
3. Practice, practice, and practice until your presentation is smooth. Although legislators do not expect health care professionals to be polished lobbyists, a good presentation is much more impressive than an unprepared, bumbling attempt.

4. Never lie! If the answer is not available, promise to get it and then communicate that answer to the legislator or aide as soon as possible.

5. Be patient. Whether elected or appointed, officials have many people competing for their attention. Practice your presentation while you wait.

6. Courtesy is imperative. Officials and their aides are, above all, human. The old adage "Common courtesy never cost a dime" applies here. These individuals may respect you and respond in a more helpful manner if you treat them with courtesy and respect.

7. Be brief. Officials are often on busy schedules. Get in and out in an expedient amount of time while getting your point across.

8. Be direct. Get to the point but personalize the issue if possible. Use your own experience, or describe how the issue will affect your practice directly.

9. Keep it simple. Do not use jargon or get too detailed or too complex. Get to the point but make sure the official understands your point.

10. Keep your group small so as not to detract from your issues with the sheer numbers (not to mention the time lost in all those introductions).

11. Close effectively. Ask for the official's support or vote for your issue.

12. Follow up with a thank-you letter. Include a summary of your position and ask for the cooperation of the legislator in persuading their hard-to-convince colleagues.

Preparing for an Effective Letter-Writing Campaign

With **grass-roots lobbying** techniques, the special interest groups try to create the appearance that a large number of constituents support or oppose certain issues, bills, or legislation. Nursing lobbying programs should have a structured network that contacts nurses to tell them who to e-mail, call, or write; the position supported or opposed by the group or organization; and how to use pertinent points related to life or work experiences. Other techniques to get the attention of the legislators include attending legislative breakfasts, dinners, or receptions; visits to the legislator's office; and providing information sheets containing key points on the issues.[3] The following are suggestions for implementing a grass-roots effort that should help you and your nursing organization in planning strategies:

1. Define the goals of this grass-roots campaign.
2. Develop a plan.
3. Assess the knowledge level of your participants concerning the legislative process and the issues that impact your organization. Use this information to plan educational sessions with the goal of improving the political sophistication of your group.
4. Give interested participants information about the bill in question and how this bill would directly affect their practice. Clearly state what action the

legislative body needs to take to meet the goal, and include the specific bill number and name.

5. Set up effective telephone or e-mail networks that can contact key members quickly. Often legislative issues are scheduled and moved up quickly on that schedule, requiring an immediate change of plan.

6. Identify and set up contacts with the key legislators involved in your issue.

7. Set numerical goals for how many letters or mailings will be generated.

8. On large issues, focus groups or polls may be used to acquire information that can be analyzed and sent to the legislators.[4]

9. Get the timing right. The time to begin your campaign is just before the committee hearings begin or just prior to the vote on the floor. Too early is ineffective; too late is wasted effort. You must follow the progress of your issue closely so as to mobilize your members at the right time.

Writing to Your Legislators: Useful Tips

Letters or e-mails from constituents are the best way for legislators to feel the pulse of their district or state. The simple tips listed here will help you and your professional organization in developing and implementing a sound communication channel with your representation in the government.

Dos

1. Do write legibly or type. Handwritten letters are perfectly acceptable so long as they can be read.

2. Do use personal stationery. Indicate that you are a registered nurse. Sign your full name and address. If you are writing for an organization, use that organization's stationary and include information about the number of members in your organization, the services you perform, and the employment settings you are found in. For example, "I am a certified registered nurse anesthetist, and President of the Louisiana Association of Nurse Anesthetists. We are a 700-member group of advanced practice nurses who provide safe, cost-effective anesthesia services for the citizens of Louisiana. In this country CRNAs perform between 60% and 80% of the anesthetics in the rural sector and approximately 60% of the anesthetics for Medicare recipients."

3. Do state if you are a constituent. If you campaigned for or voted for the official, say so.

4. Do identify the issue by number and name if possible or refer to it by the common name ("Prescriptive Authority Act").

5. Do state your position clearly and state what you would like your legislator to do. "I would like you to support the reauthorization of the funding for the Center for Nursing Research."

6. Do draft the letter in your own words and convey your own thoughts.

7. Do refer to your personal experience of how a bill will directly affect you, your family, your patients, and members of your organization or your profession. Thoughtful, sincere letters on issues that directly affect the writer receive the most attention and are those that are often quoted in hearings or debates.

8. Do contact the legislator in time for your legislator to act on an issue. After the vote is too late. If your senator or representative is a member of the committee that is hearing the issue, contact him or her before the committee hearings begin. If he or she is not on the committee, write just before the bill is due to come to the floor for debate and vote.

9. Do write the governor promptly for a state issue, after the bill passes both houses, if you want to influence his or her decision to sign the bill into law or veto it.

10. Do use e-mail to state your points.

11. Do be appreciative, especially of past favorable votes. Many letters legislators receive feedback from constituents who are unhappy or displeased about actions taken on an issue. Letters of thanks are greatly appreciated.

12. Do make your point quickly and discuss only one issue per letter. Most letters should be one page long.

13. Do remember that you are the expert in your professional area. Most legislators know little about the practice of nursing and respect your knowledge. Offer your expertise to your elected representative as an advisor or resource person to his or her staff when issues arise.

14. Do ask for what you want your legislator to do on an issue. "We would like you to support HR 2143." Ask him or her to state his or her position in the reply to you.

Don'ts

1. Don't begin a letter with "as a citizen and a taxpayer." Legislators assume that you are a citizen, and all of us pay taxes.

2. Don't threaten or use hostility. "I'll never vote for you again if you…" will get no positive response. Most legislators ignore "hate" mail.

3. Don't send carbon copies of your letter to other legislators. Write each legislator individually. Don't send letters to legislators from other states—they will refer your letter to your congressional representative.

4. Don't write House members while a bill is in the Senate and vice versa. A bill may be amended many times before it gets from one house to the other.

5. Don't write postcards; they are tossed.

6. Don't use form letters. In large numbers these letters get attention only in the form that they are tallied. These letters tend to elicit a "form letter response" from the legislator.

7. Don't apologize for writing and taking their time. If your letter is short and presents your opinion on an issue, they are glad to have it.

Understanding the Process

Committees hear testimony from interested parties and then decide to recommend the **bill** as is or to amend it. If the committee opposes the bill, they will simply let it "die" in committee. (See Box 4–1 for a glossary of terms referring to the legislative process.) If a number of bills regarding the same issue are pending, the committee may report out a clean bill, which brings the features of the other similar bills in and provides totally new provisions. Amending or cleaning a bill can range from perfecting a bill to gutting the original proposal and changing the meaning of the bill. Amendments must be carefully scrutinized.

A bill reported out of committee is put on a calendar for a vote by the full House or Senate. If your bill is placed on the consent calendar, on the date specified it will be called and passed without debate if no one objects. If your bill is placed on the regular calendar, as are all major bills and nonroutine minor bills, it will be called for debate and voted on on the date indicated on the calendar. Of course, calendars are always subject to change.

As soon as your bill is out of committee, begin contacting each member of the full House or Senate. Do not wait for the date of the vote. Your group should contact each member formally.

On the day of the vote, there must be enough volunteers in the galleries and in the lobbies of the capitol so that their numbers are noticed. Wear badges identifying yourselves. Pay close attention to your bill when it is debated on the floor of the chamber because it may be amended. Amendments can improve or destroy a bill. The sponsor must be advised as to whether acceptance of an amendment is appropriate or opposition is imperative.

To become **law,** a bill must be passed by both houses in identical form (except in Nebraska, which is unicameral). When one version of a bill is passed in the Senate and a different version in the House, a conference committee composed of members of both houses irons out the differences. Unless one version is totally objectionable, there is little to be done at this time. If your group simply cannot live with one version of the bill, your group must contact the members of the conference committee and try to gain support for the appropriate version of the bill.

Once the bill clears the conference committee, it goes to the president or governor. He or she may sign it into law, let it become law without his or her signature, **veto** it and send it back to the Congress or legislature, or **pocket veto** it (that is, leave it unsigned after the legislature adjourns). Unless there is evidence that the governor or president is in opposition to your bill, do nothing, or if it is major legislation, arrange to participate in the bill signing. If you think that the executive may oppose the bill, attempt to contact him or her. If the bill is vetoed, your chance for mounting a campaign to **override** the veto is small unless the original vote was by a sizable margin

BOX 4–1

Political Glossary

Act: Term for legislation that has been passed by both houses of Congress or the legislature and has been signed into law by the President or governor or passes over his or her veto, thus becoming law.

Amendment: Proposal of a legislator to change the language or content of a bill or act. Usually amendments are handled as bills.

Bill: Legislative proposal originating in either the House or Senate. They are numbered as either HR (for House of Representatives) or S (Senate). The numbers are assigned in order of introduction in the chamber or a committee.

Chamber: Meeting place for the total membership of the House or Senate (as opposed to committee rooms).

Conference Committee: Committee composed of members of the House and Senate appointed to reconcile differences between the two houses of the proceedings of both houses with debate, statements, and so on, reported verbatim.

Filibuster: Device used only in the Senate to delay or prevent a vote by time-consuming talk. Can only be stopped by a two-thirds vote of the senators present and voting.

Joint Committee: Committee composed of a specific number of members of both the House and Senate. It is usually investigative in nature.

Law: An act of Congress or the state legislature that has been signed by the President or governor or passed over a veto.

Lobby: To influence the passage or defeat of legislation or an election.

Political Action Committee (PAC): Organization formed by a corporation or association that solicits contributions for candidates for public office.

Quorum: Number of members needed to conduct business. This is a majority of the members (in Washington: 51 in the Senate and 218 in the House, if there are no vacancies). Any member may object to conducting business without a quorum and force a roll-call vote to bring in absentees.

Rider: A provision usually not related but tacked on to a bill that its sponsor hopes to get through more easily by including it in other legislation.

Veto: Action taken by the President or governor rejecting a bill presented to him or her by Congress or the legislature for signature. When Congress overrides a veto by a $^2/_3$ majority, it automatically becomes law.

Voice vote: The presiding officer of either chamber calls for yes or no (or aye or no) and calculates the results.

and the governor does not command party loyalty. If the pocket veto is used, you can do nothing except start your planning for the next year.

Do not be discouraged if your program is defeated. Major social reform is a series of defeats—often stretching over a generation—followed by victory. Try again.

Keep Abreast of Legislation, Regulations, and Congress

When issues are important to your profession, contact the legislator and provide the important facts that support your position. Then, because legislators receive numerous calls and documentation on a variety of issues, in addition to attending lots of meetings and campaigning, be sure to follow up routinely so your opinions stay fresh in his or her memory.

Legislation

To keep in contact with the legislature, it is important to identify key committees and subcommittees in the legislative bodies, and to identify and develop communications with the members of those committees. Identifying and developing communications with staffers who work with committee members also may help keep you abreast of what is going on, and you may also consider contacting committee chairs to ask for notification of any hearings on pertinent bills. Other ways to keep abreast of new information include the following:

1. Volunteer for campaign work and develop contacts with legislators.
2. Obtain pertinent government documents using online resources.
3. Get the general telephone number for the state government and the mailing addresses for correspondence.
4. Develop liaisons with other health professionals and utilize them as information sources and allies in lobbying for health care issues.
5. Register a member of your group as a lobbyist—the fee is generally small.
6. If possible, hire a lobbyist.
7. Once you have notified your legislator about your interest in a particular issue, the legislator's office may routinely send literature outlining his or her activities throughout the sometimes arduous process.

Regulation

Because lobbying activities can significantly affect individuals and industry, regulation is essential to avoid abuse. Lobbyists have created ethics codes, guidelines for professional conduct and standards.[5]

The following will help you keep abreast of the newest regulations and standards:

1. Subscribe to the state register (which contains all state regulations under consideration).
2. Identify and develop contacts with state agencies that exert control on or impact your practice and ask to be added to their mailing lists. A limited list includes the following:

- Nurse practice act: rules and regulations
- Medical practice act: rules and regulations
- Pharmacy act: rules and regulations
- Dental practice act: rules and regulations
- Hospital licensing act: rules and regulations
- Ambulatory surgical center licensing act: rules and regulations
- Insurance statute: rules and regulations
- Trauma center statute: rules and regulations
- Department of Health
- Podiatric Act: rules and regulations

KEEP IN MIND

▶ Lobbying is defined as attempts to influence the passage or defeat of legislation or attempts to create a favorable climate toward legislation.

▶ Nurses can become involved in the political process by gathering information on issues, forming grass-roots coalitions, visiting or writing to senators and representatives, or lobbying for specific bills.

▶ Committees hear testimony from interested parties and then decide to recommend the bill as is or to amend the bill.

▶ Legislators need direct contact and exposure to their constituents and their views.

▶ Nurses should not write to House members while a bill is in the Senate and vice versa. A bill may be amended many times before it gets from one house to the other.

▶ It is important to identify and develop contacts with state agencies that exert control on or impact your practice and ask to be added to their mailing lists.

▶ To keep in contact with the legislature, it is important to identify key committees and subcommittees in the legislative bodies, and to identify and develop communications with the members of those committees.

IN A NUTSHELL

Nurses can and should play a role in formulating the laws that affect their practice. By understanding the political process, organizing into interest groups, consistently surveying new legislation and regulation, systematically contacting the appropriate individuals and agencies, and reliably following up on their efforts, nurses can work the often bureaucratic system to their advantage.

Numerous resources exist to allow nurses to keep informed and up to date and to educate themselves on how the process works. Most of the resources are inexpensive and easily accessible. Nurses should avail themselves of this information.

AFTERTHOUGHTS

1. Define lobbying.
2. What are the various ways in which a nurse can become involved in the legislative process?
3. Identify five ways a nurse can keep up to date on what has been happening in Congress.
4. What are the five tips for writing a letter to a legislator or regulator?
5. What is the role of the committees during the process of a bill becoming a law?
6. What is the difference between legislation and regulation, what bodies promulgate each, and in what documents can you find each?
7. Explain the process of a bill becoming a law.

ETHICS IN PRACTICE

Jasmine Blithe, RN, the administrator of Sleepy Valley Rest Home, sets up a meeting with Senator Jason regarding Bill 100, which is unfavorable to the nursing home industry. In her meeting with the senator, she donates $5,000 to his campaign fund and discusses Bill 100, which she asks the senator to vote against.

Ms. Blithe also "guarantees" that if he does vote against the bill she will assist the senator in finding employment opportunities for his family or friends in the future.

1. Has Ms. Blithe acted unethically? Has she broken any laws (based on your state laws)?
2. What are the implications of her actions?

References

1. Rosenthal, A: The Third House: Lobbyists and Lobbying in the States, ed 2. CQ Press, Washington, DC, 2001.
2. Guyer, RL: Guide to State Legislative Lobbying. Gainesville, Fla: Engineering the Law, Inc, 2000.
3. Rosenthal, Ibid.
4. Ibid.
5. Ibid.

Resources

Plugging in to Washington: How to Communicate with Congress
American Society of Association Executives
1575 Eye Street, NW
Washington, DC 20005
Phone: (202) 626-2723
Fax: (202) 371-8825
http://www.asaenet.org

United States Capitol Switchboard
(202) 224-3131
http://www.senate.gov for contact information for senators
http://www.house.gov for contact information for representatives
http://www.whitehouse.gov for contact information for the President

Democratic National Committee
http://democrats.org

Republican National Committee
http://www.rnc.org/

Federal Election Committee
http://www.fec.gov/

Legislative Information on the Internet
http://thomas.loc.gov/

Library of Congress
101 Independence Ave, SE
Washington, DC 20540
(202) 707-5000
http://www.loc.gov/

Bureau of National Affairs
Publisher of print and electronic news, analysis, and reference products, providing intensive coverage
    of legal and regulatory developments for professionals in business and government.
1231 25th Street NW
Washington, DC 20037
(800) 372-1033
http://www.bna.com/

Federal Government Web site
Search and view full text of Supreme Court decisions issued between 1937 and 1975; Internal
    Revenue Service information, government research, and development publications; top govern-
    ment Web sites; key government science and technology Web resource sites.
http://www.fedworld.gov/

Contacting State Representatives
Access individual state Web sites.

American Nurses Association
Government Affairs
600 Maryland Avenue, SW
Suite 100 West
Washington, DC 20024
(800) 274-4ANA
(202) 651-7000
http://nursingworld.org/gova/federal/gfederal.htm

Ethics in Nursing — 5

Key Chapter Concepts

Values
Morals
Laws
Ethics
Code of ethics
Ethical dilemma
Autonomy
Justice
Fidelity
Beneficence

Nonmaleficence
Veracity
Paternalism
Rationalism
Pragmatism
Standard of best interest
Obligations
Rights
Utilitarianism
Deontology

Chapter Thoughts

Nurses in today's health care system, where major technological advances are almost a daily occurrence, often face ethical dilemmas they may not be prepared to resolve. Rapid advancements in health care research, as well as fundamental changes in societal values and cultural norms, have outpaced the health care system's ability to solve complicated ethical issues. As a result, judges and juries are being asked to resolve ethical questions that concern life-and-death issues among patients, their families, physicians, and nurses.

The legal system is particularly unprepared to resolve sensitive ethical issues. In many ethical conflicts, no laws deal specifically with the issues at hand. In other types of conflicts, general legal principles or laws can be cited that offer guidelines; however, ethical dilemmas are often complicated by circumstances not addressed by the legal system. When the legal system does make decisions concerning ethical dilemmas, those cases can be cited later as precedents. They then take on the force of law under the common law principle found in this country.

OBJECTIVES

Upon completing this chapter, the reader will be able to:
1. Discuss the difference between law and ethics.
2. Define the key terms used in ethics.

3. Discuss the important ethical concepts.
4. Distinguish between the two most commonly used systems of ethical decision making.
5. Name the steps in the ethical decision-making process.
6. Demonstrate the use of the ethical decision-making process in the analysis of an ethical case study.
7. Discuss ethical dilemmas in various nursing settings.
8. Define the patient's bill of rights.

Introduction

Any nurse providing care for patients must understand the steps involved in ethical decision making. Sound ethical decisions are based on an understanding of the following:

- The underlying ethical principles
- The key ethical theories or systems that can be used
- The profession's code of ethics

Ethical decision making is a skill that can be learned by any nurse. However, as with all skills, it requires mastering the theoretical material and practicing the skill itself.

This chapter presents the basic information necessary to understand ethics, the code of ethics, and ethical decision making. It discusses the fundamental definitions and principles involved in understanding ethics, two key ethical systems or theories often used by health providers in resolving ethical dilemmas, and an ethical decision-making model based on the nursing process.

Law Versus Ethics

Laws are rules made by human beings to guide society and regulate human interactions. Laws usually have a sanctioned method of enforcement, such as the police. The goal of all laws is (or should be) to preserve the species and promote peaceful and productive interactions between individuals or groups of individuals.

Ethics is the discipline that deals with the rightness and wrongness of actions. The goal of ethics is similar to that of the legal system, except that in most cases there is no system of enforcement or ethical guidelines. Ideally, the ethical system is more inclusive and usually exceeds the legal system in the situations it covers. In reality, there can be and are laws that are unethical. In practice, particularly where health care is concerned, law and ethics overlap in many areas. These areas include, but are not limited to, such issues as death, dying, birth, abortion, genetics, quality of life, breach of duty, allocation of medical services, and violations of others' rights. In health care, ethical and legal issues transect each other at every point. Each interaction with a patient produces an ethical and legal situation. Although anyone can make a mistake at any given time, nurses who have a thorough understanding of the ethical code, follow that code, and stay within the guidelines for practice set by standards of care and nurses practice acts are much less likely to have a lawsuit filed against them.

Key Definitions

The study of ethics is a specialized area of philosophy, the origins of which date back to ancient Greece. In fact, ethical principles enunciated by Hypocrites still serve as the underpinnings of many of today's ethical issues. Like most specialized areas of study, ethics has its own language and terminology. The following are some key terms that are necessary for understanding health care ethics.

Values

Values are ideals or concepts that give meaning to an individual's life. Values are most commonly derived from societal norms, religion, and family orientation and serve as the framework for making decisions and taking certain actions in everyday life. Although values usually are not written down, it may be important for nurses, at some point in their careers, to make a list of their own values and attempt to rank them by priority. Value conflicts often occur in everyday life and can force an individual to select a higher priority value over a lower priority value. For example, nurses who value both their career and their family may be forced to decide between going to work or staying home with a sick child.

Morals

Morals are the fundamental standards of right and wrong that an individual learns and internalizes, usually in the early stages of childhood development. An individual's moral orientation is often based on religious beliefs, and societal influence plays an important part in this development. Moral behavior is often manifested as behavior in accordance with a group's norms, customs, or traditions. For example, in the Mormon tradition, polygamy is an accepted practice (and therefore considered morally correct), whereas most Christian religions consider polygamy an immoral activity.

Laws

Laws are generally defined as rules of social conduct devised by people to protect society. Laws are based on concerns for fairness and justice. The fundamental goal of society's laws is the preservation of the species, which can be achieved by the promotion of peaceful and productive interactions between individuals and groups of individuals. Laws achieve this goal by preventing the actions of one citizen from infringing on the rights of another citizen. Importantly, laws are enforceable through some type of police force.

Ethics

Ethics are declarations of what is right or wrong and what ought to be. Ethics, which are usually presented as systems of valued behaviors and beliefs, govern conduct to ensure that individuals' rights are protected. Ethics exist on several levels, ranging from the individual or small group to the society as a whole. The concepts of ethics and morals are similar in both their development and purposes. In one sense, ethics can be considered a system of morals for a particular group.

Code of Ethics

A **code of ethics** is a written list of a profession's values and standards of conduct. The code of ethics provides a framework of decision making for the profession and should be oriented toward the day-to-day decisions made by members of the profession. Codes of ethics are presented in general statements and do not give specific answers to every possible ethical dilemma that might arise. However, these codes do offer guidance to the individual practitioner making a decision. Ideally, codes of ethics should undergo periodic revision to reflect changes in the profession and society as a whole. Although codes of ethics are not legally enforceable as laws, consistent violations of a professional code of ethics indicate an unwillingness by the individual to act in a professional manner, which often results in disciplinary actions ranging from reprimands and fines to suspension and revocation of licensure.

Although similar, there are several different codes of ethics that nurses may adopt. In the United States, the American Nurses Association's Code of Ethics for Nurses is the generally accepted code. There is a Canadian Nurses Association Code of Ethics for Registered Nurses and an International Council of Nurses Code of Ethics for Nurses. (See Box 5–1 for a summary of each of the codes for nurses.)

Ethical Dilemma

An **ethical dilemma** is a situation that requires an individual to make a choice between two equally unfavorable alternatives. When ethical dilemmas are reduced to their elemental aspects, conflicts between one individual's rights and those of another, between one individual's obligations and the rights of another, or any combination of obligations and rights conflicting usually form the basis of the dilemma. By the very nature of an ethical dilemma, there is no one good solution, and the decision made often has to be defended against those who disagree with it.

Ethical Decision-Making Process

Nurses, by definition, are problem solvers. The primary focus of nursing education is to learn to solve patient nursing care problems. One of the important problem-solving tools is the nursing process itself, which is a systematic, step-by-step approach to resolving problems that arise when dealing with a patient's health and well-being.

BOX 5–1

Code of Ethics for Nurses

American Nurses Association Code of Ethics for Nurses*

1. The nurse, in all professional relationships, practices with compassion and respect for the inherent dignity, worth, and uniqueness of every individual, unrestricted by considerations of social or economic status, personal attributes, or the nature of health problems.
2. The nurse's primary commitment is to the patient, whether an individual, family, group, or community.
3. The nurse promotes, advocates for, and strives to protect the health, safety, and rights of the patient.
4. The nurse is responsible and accountable for individual nursing practice and determines the appropriate delegation of tasks consistent with the nurse's obligation to provide optimum patient care.
5. The nurse owes the same duties to self as to others, including the responsibility to preserve integrity and safety, to maintain competence, and to continue personal and professional growth.
6. The nurse participates in establishing, maintaining, and improving health care environments and conditions of employment conducive to the provision of quality health care and consistent with the values of the profession through individual and collective action.
7. The nurse participates in the advancement of the profession through contributions to practice, education, administration, and knowledge development.
8. The nurse collaborates with other health professionals and the public in promoting community, national, and international efforts to meet health needs.
9. The profession of nursing, as represented by associations and their members, is responsible for articulating nursing values, for maintaining the integrity of the profession and its practice, and for shaping social policy.[1]

*Reprinted with permission from American Nurses Association, Code of Ethics for Nurses with Interpretive Statements. © 2001 American Nurses Publishing, American Nurses Foundation/American Nurses Association, Washington, DC.

(continued)

BOX 5–1

Code of Ethics for Nurses *(continued)*

Canadian Nurses Association Code of Ethics for Registered Nurses[†]

Values: A value is something that is prized or held dear; something that is deeply cared about. This code is organized around eight primary values that are central to ethical nursing practice:

Safe, competent and ethical care: Nurses value the ability to provide safe, competent and ethical care that allows them to fulfill their ethical and professional obligations to the people they serve.

Health and well-being: Nurses value health promotion and well-being and assisting persons to achieve their optimum level of health in situations of normal health, illness, injury, disability or at the end of life.

Choice: Nurses respect and promote the autonomy of persons and help them to express their health needs and values, and also to obtain desired information and services so they can make informed decisions.

Dignity: Nurses recognize and respect the inherent worth of each person and advocate for respectful treatment of all persons.

Confidentiality: Nurses safeguard information learned in the context of a professional relationship, and ensure it is shared outside the health care team only with the person's informed consent, or as may be legally required, or where the failure to disclose would cause significant harm.

Justice: Nurses uphold principles of equity and fairness to assist persons in receiving a share of health services and resources proportionate to their needs and in promoting social justice.

Accountability: Nurses are answerable for their practice, and they act in a manner consistent with their professional responsibilities and standards of practice.

Quality Practice Environments: Nurses value and advocate for practice environments that have the organizational structures and resources necessary to ensure safety, support and respect for all persons in the work setting.[2]

[†] Reprinted with permission from the Canadian Nurses Association.

Despite this ability to deal with patients' physical problems, many nurses feel inadequate when confronted with ethical dilemmas associated with patient care. These feelings may stem from their unfamiliarity with a systematic problem-solving technique for ethical dilemmas. However, nurses in any health care setting can develop the decision-making skills necessary to make sound ethical decisions if they learn and practice using an ethical decision-making model.

BOX 5–1

Code of Ethics for Nurses

The International Council of Nurses Code of Ethics for Nurses[†]

Nurses and people: The nurse's primary professional responsibility is to people requiring nursing care.

In providing nursing care, the nurse promotes an environment in which the human rights, values, customs and spiritual beliefs of the individual, family and community are respected.

The nurse ensures that the individual receives sufficient information on which to base consent for care and related treatment.

The nurse holds in confidence personal information and uses judgement in sharing this information.

The nurse shares with society the responsibility for initiating and supporting action to meet the health and social needs of the public, in particular those of vulnerable populations.

The nurse also shares responsibility to sustain and protect the natural environment from depletion, pollution, degradation and destruction.

Nurses and practice: The nurse carries personal responsibility and accountability for nursing practice, and for maintaining competence by continual learning.

The nurse maintains a standard personal health such that the ability to provide care is not compromised.

The nurse uses judgement regarding individual competence when accepting and delegating responsibility.

The nurse at all times maintains standards of personal conduct which reflect well on the profession and enhance public confidence.

The nurse, in providing care, ensures that use of technology and scientific advances are compatible with safety, dignity and rights of people.

Nurses and the profession: The nurse assumes the major role in determining and implementing acceptable standards of clinical nursing practice, management, research and education.

The nurse is active in developing a core research-based professional knowledge.

The nurse, acting through professional organization, participates in creating and maintaining equitable social and economic working conditions in nursing.

Nurses and coworkers: The nurse sustains a co-operative relationship with coworkers in nursing and other fields.

The nurse takes appropriate action to safeguard individuals when their care is endangered by a coworker or any other person.[3]

[†] Used with permission, International Council of Nurses, Geneva, Switzerland, 2000. Approved 2000; see http://www.icn.ch/ethics.htm.

The ethical decision-making process provides a method for nurses to answer key questions about ethical dilemmas and to organize their thinking in a more logical and sequential manner. The problem-solving method presented here, unlike some others, is based on the nursing process. It should be relatively easy for the nurse to move from the nursing process used in resolving patient physical problems to the ethical decision-making process used in resolving ethical problems.

The chief goal of the ethical decision-making process is determining right from wrong in situations where clear demarcations do not exist or are not apparent to the nurse faced with the decision. The ethical decision-making process also presupposes that the nurse making the decision knows that a system of ethics exists, knows the content of that ethical system, and knows that the system applies to similar ethical decision-making problems despite multiple variables. At some point, nurses need to undertake the task of clarifying their own values if this has not been done or has not been done recently.

The following five-step ethical decision-making process is presented as a tool for resolving ethical dilemmas.

Step 1: Collect, Analyze, and Interpret the Data

Obtain as much information as possible about the particular ethical dilemma to be decided. Unfortunately, information is sometimes limited, which complicates the analysis and interpretation. Among the things that are important to know are the patient's wishes, the family's wishes, and the extent of the physical or emotional problems causing the dilemma.

A common ethical situation that many nurses must face at some time is whether to resuscitate a hospital patient with a terminal disease. Physicians often leave instructions for the nursing staff not to code or resuscitate the patient but to go through the motions to make the family feel better. The nurse's dilemma is whether to attempt seriously to revive the patient in the event of cardiac or respiratory cessation.

Some of the questions nurses need answered in these cases include how mentally competent the patient is to make a no-resuscitation decision, what the patient's desires are, what the family thinks about the situation, and whether the physician has sought input from the patient and the family. Many institutions have policies concerning no resuscitation, and it is wise to consider these in the data collection stage. After collecting information, the nurse needs to bring the pieces of information together in a manner that gives the clearest and sharpest focus to the dilemma.

Step 2: State the Dilemma

After collecting and analyzing all available information, the nurse needs to state the dilemma as clearly as possible. Most of the time, the dilemma can be reduced to a statement or two that revolves around the key ethical issues. These ethical issues often involve a question of conflicting rights or basic ethical principles.

In the resuscitation situation just posed, where the situation is a question of slow resuscitation or no resuscitation, the statement of the dilemma might be: "The patient's right to death with dignity versus the nurse's obligation to preserve life and do no harm."

Step 3: Consider the Choices of Action

After stating the dilemma as clearly as possible, list all the possible courses of action that can resolve the dilemma without considering the consequences. This undertaking needs to be a real brainstorming activity in which all possible courses of action are considered. The consequences of the different actions are considered later. This process of idea development may require input from outside sources such as colleagues, supervisors, or even experts in the ethical field.

Some of the options for the nurse dealing with the patient who is a questionable resuscitation candidate include the following:

- Resuscitating the patient to the nurse's fullest capabilities despite what the physician has requested
- Not resuscitating the patient at all, just going through the motions without any real attempt to revive the patient
- Seeking another assignment to avoid dealing with the situation
- Reporting the problem to a supervisor
- Attempting to clarify the question with the patient
- Attempting to clarify the question with the family
- Confronting the physician about the question

Step 4: Analyze the Advantages and Disadvantages of Each Course of Action

Some of the courses of action developed during the previous step in the process are more feasible than others. That will become readily apparent during this step, when the nurse considers the advantages and the disadvantages of each action, along with the consequences of taking each course of action.

In the ethical dilemma described earlier, discussing the decision with the physician might lead to an angry physician who will no longer trust the nurse involved. A nurse who successfully resuscitates a patient despite orders to the contrary may face disciplinary action ranging from a reprimand to termination. Not resuscitating the patient at all has the potential to produce a lawsuit and disciplinary action if there is no clear do not resuscitate order. Presenting the situation to a supervisor may, if the supervisor supported the physician, label the nurse as a troublemaker and have a negative effect on future evaluations. The same process, enumerating the advantages and disadvantages, should be applied to the other courses of action.

By considering the advantages and disadvantages, the nurse should be able to pare the options down to the few realistic choices of action. Other relevant issues need to be examined while attempting to weigh the choices of action. The American Nurses

Association (ANA) Code of Ethics for Nurses is an important source for guidance when making many patient care decisions where ethical dilemmas exist.

Step 5: Make the Decision

The most difficult part of the process is actually making the decision and, as a corollary, living with the consequences. By their nature, ethical dilemmas produce differences of opinion. Not everyone will be pleased with the decision. The best decision is one that is based on a sound ethical decision-making process.

In resolving any ethical dilemma, questions will always remain regarding the correct course of action.

AUTHOR TIP: *Keep in mind that the patient's wishes almost always supersede independent decisions on the part of health care professionals. Collaborative decision making among the patient, physician, nurses, and family about resuscitation is the ideal and tends to produce fewer complications in the long run.*

An Ethics Primer

In addition to the terminology used in the study and practice of ethics, there are several important concepts, or principles, that often underlie ethical dilemmas. Although the following list is by no means comprehensive, it does present several key principles that often serve as the underpinnings for ethical dilemmas.

Autonomy

Autonomy is the right of self-determination, independence, and freedom. Autonomy in the health care setting involves the health care provider's willingness to respect patients' rights to make decisions about and for themselves, even if the provider does not agree with those decisions.

As with most rights, autonomy is not an absolute right. Under certain circumstances, limitations can be imposed on it, such as when one individual's autonomy interferes with another's rights, health, or well-being. For example, patients generally can use their right to autonomy by refusing any or all treatments. However, in the case of contagious diseases that affect society, such as tuberculosis (TB), the individual can be forced by the health care and legal systems to take medications to cure the disease. The individual can also be forced into isolation to prevent the spread of the disease.

Justice

Justice is the obligation to be fair to all people. The concept is often expanded to what is called distributive justice, which specifically states that individuals have the right to

? What Would You Do?

Reporting Incidents

What is your ethical and legal duty with regard to reporting incidents?

As a professional, you must report incidents of which you have firsthand knowledge. Failure to report could result in termination of your job or disciplinary actions. Also, professional liability and involvement in litigation could occur if you fail to report an incident that causes harm to a patient.

What is your ethical and legal duty with regard to reporting unsafe or impaired health care professionals?

As a professional you must report the unsafe or impaired health care provider. This person may cause injury to the patient or provide an unsafe environment that could result in injury or even death. Moreover, if this person causes harm to a patient and the Board of Nursing learns that you had knowledge that the nurse was unsafe or impaired and you failed to do anything or report the person, then you may also be brought before the Board for disciplinary actions.

To Code or Not to Code

Mrs. Lynn's cardiac monitor shows a heart rate of 52, blood pressure of 76/52 mm/Hg, and respiration of 32.

Mrs. Julie Lynn is 75 years old with a history of uncontrolled diabetes, hypertension, emphysema, and advanced lung cancer. She has had bilateral amputations and has partial paralysis from a stroke. The cancer has metastasized. Two days ago she became disoriented and less responsive. Her physician discontinued dialysis and considered her death "just a matter of time." The patient wants everything done. She will not sign a do not resuscitate (DNR) order, but the physician has talked to her two sons and is awaiting their reply.

Apply the decision-making process to determine what action you should take. What are the legal and ethical implications?

Some questions to investigate:

1. Does the patient have a living will?
2. Does the patient have a health care agent?
3. Can the sons override their mother's wishes to have everything done for her?

be treated equally regardless of race, sex, marital status, medical diagnosis, social standing, economic level, or religious belief. The principle of justice underlies the first statement in the ANA Code of Ethics for Nurses. Distributive justice is sometimes expanded to include ideas such as equal access to health care for all. As with other rights, limits can be placed on justice when it interferes with the rights of others.

Justice requires that the person or patient be treated according to what is fair. This implication is that patients with the same diagnosis should receive the same level of care. However, nurses are often challenged to fairly allocate scarce resources and supplies.

? What Would You Do?

Justice

Mr. Brett Hunter, an 80-year-old welfare patient, developed respiratory distress and high fever and has compromised arterial blood gases. Respirations are 32 and labored. He has consolidation of right lower lobe (pneumonia) and is deteriorating quickly. Dr. Maken feels he would benefit from being in the intensive care unit (ICU) but knows that the two beds will be needed for two new post-operative patients tomorrow. He asks your opinion as the charge nurse.

Gather information on the following:

1. Would ICU admission prolong suffering?
2. Is Mr. Hunter being treated differently because of age or ability to pay?
3. Is it unfair to deny an ICU bed to Mr. Hunter today just because beds will be needed the next day?
4. How many ICU beds are available?
5. Has Mr. Hunter signed a DNR?
6. How long will he be in ICU?
7. Does he have a living will?
8. Is his condition life threatening?
9. Is his condition acute?
10. Is there an option to transfer Mr. Hunter to another facility?
11. What are the potential legal implications of denying an ICU admission to a patient who can benefit from it on the basis that the bed will be needed the following day?

Evaluate your options without regard to the consequences:

1. Admit to ICU tonight and re-evaluate the situation in the morning.
2. Admit for aggressive pulmonary treatment tonight and transfer Mr. Hunter tomorrow.
3. Cancel one of the other patients' surgeries.
4. Use additional staffing to provide one-on-one care.
5. Transfer to another facility with ICU beds.
   What would you do?

Fidelity

Fidelity is the individual's obligation to be faithful to commitments made to self and others. In health care, fidelity includes the professional's faithfulness or loyalty to agreements and responsibilities accepted as part of the practice of the profession. Fidelity is the main support for the concept of accountability, although conflicts in fidelity might arise because of obligations owed to different individuals or groups. For example, a nurse who is just finishing a very busy and tiring 12-hour shift may experince a conflict of fidelity when asked by a supervisor to work an additional shift because of "call-ins." The nurse has to weigh fidelity to the employing institution against fidelity to the profession and patients to do the best job possible, particularly if the nurse feels that fatigue would interfere with the performance of those obligations.

Beneficence

Beneficence is a very old requirement for health care providers who view the primary goal of health care as doing good for patients under their care. In general, the term *good* includes more than just technically competent care for patients. Good care requires that the health care provider approach the patient in a holistic manner, including the patient's beliefs, feelings, and wishes, as well as those of the patient's family and significant others. However, the difficulty that sometimes arises in implementing the principle of beneficence lies in determining what exactly is good for another and who can best make that decision.

Nonmaleficence

Nonmaleficence is the requirement that health care providers do no harm to their patients, either intentionally or unintentionally. In a sense, it is the opposite side of the coin of beneficence, and in fact, it is difficult to speak of one term without mentioning the other. In current health care practice, the principle of nonmaleficence is often violated in the short run to produce a greater good in the long-term treatment of the patient. For example, a patient may undergo a very painful and debilitating surgery to remove a cancerous growth to prolong his life in the future.

By extension, the principle of nonmaleficence also requires that health care providers protect from harm those who cannot protect themselves. This protection from harm is particularly evident in such groups as children, the mentally incompetent, the unconscious, and those who are too weak or debilitated to protect themselves. For example, very strict regulations have developed around situations involving child abuse and the health care provider's obligation to report suspected child abuse.

Veracity

Veracity, or truthfulness, requires that the health care provider tell the truth and not intentionally deceive or mislead patients. As with other rights and obligations, there are limitations to this principle, for example, in situations where telling patients the truth would seriously harm (principle of nonmaleficence) their ability to recover or would produce greater illness. Many times health care providers feel uncomfortable giving patients the "bad news" and have a tendency to avoid answering questions truthfully. Feeling uncomfortable is not a good enough reason to avoid telling patients

? What Would You Do?

Autonomy Versus Beneficence

Mr. Lamy, 90 years old, has been hospitalized due to dehydration, nausea, vomiting, and a urinary tract infection. He also has Alzheimer's, is a high risk for falls, has a history of falls with two broken hips, and has a tendency to wander. He was found in the parking lot on three separate occasions.

Mr. Lamy has an intravenous (IV) line. Concerned that he may fall, dislodge his IV, or wander off somewhere, the staff believes it is best to restrain him. Mr. Lamy is adamant that he does not want to be restrained.

Apply the ethical decision-making process:

1. *Clarify the ethical dilemma.* The scenario presents a common ethical dilemma. As the nurse responsible for Mr. Lamy, you need to decide whether to act on the basis of beneficence (specifically, nonmaleficence—avoiding the possibility of a fall and injury to the patient) or on the basis of autonomy (supporting the patient's decision or request not to be restrained).
2. *Gather additional data.* Your course of action depends on the additional information you gather. Is Mr. Lamy able to understand that he could harm himself getting out of bed without assistance? How does the family feel about restraints? What facility policies relate to this situation? What is the position of the treating physician?
3. *Identify options.* Have all other attempts to help Mr. Lamy maintain his independence failed? For example, has the staff tried keeping the bed's four side rails up and the call bell within reach? Are they making frequent checks and reminding him to call for assistance? Is there staff available to perform checks every half hour? Can a sitter be provided? Are there available family or friends who might be able to stay with Mr. Lamy? How long will the IV be necessary?
4. *Make a decision.* The family says they can stay with Mr. Lamy as long as he needs the IV. When the IV is no longer necessary, it is hoped that Mr. Lamy can be discharged to more familiar surroundings.
5. *Act.* In this situation, it is essential for the staff physician and the family members to work together to provide patient safety. If the family members are available to stay with Mr. Lamy around the clock, create a schedule and notify all staff.

the truth about their diagnosis, treatment, or prognosis. The patient has a right to know this information.

Paternalism

Paternalism refers to practices that limit the liberty of individuals without their consent. A paternalistic attitude does not prioritize individuals' choices or wishes. Those acting in a paternalistic way assume that they know better what is good for the patient.

? What Would You Do?

Veracity

Mrs. Alexes Beam's intravenous (IV) line infiltrated. The doctor agrees to change the route for the antibiotics. You suggest the oral route; the doctor orders intramuscular because she feels oral antibiotics may not be absorbed as well. Mrs. Beam and her family ask if the antibiotics can be given any other way other than intramuscularly (IM) because she is so frail and they do not want her to receive the painful injections.

What steps should you take?

1. Gather additional information:
   Is the oral medication as effective as the IM?
   Call the pharmacy for information.
   Check a reputable drug information resource, such as the *Physicians' Desk Reference.*
   Does the doctor realize that the patient is very thin and frail?
   Does the doctor know about the request for oral medication?
   Does the doctor know about the feelings of the family?
   Has someone spoken to the patient about the route of treatment?
2. Clarify the ethical dilemma.
3. Brainstorm your options.
   Talk to the doctor to re-evaluate the situation.
   Tell the patient and family that this is the best way to administer the antibiotics.

What would you do?

Rationalism

Reason is the basis for how things or conditions appear for decision making. **Rationalism** focuses on logical sequencing.

Pragmatism

Pragmatism is the process of clarifying ideas objectively through problem solving.

Standard of Best Interest

The **standard of best interest** is a decision made about individual patients' health care when they are unable to make an informed decision for their own care. The standard of best interest is based on what the health care providers and the family decide is best for that individual. It is important to consider the individual's expressed wishes, either formally in a written declaration (such as a living will) or informally in what may have been said to family members.

The standard of best interest should be based on the principle of beneficence. Unfortunately, in situations where patients are unable to make decisions for themselves, the resolution of the dilemma often appears to be a unilateral decision made about the individual's health care by the health care providers. This type of unilateral decision by health care providers, disregarding the patient's wishes and implying that the health care provider knows best, is paternalistic.

Obligations

Obligations are demands made on individuals, professions, society, or government to fulfill and honor the rights of others. Obligations are often divided into two categories:

Legal Obligations

Legal obligations are those obligations that have become formal statements of law and are enforceable under the law. For example, nurses have a legal obligation to provide safe and adequate care for patients assigned to them.

Moral Obligations

Moral obligations are those obligations that are based on moral or ethical principles but are not enforceable under the law. For example, in most states there is no legal obligation for a nurse who is not on duty to stop and help an automobile accident victim.

Rights

Rights are generally defined as just claims or titles or as something that is owed to an individual according to just claims, legal guarantees, or moral and ethical principles. Although the term *right* is often used in both the legal and ethical systems, its meaning is often blurred in everyday usage. Those things that individuals tend to claim as "rights" are really privileges, concessions, or freedoms. There are several classification systems for rights in which different types of rights are delineated. The following three types of rights cover the range.

Welfare Rights

Welfare rights, also called legal rights, are rights that are based on a legal entitlement to some good or benefit. These rights are guaranteed by laws (such as the Bill of

Rights) and, if violated, can lead to punishment within the legal system. For example, citizens of the United States have a right to equal access to housing regardless of race, sex, or religion.

Ethical Rights

Ethical rights, also called moral rights, are based on a moral or ethical principle. Ethical rights usually do not have the power of law behind them for enforcement. In reality, they are often privileges allotted to certain individuals or groups of individuals. Over time, popular acceptance of an ethical right can give it the force of a legal right. For example, access to health care is really a long-standing privilege for Americans that is sometimes viewed as a right.

Option Rights

Option rights are based on a fundamental belief in the dignity and freedom of human beings. Option rights are particularly evident in free and democratic countries and much less evident in totalitarian and restrictive societies. Option rights give individuals the freedom of choice and the right to live their lives as they choose, as long as they stay within a set of prescribed boundaries. For example, people may wear whatever clothes they choose, as long as they wear some type of clothing.

Comparing Two Ethical Systems

An ethical situation exists every time a nurse interacts with a patient in a health care setting. Nurses are continually making ethical decisions in their daily practices, whether or not they recognize it. The types of ethical decisions they make are known as normative decisions. Normative decisions deal with questions and dilemmas requiring a choice of actions where there is a conflict of rights or obligations between the nurse and the patient, the nurse and the patient's family, the nurse and the physician, or any other combination. In resolving these ethical questions, nurses often use one, or perhaps a combination, of the ethical systems.

When ethical theories are applied to information the nurse already possesses, they form an essential structure for the practicing nurse to use as a means of resolving a particular ethical dilemma. Depending on which theory or system of ethics is used, a nurse may reach similar or different decisions for an action. Ethical theories do not provide cookbook solutions for ethical dilemmas. Instead, they provide a framework for decision making that the nurse can apply to a particular situation.

At times, ethical theories may seem too abstract or general to be of much use to specific ethical situations. Without them, however, ethical decision making often becomes an exercise in personal emotions. Using the theories helps pinpoint the important aspects of the ethical decision making process.

? What Would You Do?

A Question of Discharge

ABC Insurance Company has determined that they will cover only 2 more days of hospitalization for your patient. You are concerned because Mr. Kyle Wayne lives alone and bedrest has left him very weak, limiting his ambulation. In addition, his mental status appears to be deteriorating. You are also concerned that he won't remember to take the remaining doses of his medication for the next ten days. Yesterday, the staff was notified that your facility has opened some beds.

Based on the principle of beneficence, you feel it is in Mr. Wayne's best interest to stay in the facility until he has had a chance to finish his medication course and attend physical therapy to increase his strength.

1. Pursue answers to these questions:

   Is Mr. Wayne's changing mental state due to organic process? Medications? Hospitalization and an unfamiliar environment?

   Has a physical therapist determined whether he can safely ambulate?

   Does he have resources to go to a long-term care facility?

   Can family or friends stay with him at home for several days? Can he stay with family or friends? How many beds are available in the facility? Are there any other resources available to care for him at home?

   Has the physician spoken to the insurance company or appealed the decision to limit the patient to only 2 additional days of hospitalization?

2. Brainstorm your options:

   Continue with the discharge plan as indicated because Mr. Wayne's insurance will not pay for additional days and his condition is no longer acute.

   Encourage Mr. Wayne's transfer to a long-term care facility until he regains some strength. Attempt to contact family and friends to explain the situation and ask whether they will provide supervision at home.

   Speak to the social worker who may be aware of other resources.

   Speak to Mr. Wayne's physician to determine if he has spoken to the insurance company.

   Consider these points:

   ▪ Although the option to discharge Mr. Wayne might be justifiable in the sense that it allows other patients to receive acute care, this option doesn't take into consideration any acts of beneficence toward Mr. Wayne.

   ▪ No arrangements for long-term care have been made.

   ▪ In the past both Mr. Wayne and his family have opposed going to a long-term care facility. What are their feelings now?

   Which option seems to respect all ethical principles involved?

A detailed, comprehensive presentation of all the existing systems of ethics is beyond the scope of this chapter. The two fundamental and predominant systems that are most directly implicated by ethical decision making in the health care arena are addressed. These systems are utilitarianism and deontology. The following discussion of these two systems of ethics is undertaken within the context of bioethics—the ethics of life, or death in some cases. *Bioethics,* a word that is in common use, has become synonymous with health care ethics. It includes not only questions concerning life and death but also questions of quality of life, life-sustaining and life-altering technologies, and bioscience in general.

Utilitarianism

Ethical Precepts

Utilitarianism (also called teleology, consequentialism, or situation ethics) is referred to as the ethical system of utility. As a system of normative ethics, utilitarianism defines *good* as happiness or pleasure. It is based on two underlying principles. The first principle is stated as "The greatest good for the greatest number." The second principle is "The end justifies the means." Because of these two principles, utilitarianism is sometimes subdivided into rule utilitarianism and act utilitarianism. According to rule utilitarianism, the individual draws on past experiences to formulate rules that are the most useful in determining the greatest good. With act utilitarianism, the particular situation that an individual finds himself or herself in determines the rightness or wrongness of a particular act. In practice, the true follower of utilitarianism does not believe in the validity of any system of rules because the rules can change depending on the circumstances surrounding the decision to be made.

Situation ethics is probably the most publicized form of act utilitarianism. Joseph Fletcher, one of the best-known proponents of act utilitarianism, outlines a method of ethical thinking in which the situation or outcome determines whether an act is morally right or wrong. An act, then, is good to the extent that it promotes happiness and wrong to the degree that it promotes unhappiness.

Based on the concept that moral rules should not be arbitrary but should serve a purpose, ethical decisions derived from a utilitarian framework weigh the effect of alternative actions that influence the overall welfare of present and future populations. As such, this system is oriented toward the good of the population in general and the individual as a member of that population.

Advantages

The major advantage of the utilitarian system of ethical decision making is that many individuals find it easy to apply to most situations because it is built around their own need for happiness, about which they have an immediate and vested knowledge. Another advantage is that utilitarianism fits well into a society that shuns rules and regulations. The follower of utilitarianism can justify almost any decision based on the "happiness" principle. Also, its utility orientation fits well into Western society's belief in the work ethic and the behavioristic approach to education, philosophy, and life. For example, the follower of utilitarianism would agree with a general prohibition against lying and deceiving because, ultimately, the results of truth telling lead to more happiness than the results of lying. Yet truth telling is not an absolute requirement for the follower of utilitarianism. If telling the truth would produce widespread unhappiness for a great number of people and future generations, then it would be ethically better to tell a lie that would yield more happiness. Although such behavior might appear to be unethical at first glance, the follower of strict act utilitarianism would have little difficulty in deriving this result as a logical conclusion of utilitarian ethical thinking.

Disadvantages

Pure utilitarianism, although easy to use as a decision-making system, does not work well as an ethical system for decision making in health care because of its arbitrary, situation-based nature. In the everyday delivery of health care, utilitarianism is often combined with other types of ethical decision making in the resolution of ethical dilemmas.

There are some serious limitations to utilitarianism as a system of health care ethics or bioethics. For example, does "happiness" refer to the average happiness of all or to the total happiness of a few? Because individual happiness is also important, how does one make decisions when the individual's happiness conflicts with the larger group's happiness? Perhaps more important are the basic questions of what constitutes "happiness" or "the greatest good for the greatest number"? Who determines what is "good" in the first place? Society in general? The government? Governmental policy? The individual? In health care delivery and the formulation of health care policy, the general guiding principle often seems to be the greatest good for the greatest number. Yet where do minority groups fit into this taxonomy? And what happens when a minority group becomes a majority group, as is happening in parts of this country today?

In addition, the "ends justify the means" principle has been consistently rejected as a method of achieving ideals. This aphorism has been invoked in the past to justify brutal and repressive acts that are difficult to view as "good." It is generally not considered acceptable to do whatever you want just as long as the end result or purpose is good. When dealing with health care issues that involve individuals' lives, applying reality to such concepts as "good," "harmful," "beneficial," or "greatest" is especially difficult.

In day-to-day health care situations, individuals who espouse utilitarianism as a system of ethical decision making usually combine it with the principle of distributive justice. Distributive justice has several levels of meaning. In the broadest sense, distributive justice is an ethical principle that advocates equal allocation of benefits and burdens to all members of society. At this level, the main concerns of distributive justice become (1) how the country as a whole should allocate its resources and (2) who should pay for these resources. The United States tax code, to some degree, is based on the principle of distributive justice. It is easy to see that utilitarianism and distributive justice share some common goals at the theoretical level.

Most nurses have little time or desire to consider all the broad theoretical underpinnings and implications of their daily patient care decisions. At a more practical level, distributive justice simply means treating all patients equally regardless of their backgrounds, beliefs, or diagnoses. The principle of distributive justice presumes that people are very similar in the most important aspects of life, such as basic needs (food, housing, health care), freedoms, (self-determination, self-expression, self-government), and goals (life, liberty, and the pursuit of happiness). When the principle of distributive justice is combined with utilitarianism as a system of ethical decision making, the decisions made will more often than not approximate the decisions made by the follower of the deontological system. Indeed, using the principle of distributive justice with utilitarianism contradicts the most basic principle of pure utilitarianism, namely that there are no fixed or unchanging rules.

Deontology

Ethical Precepts

Deontology is a system of ethical decision making that is based on moral rules and unchanging principles. This system is also referred to as the formalistic system, the principal system of ethics, or duty-based ethics. A follower of a pure form of the deontological system of ethical decision making believes in the ethical absoluteness of principles regardless of the consequences of the decision. This strict adherence to an ethical theory in which the moral rightness or wrongness of human actions is considered separately from the consequences is based on a fundamental principle called the categorical imperative. It is not the results of the act that make it right or wrong, but the principles on which the act is carried out. These fundamental principles are ultimately unchanging and absolute and are derived from the same universal values that underlie all major religions. Focusing on a concern for right and wrong in the moral sense, the system is based on the need for survival of the species and social cooperation.

Deontology is based on the belief that there are standards for the ethical choices and judgments that an individual makes. These standards are fixed and do not change when the situation changes. Although the number of standards or rules is potentially unlimited, in reality, and particularly in dealing with bioethical issues, many of these principles can be grouped together into a few general or cover principles. These principles can also be arranged into a type of hierarchy of rules, including such maxims as "Humans should always be treated as ends and never as means"; "Human life has value"; "One is always to tell the truth"; "Above all in health care, do no harm"; "The human person has a right to self-determination"; "All persons are of equal value"; and so on. The similarity among these principles and fundamental documents such as the Bill of Rights and the American Hospital Association's Patient's Bill of Rights is immediately evident (Box 5–2).

BOX 5–2

American Hospital Association Patient's Bill of Rights

These rights can be exercised on the patient's behalf by a designated surrogate or proxy decision maker if the patient lacks decision-making capacity, is legally incompetent, or is a minor.

1. The patient has the right to considerate and respectful care.
2. The patient has the right to and is encouraged to obtain from physicians and other direct caregivers relevant, current, and understandable information concerning diagnosis, treatment, and prognosis.

   Except in emergencies when the patient lacks decision-making capacity and the need for treatment is urgent, the patient is entitled to the opportunity to discuss and request information related to the specific procedures and/or treatments, the risks involved, the possible length of recuperation, and the medically reasonable alternatives and their accompanying risks and benefits.

   Patients have the right to know the identity of physicians, nurses, and others involved in their care, as well as when those involved are students, residents, or other trainees. The patient also has the right to know the immediate and long-term financial implications of treatment choices, insofar as they are known.
3. The patient has the right to make decisions about the plan of care prior to and during the course of treatment and to refuse a recommended treatment or plan of care to the extent permitted by law and hospital policy and to be informed of the medical consequences of this action. In case of such refusal, the patient is entitled to other appropriate care and services that the hospital provides or transfer to another hospital. The hospital should notify patients of any policy that might affect patient choice within the institution.
4. The patient has the right to have an advance directive (such as a living will, health care proxy, or durable power of attorney for health care) concerning treatment or to designate a surrogate decision maker with the expectation that the hospital will honor the intent of that directive to the extent permitted by law and hospital policy.

   Health care institutions must advise patients of their rights under state law and hospital policy to make informed medical choices, ask if the patient has an advance directive, and include that information in patient records. The patient has the right to timely information about hospital policy that may limit its ability to implement fully a legally valid advance directive.
5. The patient has the right to every consideration of privacy. Case discussion, consultation, examination, and treatment should be conducted so as to protect each patient's privacy.

BOX 5–2

American Hospital Association Patient's Bill of Rights

6. The patient has the right to expect that all communications and records pertaining to his/her care will be treated as confidential by the hospital, except in cases such as suspected abuse and public health hazards when reporting is permitted or required by law. The patient has the right to expect that the hospital will emphasize the confidentiality of this information when it releases it to any other parties entitled to review information in these records.

7. The patient has the right to review the records pertaining to his/her medical care and to have the information explained or interpreted as necessary, except when restricted by law.

8. The patient has the right to expect that, within its capacity and policies, a hospital will make reasonable response to the request of a patient for appropriate and medically indicated care and services. The hospital must provide evaluation, service, and/or referral as indicated by the urgency of the case. When medically appropriate and legally permissible, or when a patient has so requested, a patient may be transferred to another facility. The institution to which the patient is to be transferred must first have accepted the patient for transfer. The patient must also have the benefit of complete information and explanation concerning the need for, risks, benefits, and alternatives to such a transfer.

9. The patient has the right to ask and be informed of the existence of business relationships among the hospital, educational institutions, other health care providers, or payers that may influence the patient's treatment and care.

10. The patient has the right to consent to or decline to participate in proposed research studies or human experimentation affecting care and treatment or requiring direct patient involvement, and to have those studies fully explained prior to consent. A patient who declines to participate in research or experimentation is entitled to the most effective care that the hospital can otherwise provide.

11. The patient has the right to expect reasonable continuity of care when appropriate and to be informed by physicians and other caregivers of available and realistic patient care options when hospital care is no longer appropriate.

12. The patient has the right to be informed of hospital policies and practices that relate to patient care, treatment, and responsibilities. The patient has the right to be informed of available resources for resolving disputes, grievances, and conflicts, such as ethics committees, patient representatives, or other mechanisms available in the institution. The patient has the right to be informed of the hospital's charges for services and available payment methods.

(continued)

BOX 5–2

American Hospital Association Patient's Bill of Rights (continued)

The collaborative nature of health care requires that patients, or their families/surrogates, participate in their care. The effectiveness of care and patient satisfaction with the course of treatment depend, in part, on the patient fulfilling certain responsibilities. Patients are responsible for providing information about past illnesses, hospitalizations, medications, and other matters related to health status. To participate effectively in decision making, patients must be encouraged to take responsibility for requesting additional information or clarification about their health status or treatment when they do not fully understand information and instructions. Patients are also responsible for ensuring that the health care institution has a copy of their written advance directive if they have one. Patients are responsible for informing their physicians and other caregivers if they anticipate problems in following prescribed treatment.

Patients should also be aware of the hospital's obligation to be reasonably efficient and equitable in providing care to other patients and the community. The hospital's rules and regulations are designed to help the hospital meet this obligation. Patients and their families are responsible for making reasonable accommodations to the needs of the hospital, other patients, medical staff, and hospital employees. Patients are responsible for providing necessary information for insurance claims and for working with the hospital to make payment arrangements, when necessary.

A person's health depends on much more than health care services. Patients are responsible for recognizing the impact of their life-style on their personal health.

Conclusion

Hospitals have many functions to perform, including the enhancement of health status, health promotion, and the prevention and treatment of injury and disease; the immediate and ongoing care and rehabilitation of patients; the education of health professionals, patients, and the community; and research. All these activities must be conducted with an overriding concern for the values and dignity of patients.[4]

§ Adapted from "A Patient's Bill of Rights," copyright 1992, American Hospital Association.

The terminology and concepts used in the deontological approach to ethics are similar to those used by the legal system. Like the deontological system, the legal system stresses rights and duties, principles and rules. However, it is important to remember that there are significant differences between the two. Legal rights and duties are enforceable under the law; ethical rights and duties usually are not. In general, ethical systems are much wider and more inclusive than the system of laws to which they relate. An ethical perspective on law by health care professionals ultimately leads to an interest in making laws that govern health care and nursing practice. Evaluating and revising laws from an ethical perspective prevents professional nurses from being placed in practice situations where there is no legal support for their ethical practice.

Advantages

Nurses who espouse the deontological system of ethical thinking believe that duties and obligations, rather than mere actions, bring about the best ends. When the concepts of rights and duties are added to moral and ethical thinking, the result is a decision-making process that also takes into account a larger and often interwoven system of duties. These guiding principles affect nurses' behavior and consequently their relationships with patients. The deontological system is useful in making ethical decisions in health care because it holds that an ethical judgment based on principles is the same in a variety of similar situations regardless of time, location, or particular individuals involved.

Disadvantages

The deontological system of ethical decision making is not free from imperfection. Some of the more troubling questions include: What do you do when the basic guiding principles conflict with each other? What is the source of the principles? Is there ever a situation where an exception to the rule will apply? Although various approaches have been proposed to circumvent these limitations, it may be difficult for the nurse to resolve situations where duties and obligations conflict, particularly where the consequences of following a rule may end in harm or hurt to a patient. In reality, there are probably few followers of pure deontology because most people do consider the consequences of their actions in the decision-making process.

KEEP IN MIND _____

- ▶ Autonomy is the right to choose one's own health care and may be the most important principle to consider in resolving ethical dilemmas.
- ▶ Values are concepts that give meaning to an individual's life and serve as the framework for making decisions.
- ▶ Morals are fundamental standards of right and wrong that an individual internalizes.
- ▶ Laws are rules of societal conduct devised by people to protect society at large.
- ▶ Ethics are declarations of what is right and what is wrong, systems of valued behaviors and beliefs.

▶ Codes of ethics are written lists of a profession's values and standards of conduct.

▶ Beneficence, the obligation to do good for patients, and nonmaleficence, the obligation to do no harm to patients, are the minimal ethical requirements for nurses.

▶ Rights are just claims to something. Many times individuals claim something as a right that may really be a privilege, concession, or freedom. Only legal rights have the force of law behind them.

▶ Utilitarianism is a system of ethics that is based on the principle of greatest good. As a system, utilitarianism may not be appropriate for some health care decisions.

▶ Deontology is a system of ethics that is based on unchanging principles. This system parallels the legal and moral systems most people follow growing up in today's world.

▶ The ethical decision-making process is a step-by-step approach for reaching resolutions of ethical dilemmas:

1. Collect, analyze, and interpret the data.
2. State the dilemma.
3. Consider the choices of action.
4. Analyze the advantages and disadvantages of each choice of action.
5. Make a decision about the action to resolve the dilemma.

IN A NUTSHELL

Ethics deals with the rightness and wrongness of situations and has no mechanism of enforcement, whereas laws are man-made rules that regulate society and are enforceable. Ethical dilemmas are situations that require an individual to choose between two equally unfavorable alternatives. Often there are no clear or ideal solutions, and differences of opinion often exist.

AFTERTHOUGHTS

1. Compare and contrast ethics with law by delineating the purposes, scope, and methods of enforcement.
2. Define and explain ethics, law, values, morals, ethical code, and ethical dilemma.
3. Define and explain the concepts of autonomy, justice, fidelity, beneficence, nonmaleficence, veracity, obligations, and rights.
4. Distinguish between the two types of obligations.
5. Distinguish between the three categories of rights.

6. Define utilitarianism and list its advantages and disadvantages as an ethical decision-making system.

7. Define deontology and list its advantages and disadvantages as an ethical decision-making system.

8. Define and give an example of paternalism in the health care setting.

9. Name and explain the steps in the ethical decision-making process.

10. List five rights designated in a patient's bill of rights.

11. Compare the Canadian Nurses Association Code of Ethics, the International Counsel of Nurses Code of Ethics and the ANA's Code of Ethics. How are they similar? How do they differ?

12. Discuss with the class an ethical dilemma that you have witnessed or have encountered recently.

13. Can ethical dilemmas end in litigation? Explain and give an example.

ETHICS IN PRACTICE

Ruth Rigid, RN, began her career in home health care some 7 years ago after having worked as an assistant head nurse on a busy medical-surgical unit for almost 10 years at a Veterans' Administration (VA) hospital. Ruth has proved to be a hard-working, very responsible, and reliable home health care nurse with excellent assessment and nursing skills. In general, she communicates well with patients and provides a high level of care to the patients she is assigned. Ruth has a reputation among the other nurses working in the agency as being competent and hard working but rather inflexible when it comes to the interpretation of protocols, procedures, and standing orders. This by-the-book philosophy is an essential part of Ruth's psychological makeup and pervades all aspects of her life, including her religious beliefs and value system.

This past week a new patient has been referred to the agency for home care. He is a 38-year-old admitted homosexual male who is human immunodeficiency virus (HIV) positive and in the terminal stages of acquired immunodeficiency syndrome (AIDS). He has decided to spend his final days at home rather than in a hospital intensive care unit (ICU). Because of the rural location of this agency, this is its first referral of a person with AIDS.

After consideration of the various qualifications and experience levels of the nurses available, as well as their patient loads, the director of the agency decides that Ruth would be the most qualified nurse to care for this patient. The agency director places the referral form and chart on Ruth's desk with a note to see the patient before the end of the week.

Later that day when Ruth returns from her morning visits, she discovers the referral and chart on her desk. After reviewing the chart and referral form, she storms into the director's office, throws the chart down on the director's desk, and states in a loud voice: "I cannot take care of a patient who has AIDS. My religion teaches that homosexuality is a sin against nature and God and I believe that AIDS is a punishment for that sin!"

If you were the director, how would you handle the situation? Use the ethical decision-making model in solving this problem.

- What are the important data in relation to this situation?
- What is the ethical dilemma? State it clearly and simply.
- What are the choices of action, and how do they relate to specific ethical principles?
- What are the consequences of these actions?
- What decision can be made?

Other factors to consider:

- Are there ever any situations when a nurse can ethically (and legally) refuse a work assignment?
- What effect will the final decision have on the other staff members?

References

1. American Nurses Association: Code of Ethics for Nurses. American Nurses Publishing, American Nurses Foundation/American Nurses Association, Washington, DC, 2001.
2. Canadian Nurses Association: Code of Ethics for Registered Nurses. CNA, Ottawa, Canada, 1997.
3. International Council of Nurses: Code of Ethics for Nurses. ICN, Geneva, Switzerland, 2000.
4. American Hospital Association: Patient's Bill of Rights. AHA, Chicago, Ill, 1992.

Resources

Ellis, RE, and Hartley, CL: Nursing in Today's World: Challenges, Issues, and Trends. Philadelphia, Lippincott Williams and Wilkins, 2001.
Fletcher, J: Situation Ethics. Philadelphia, Westminster, 1966.

Part 4

Liability in Professional Practice

Intentional and Quasi-intentional Torts 6

Key Chapter Concepts

Tort

Tortious

Intentional tort

Strict liability

Intent

Assault

Battery

Medical battery

False imprisonment

Trespass to land

Intentional infliction of emotional
distress

Quasi-intentional tort

Defamation

Libel

Slander

Truth

Absolute privilege

Qualified privilege

Consent

Invasion of privacy

Chapter Thoughts

Nurses are viewed by the public as the one group of health care providers whose primary goal is to understand, provide comfort, and help patients under their care. The vast majority of lawsuits brought against nurses involve acts of negligence and are, by definition, unintentional torts. Very few lawsuits brought against nurses fall into the category of intentional torts—that is, torts that require an act of intentional wrongdoing against a patient.

The ethical concept of nonmaleficence—the obligation to "do no harm" to a patient—is the underlying principle pitted against an intentional tort. If no one ever violated the principle of nonmaleficance, then no harm would ever come to patients through the commission of intentional torts. Unfortunately, in the real world of health care, problems begin to arise when this principle is applied to actual health care situations. The principle of nonmaleficance presumes that there is a more or less unchanging set of criteria for determining what constitutes harm to a patient. Realistically, the term *harm* has a range of degrees and multiple meanings. For example, if nurses were to never "harm" their patients, they would never be able to start intravenous lines (IVs), place nasogastric tubes, insert urinary catheters, or perform the numerous other procedures necessary to help cure patients or even keep them alive.

Similarly, the principle of nonmaleficance has a tendency to conflict with other important ethical principles. Ethical principles such as patient autonomy, the nurse's obligation to truthfulness, and even beneficence can create situations in which the nurse has to make a decision about which principle should outweigh another. It is at this ethical juncture—when various ethical principles conflict and "harm" is a matter of opinion—that a nurse becomes vulnerable to the legal system and to liability for intentional torts. Yet nurses are faced with these types of decisions on a daily basis. Often making the decision not to act or treat can produce worse results than making an informed, thoughtful decision and accepting the consequences.

OBJECTIVES

Upon completing this chapter, the reader will be able to:
1. Describe the concept of intentional torts and distinguish intentional tortious conduct from negligent conduct.
2. Discuss the elements of the intentional torts of assault, battery, medical battery, false imprisonment, trespass to land, and intentional infliction of emotional distress, including the rights protected by each.
3. Give examples of each of the intentional torts described in the chapter.
4. Discuss the quasi-intentional torts of defamation, invasion of privacy, and breach of confidentiality.
5. Describe the defenses available to allegations of defamation.
6. Describe the four types of invasion of privacy and the media's right to patient information.
7. Discuss a health facility's right to eject a patient or visitor from the premises and the type of intentional tort involved.

Introduction

A **tort** is a wrong that harms, and a **tortious** act is a wrongful act.[1] Three types of torts exist:

1. Intentional torts
2. Negligence
3. Strict liability

The law of torts includes a variety of wrongs that have as their common principle the idea that injuries are to be compensated and antisocial behavior is to be discouraged. For purposes of this discussion, torts may be divided into two classifications: those arising from intentional conduct and those arising from negligent conduct.

Intentional torts are willful or intentional acts that violate another person's rights or property. Intentional torts that can involve nurses include, among others, assault, battery, and false imprisonment. The most critical distinction between an intentional tort and a negligent tort is the intent of the person committing the tort. (See Box 6–1 for the difference between negligence and an intentional tort.) Proof of an intentional tort requires that the person committing it have the requisite knowledge and will to be committing the wrong.

The basis of an intentional tort centers on the issues of intent and, in the health care arena in particular, consent. Examples of intentional torts include assault, battery, false imprisonment, intentional infliction of emotional distress, and trespass to land. The principles of negligence are discussed in another chapter. The **strict liability** principle is applied when the party is participating in specified activities, such as possession or use of material of equipment inherently dangerous (e.g., explosives and assault weapons). Negligence does not have to be proven because there is an automatic responsibility when this doctrine is used. The person participating in the activities has committed a tort (regardless of negligence or intentional wrongdoing) just by

---

BOX 6–1

Differences Between Negligence and Intentional Torts

There are several distinct differences between intentional and nonintentional (negligent) torts. These can be characterized as differences in intent, injury, duty, and consent.

1. *Intent.* Whereas negligence can occur without any intent to act, the person charged with an intentional tort must have intended to interfere with another person's rights, although not necessarily with a hostile motive. For example, a patient who did not consent to a surgical procedure may bring a legal action for battery, based on unauthorized touching, even if the surgical procedure was necessary and correctly done. The health care provider, in performing the surgery, had the intent to touch the patient.
2. *Proof of damages.* Because intentional torts interfere with a person's rights, the plaintiffs do not have to prove that any actual injury occurred. The harm is the actual invasion of a right, rather than a specific injury as required in negligence cases.
3. *Duty or standards of care.* Duty or standards of care are only relevant in negligence actions, not intentional torts. Likewise, expert witnesses are unnecessary in proving intentional torts but are usually required to establish standards of care in malpractice cases. (Experts may be retained to prove the extent of damages caused by intentional torts.)
4. *Consent.* Consent is always a defense to intentional torts but not necessarily in negligence. For example, although patients may consent to a surgical procedure, they may still sue for negligence if injury occurs. On the other hand, no legal action for battery can arise if a patient has consented to surgery because battery, by definition, is nonconsensual touching.

virtue of participating in that activity. Strict liability also applies to certain specific behaviors such as distributing abnormally dangerous objects.[2]

The concept of torts evolved from the fundamental principle that every person is bound to abstain from injuring the person or property of another or from infringing on that other person's rights.[3] The same act may constitute both a crime and a tort. However, a crime is an offense against the public that is prosecuted by the state, whereas a tort is a private injury that may be pursued in civil court by the injured party. Tort law focuses on compensating individuals for injuries they sustained because of the conduct of another.

AUTHOR TIP: *The distinction between negligent and intentional acts is also significant because most Good Samaritan statutes[4] do not protect the nurse from liability for harm caused by intentional tortious conduct.*

Intentional Torts

The concept of intent distinguishes between intentional tortious acts and negligent tortious acts. (See Box 6–2 for types of intentional torts.) **Intent** means that either the person acted for the purpose of causing an injury (or violating a right) or that the person knows or is reasonably certain that an injury or violation will result from the act. For example, if a nurse picks up the wrong syringe during an emergency situation and administers epinephrine instead of aminophylline, causing cardiac arrest, there is no evidence that the nurse intended to cause the cardiac arrest. This would be an example of negligence, not the intentional tort of battery. However, if a nurse slaps or kicks a geriatric patient or pinches a pediatric patient, assault and battery have occurred.

The motive or purpose behind an act plays an important role in determining tort liability. For example, a motive such as self-defense may justify an action that otherwise would be considered an intentional tort. On the other hand, an improper motive, such as the desire to harm the person, may support not only liability and compensatory damages but an additional jury award of punitive damages.

To recover monetary damages from the person committing the tort, the victim must show injuries and damages resulting from the tortious actions. After all, a wrong

---

BOX 6–2

Types of Intentional Torts

1. Assault
2. Battery
3. False imprisonment
4. Intentional infliction of emotional distress
5. Trespass to land

A CASE IN POINT

Assault

The Facts

In *Baca v. Velez*,[5] an operating room nurse in a New Mexico hospital had a disagreement with an orthopedic surgeon, during which the nurse alleged that the doctor jabbed her in the back with the sharp end of a bone chisel. Subsequently, she brought suit against the doctor for assault and battery.

The Court Decides

The appeals court found no evidence of conduct that would substantiate an assault charge, even though the physician could be found to have committed a battery on the nurse. The court explained that all batteries do not include an assault. For there to be an assault, there must have been an "act, threat or menacing conduct that causes another person to reasonably believe that he is in danger of receiving an immediate battery." Because the injury occurred to the nurse's back, the court found that there was no evidence to prove that she feared for her safety before the "touching" with the bone chisel took place.

without any injury cannot be the basis of a lawsuit. However, in circumstances where there is a wrongful invasion of a clear legal right, the law presumes damage sufficient to support the lawsuit.

Assault and Battery

Is this assault and battery? A nurse overhears a patient cursing and making derogatory comments about the staff. To teach the patient a lesson, the nurse forces her to drink a cup of soap.

Assault and battery, terms that are often used together, are distinctly different legal actions. **Assault** is the threat or attempt to inflict effective physical contact to a person, and **battery** is the invasion of a person's privacy by unpermitted touching. To bring a suit claiming assault, the plaintiff must feel fear or apprehension of an immediate harmful or threatening contact. The harm is not the actual contact (which would then give rise to a battery charge), but the mental fear caused by the threatened contact. However, most suits in which an assault has occurred also include a charge of battery.

When force is used to restrain a person, the person exerting the force may be liable for both false imprisonment and assault and battery. However, treatment administered to a person who has been improperly detained in the hospital does not always constitute assault or battery. If the treatment itself is proper, it does not become unlawful merely because it is given while a person is improperly detained.

The most common example of battery in the hospital setting occurs when surgical procedures are performed without patient consent and is called **medical battery.** For example, the surgeon has obtained informed consent to amputate the right leg but instead amputates the left leg. The patient could make claims based on medical malpractice and medical battery.

The following case illustrates how a nurse can be held liable for battery against a patient: In a nursing home, a quadriplegic patient with an external catheter also had an as-needed (PRN) order for an indwelling catheter. When the nurse inserted the indwelling catheter, the patient objected but was told to "shut up." After requests from the patient and family, the catheter was removed but subsequently reinserted. The patient begged that it not be put in because of past complications and pain, but his objections were ignored. Finally a nurse jerked the catheter out, causing injury. The family sued for damages. The court found that "a nurse commits a battery upon a patient when she performs an invasive procedure like the insertion of an indwelling catheter over the objections of the patient." The patient recovered $25,000 for pain and suffering.[6]

Consent and Its Role in Assault and Battery

The goal of the torts of assault and battery in the medical context is to protect the sanctity of the human body. As stated by the eminent jurist Justice Benjamin Cardozo:

> Every human being of adult years and sound mind has a right to determine what shall be done with his own body, and a surgeon who performs an operation without his patient's consent commits an assault for which he is liable in damages.[7]

Any kind of medical, surgical, or nursing procedure that is performed without the patient's consent is considered a battery. A claim of battery may be brought against a

---

? What Would You Do?

You are a nurse who is pregnant and working on a medical-surgical unit. On your 11 to 7 shift, a new patient who has attempted suicide is admitted to your unit because there are no available beds on the psychiatric unit. You enter the room and the patient looks at you and yells "I hate you!" and then kicks you in the abdomen.

Both you and your unborn child sustain injuries.

1. What actions, if any, can be filed on your behalf?
2. What are potential defenses?
3. Can you file a civil or criminal action?
4. What other remedies may be available?

A Case in Point

Battery

The Facts

In *Berkey v. Anderson,*[9] the patient thought he was consenting to a procedure no more complicated than the electromyograms that he had previously undergone. However, the actual procedure performed was a myelogram involving a spinal puncture.

The Court Decides

The court classified the situation as a battery because there was a deliberate intent to deviate from the given consent.

physician or other health professional assisting the physician, such as a nurse or technician, who performs a medical procedure on the patient, however slight the physical contact may be, without the patient's consent. A battery may also occur if the health care provider exceeds the scope of the consent or performs a different procedure than that for which consent was obtained.

With the evolution of informed consent principles and the inquiry that many courts now make into the adequacy and quality of the physician's disclosure of information, patients are now alleging medical negligence, as well as the intentional torts of assault and battery.

The difference between negligence and battery can be explained by considering the concept of informed consent. If the health care practitioner performs the treatment that the patient consented to but fails to make a proper disclosure when obtaining that consent, the tort is negligence; if the procedure was different from the one the patient consented to, the tort is battery.[8]

Failure to obtain the patient's consent in accordance with applicable legal standards may result in a charge of battery or negligence, or even unprofessional conduct, against the health care provider. The principles of informed consent are discussed at length in Chapter 11.

Clearly, performing a surgical or medical procedure without consent constitutes a battery. In one case, an oral surgeon removed the lower teeth of his patient without reviewing the patient's charts, which indicated that the patient wanted to retain his five lower teeth. He was accused of battery.[10]

Special Consideration with Psychiatric Patients

Assertions of assault and battery can be an issue in the treatment of psychiatric patients. The validity of these allegations depends on the nature of the common and statutory law of the individual state where the treatment occurred.

Here's an example. After initial drug detoxification in the hospital, a mentally ill patient was committed to the psychiatric unit, where he was forcibly given antibiotics for treatment of life-threatening urinary failure. Although he charged assault and battery and false imprisonment, the court found that the treatment given to him was authorized by both the common and the statutory law of the state.[11]

Admission to a mental health facility alone, either voluntarily or involuntarily, is not the deciding factor when analyzing whether the patient is capable of making informed decisions about health care. Even if a person is involuntarily committed to a facility, he or she is considered to be capable of consenting to treatment unless there has been a judicial determination to the contrary. Involuntary commitment does not automatically deprive a person of the right to reasonably safe conditions of confinement, the right to freedom from unreasonable bodily restraints, or the right to refuse psychotropic or antipsychotic medications.[12] Disregard of a competent mental health patient's wishes may constitute assault and battery. (See Box 6–3 for some commonly asked questions about assault and battery.)

Defenses for Assault and Battery

An exception to the duty to adequately inform patients of the risk of treatment exists in the case of an emergency when the patient's wishes are not known. If the patient is unconscious or otherwise unable to give informed consent and the medical procedure is immediately necessary to protect the health or life of the patient, informed consent

---

BOX 6–3

Commonly Asked Questions About Assault and Battery

1. *Can I sue a patient if he or she commits assault and battery on me?*
   Yes. However, the courts will look at the medical records to see if the patient could have the requisite *intent* to cause harm. Was the patient on medications? Did the patient have an emotional or mental illness that would prevent the patient from having intent? What was the patient's state of mind when the assault and/or battery occurred?
2. *What are the remedies available if I am injured by a patient as a result of an assault and battery?*
   a. You can file suit for civil money damages.
   b. You can file criminal charges against the patient.
   c. You can file a workers' compensation claim because you were injured on the job.

? What Would You Do?

You work at a long-term care facility in a rural area of the state. Several patients have been there for years without any incident. A new nursing assistant is hired, and patient and family members complain about her rudeness and erratic behavior.

You are assigned to patients she has recently cared for and notice unexplained bruises and scratches on several patients.

You walk into a patient's room one night and discover a family member attempting to secretly insert a miniature video camera. He explains that he wants to catch the person abusing his mother.

1. What should you do?
2. What are the potential legal implications?

is not required.[13] The emergency treatment exception is discussed in greater detail in Chapter 11.

The principle of self-defense is also available to avoid liability for acts that would otherwise constitute assault or battery. The person claiming self-defense must reasonably believe that a danger exists to himself or herself or to others and must use only the force that is reasonably necessary.

False Imprisonment

False imprisonment is defined as the unlawful intentional confinement of another within fixed boundaries so that the confined person is conscious of or harmed by the confinement.[15]

The restraints used to confine another may be chemical, physical, or emotional (e.g., intimidation). There must be a direct restraint of the person for some appreciable length of time, however short, compelling the person to stay or go somewhere against the person's will. Merely preventing a person from going to a particular place is not false imprisonment.

Many specialty treatment facilities, such as mental health and nursing home facilities, have rules and policies that require the patient to agree to remain in the facility until discharge. Confinement of a patient against his or her will pursuant to such policies has been ruled to be false imprisonment.

AUTHOR TIP: *If a patient must be detained because he or she is a danger to self or others (e.g., the patient received narcotics in the Emergency Department and wants to drive home), document the reason the patient is being kept at the facility, notify security or the police in the facility, and notify the Emergency Department or attending physician so that if the matter goes to court, witnesses can testify as to the reasons for detaining the patient.*

A CASE IN POINT

Self-Defense

The Facts

In *Mattocks v. Bell*,[14] a 23-month-old child clamped her teeth on the finger of a medical student as he was treating her for a lacerated tongue. When he was unable to extricate his finger, he slapped the child on the cheek with his other hand.

The Court Decides

The court denied recovery for assault and battery, finding that the force was required and not applied in an improper manner. Although the court considered the medical student's action to be rash, it found it neither malicious nor severe and the child was not injured.

Vulnerable Patients

Many times, allegations of false imprisonment arise from circumstances involving particularly vulnerable patients, such as elderly, impaired, or mentally ill persons. Nurses must be especially aware of the rights of patients who may not be able to speak up and defend themselves.

For instance, preventing a voluntary nursing home patient from leaving the premises may result in liability for false imprisonment, and in certain circumstances, confinement of intoxicated patients may be found to be appropriate to protect them from harming themselves.

The involuntary confinement of persons who are mentally ill or who are considered to be a danger to themselves or others is highly regulated by state laws. The involuntary hospitalization of a person in a mental institution in violation of the statute constitutes false imprisonment.[20] Nurses must be familiar with these laws because they can be quite specific in some states regarding the responsibilities of the hospital and health care providers. Failure to understand and comply with the applicable laws can lead to liability for false imprisonment.

Trespass to Land

Trespass to land is the unlawful interference with another's possession of land. The tort may be committed by an intentional or a negligent act.[21] Trespass to land may occur when a person intrudes onto a property, fails to leave a property, throws or places something on the land, or causes another person to enter the property.[22]

Trespass is most commonly encountered in the health care field when a patient

A Case in Point

False Imprisonment

The Facts

In *Cook v. Highland Hospital*,[16] the patient was admitted to a private hospital for rehabilitative treatment. Upon admission, she signed an agreement obligating her to abide by the rules and regulations of the facility; she believed she would be free to leave whenever she wanted. However, when she refused to comply with the hospital authorities, she was confined for 32 days and was locked in a room despite her demand to leave.

The Court Decides

Even though the patient had agreed to abide by the hospital rules, the court said that this agreement did not justify detaining her against her will.

refuses to leave on discharge or a visitor refuses to comply with visiting policies. (See Box 6–4 for definition of trespass.) Trespass may also occur in the context of protest actions (such as animal rights, antiabortion protests, or labor disputes).

In *Fardig v. Municipality of Anchorage*,[23] antiabortion protesters were convicted of criminal trespass for refusing requests to cease distributing literature to patrons of a women's clinic and to leave its parking lot.

A private health care facility is considered private property, and people do not have the absolute right to remain on the premises. When a patient, family member, or visitor refuses to leave the facility, staff should attempt to reason with the person. If reasoning is unsuccessful, then it may be necessary to pursue legal remedies such as arresting the individual for trespass or obtaining a court order directing the person to leave the facility.

Some state laws make it a crime for a patient to trespass by refusing to leave a hospital once he or she has been discharged by the attending physician. A patient found guilty of criminal trespass may be fined or imprisoned.

During labor disputes, only peaceful, lawful strike and picketing activities are permitted. Although the federal National Labor Relations Act provisions govern most aspects of strikes and picketing activities, state criminal statutes regulating strike violence and trespass may be enforced to maintain order.

Intentional Infliction of Emotional Distress

Intentional infliction of emotional distress is the intentional invasion of a person's peace of mind. The conduct must be outrageous and beyond all bounds of decency. Ordinary rude or insulting behavior is not enough.

A CASE IN POINT

Vulnerable Patients

The Facts

In *Big Town Nursing Home, Inc. v. Newman*,[17] a 67-year-old man was kept against his will for 51 days. Three days after he was admitted by a nephew, the man attempted to leave but was forcibly returned to the facility by employees. Following his five or six escape attempts, he was confined to a "restraint chair" and denied the use of the telephone and his own clothes.

The Court Decides

The court found that the actions of the nursing home staff were in utter disregard of the man's legal rights and that the staff acted recklessly, willfully, and maliciously in unlawfully detaining him.

In certain circumstances, confinement of intoxicated patients may be found to be appropriate to protect them from harming themselves.

The Facts

In *Blackman for Blackman v. Rifkin*,[18] the plaintiff's extreme intoxication, coupled with her head trauma, warranted her retention in an emergency room to prevent further harm to herself or others. The plaintiff alleged false imprisonment.

The Court Decides

The court ruled that the hospital could assume that she would have consented to treatment if she had not been in that condition and dismissed the patient's false imprisonment claims.

The Facts

In *Hapgood v. Biloxi Regional Medical Center*,[19] the patient charged that she was falsely imprisoned when the hospital failed to follow statutory commitment procedures and improperly subjected her to 10 weeks of involuntary treatment at the hospital, including 15 episodes of electroconvulsive therapy, after she was diagnosed as exhibiting acute schizophrenic reaction.

The Court Decides

The court ruled in favor of the plaintiff, and the defendant appealed.

The Appeals Court Decides

The appellate court affirmed the false imprisonment claim.

> **BOX 6–4**
>
> ## Defining Trespass
>
> Trespass is the ...
>
> 1. Intentional or negligent ...
> 2. Interference ...
> 3. With another's possession ...
> 4. Of land.

Quasi-intentional Torts

Quasi-intentional torts are based on speech and are not intentional in the same sense that assault, battery, and false imprisonment may be.[25] Quasi-intentional torts include defamation (libel and slander), invasion of privacy, and breach of confidentiality. (See Box 6–5 for types of quasi-intentional torts.)

Defamation

Defamation is defined as an oral or written communication to a third party about the plaintiff that is false and that tends to injure the plaintiff's reputation. To clarify "injuring reputation," the common law has said that the communication has the tendency to diminish the esteem, respect, goodwill, or confidence in which the plaintiff was held or to cause adverse, derogatory, or unpleasant feelings or opinions against him or her.[26] **Libel** is defamation in written form, whereas **slander** is oral defamation. Because of the damaging nature of written documents, the libeled individual does not have to prove any actual damages to prevail. Certain types of slander, such as imputation of a crime or a sexually transmitted disease, also do not require proof of actual damages, but most forms of slander do require such proof.

Often, defamatory remarks are made in the context of a joke. If a reasonable person understands the statement to be a joke, it is not actionable. In situations where words have an ambiguous meaning or seem innocent, it must be proved that they contain an "innuendo" or meaning that makes them defamatory.[28]

Any living person may be defamed; however, a plaintiff cannot file a lawsuit based on the defamation of a third party, and there are no grounds for a lawsuit for the defamation of a deceased person. A parent cannot sue for defamation of a child.

It is possible, however, to defame a corporation or other legal entity, such as a partnership or an unincorporated association, if the statements prejudice the public against the entity or injure its business reputation.

A CASE IN POINT

Intentional Infliction of Emotional Distress

The Facts

In *Adams v. Murakami,*[24] a patient of low intelligence with chronic schizophrenia gave birth to an autistic child while she was under a doctor's care residing in a convalescent hospital. She alleged that while she resided in the hospital, the doctor knew she was of childbearing age, had been sexually active, and was in an environment where sexual relations frequently occurred. The plaintiff further alleged that the doctor failed to prescribe birth control pills, even though he knew she had requested them, and failed to examine her when she began exhibiting symptoms of pregnancy. On later determining that she was pregnant, he did not counsel her that her mental condition was genetically linked and could be passed to a child, nor did he discuss abortion or inform the patient that the stress of having a child often exacerbates the mental problems of schizophrenics. The doctor also did not take the patient off the strong psychotropic medications or inform her that these drugs were contraindicated for pregnancy and could seriously harm the fetus.

The Court Decides

The jury found that this evidence was proof of medical negligence and intentional infliction of emotional distress and awarded the patient $1,024,266, of which $750,000 were punitive damages intended to punish the physician.

Publication/Communication

To be defamatory, the material or information must be published or communicated to some third party who understands the defamatory meaning and recognizes that it applies to the defamed individual or entity. A statement made only to the defamed person is not considered a publication. The publication or communication may be

---

BOX 6–5

Quasi-intentional Torts

1. Defamation
2. Libel
3. Slander
4. Breach of confidentiality
5. Invasion of privacy

A Case in Point

Slander

The Facts

In *Schessler v. Keck*,[27] an unmarried female chef had a false-positive reaction to a syphilis blood test, although she had never had the disease. During treatments by a physician, a nurse had access to the medical record and was told about the false-positive condition. Despite knowing that it was a false positive, the nurse told various friends that the physician was treating the woman for syphilis. This information led to economic losses to the woman's cooking and catering business.

The Court Decides

In the suit that followed, the appeals court found that the plaintiff had a cause of action for slander.

oral, printed, or written or conveyed by means of a picture, statement, or even gestures.

Publication may occur unintentionally, such as sending a defamatory personal letter knowing that the addressee is often absent and that others may read his or her mail. No publication occurs if the letter is stolen or opened despite the "personal" mark on the envelope and letter.

Repetition of defamatory publication or communication is itself defamation. The person who repeats the defamation is liable for the injury it causes to the defamed person's reputation even if he or she states the source of the information or indicates that it is only a rumor. The person who initially published or communicated the defamatory remarks also may be liable for the repetition of them if the person had reason to expect that the remarks would be repeated. An example would be if nurse A tells the supervisor that she "heard" that nurse B is human immunodeficiency virus (HIV) positive and a cocaine abuser, when in fact this is not true.

Defenses to Defamation

There are several defenses to the charge of defamation (Box 6–6).

Truth

Truth is considered an absolute defense to claims of defamation. Out of a strong regard for reputations, the law presumes that all defamation is false and the person making the statement has the burden of proving its truth.

BOX 6–6

Defenses to Defamation

1. Truth
2. Absolute privilege
3. Qualified privilege
4. Consent
5. Duty to disclose imposed by law

A person may not avoid liability by proving that the defamatory inference is true in part, nor can the proof of a single incident be a defense when the accusation alleged multiple acts of misconduct. If the accusations address specific misconduct, other acts of misconduct cannot be used to prove the truth of the accusations. The person making the statement must prove that the content of the statement itself is true.

If a nurse is accused of stealing drugs, the fact that the same nurse was also caught stealing a patient's watch does not prove the truth of the accusation about the drugs and does not absolve the defendant of the defamation claim.

Information contained in medical records may, on occasion, be inaccurate and may adversely affect the patient's reputation. Allowing an unauthorized person access to records may precipitate an action alleging defamation.

Absolute Privilege

The law recognizes that publications made in certain legislative, judicial, and administrative proceedings are **absolutely privileged** and do not give rise to an action for defamation. For example, release of medical record information pursuant to a subpoena or court order is not actionable even if the medical records contained false and defamatory information.

In *Mickens v. Davis,*[29] the physician's written report stating that the plaintiff was suffering from a sexually transmitted disease (syphilis) was prepared in response to a court order entered in workers' compensation proceedings. The court determined that the report was privileged.

Also, testimony given in open court or during the course of official proceedings before legislative bodies, even if defamatory, is protected by the absolute privilege.

Qualified Privilege

A **qualified privilege** is an exemption from liability for defamatory statements that are made in good faith, and without malice, concerning subjects in which the person has an interest or a duty to communicate to another with a corresponding interest or responsibility. For a qualified privilege to apply, the person must believe the statement to be true or have reasonable grounds for believing it to be true. Most states have laws that specify when a qualified privilege applies.

For example, medical records may contain inaccurate information that, if published, could adversely affect a person's reputation. Release of information concerning the medical condition or medical record of a patient must always be approached cautiously and must only occur in compliance with applicable state and federal laws, such as Health Insurance Portability and Accountability Act of 1996 (HIPAA). When a specific state law addresses the release of medical record information, the qualified privilege described here provides no protection if the disclosure is made in violation of the law.

The most common example of a qualified privilege occurs in employment situations. If a prospective employer asks a former employer about a job applicant and the prior employer divulges information about the applicant's work history, it is clear that both the potential employer and the prior employer have a legitimate interest in the exchange of information. If the information given is reasonably believed to be true, the disclosure would be protected by a qualified privilege.

When considering whether to disclose information, it is usually wiser to wait for a legitimate inquiry than to volunteer information. Also, follow the facility policy and procedures regarding divulging employee information.

Consent

If the defamed person gives **consent** to the publication of the defamatory material, then the person cannot later complain that it damaged his or her reputation. However, the scope of this consent may be limited, and consent to one form of publication does not imply consent to publish the defamation in a different manner. For example, permission to disclose information to a patient's spouse does not imply permission to disclose the information to the patient's employer. And permission to write the information in a letter to another individual is not permission to post the information on an Internet Web site.

Invasion of Privacy

Another quasi-intentional tort, **invasion of privacy,** violates a person's right to be left alone and not be subjected to unreasonable interference with his or her personal life. In contrast to some defamation actions, in an action for invasion of privacy, the plaintiff does not have to prove any actual damage or demonstrate that information was false. Rather, the plaintiff must show the following:

1. The privacy right has been violated.
2. The public disclosure has occurred.
3. A reasonable person would object to the intrusion.

Examples of invasion of privacy in medical settings include using a patient's name or picture without consent in commercials or other publications, or revealing names of persons in mental hospitals or drug rehabilitation centers.

A CASE IN POINT

Qualified Privilege

The Facts

In *Bolling v. Baker*,[30] a nurse alleged defamation because, immediately after firing her, the doctor told his five office employees at a staff meeting that he could not work with her because she was a liar, not trustworthy, and not loyal to his practice.

The Court Decides

Qualified privilege did not cover the doctor because he did not communicate the information to parties with a legitimate interest in the information. The nurse recovered $65,000.

The Facts

In *Murphy v. Herfort*,[31] a hospital official used qualified privilege as a defense against defamation claims by an anesthesiologist whose staff privileges had been suspended.

The Court Decides

The court ruled that statements made by the hospital official to colleagues about matters of concern to the hospital fell under the principle of qualified privilege. Although such privilege is not absolute, the anesthesiologist was not able to show that the hospital official had doubted the truth of any of his statements or that he had been motivated by a desire to injure the anesthesiologist.

The tort of invasion of privacy is fundamentally different from the tort of defamation. Defamation causes an injury to the character or reputation, which is where proof of actual damages may come in. Invasion of privacy, on the other hand, harms the feelings without regard to any effect on (or actual damages to) the property, business interest, or standing of the individual in the community.[32] The publicity, the breach of privacy, is the harm in and of itself, regardless of tangential injuries or damages that may or may not have flowed from it. The right to privacy concerns one's peace of mind, the right to be left alone without being subjected to unwarranted or undesired publicity. The right to privacy is personal; it applies to the individual and does not extend to family members or businesses. Invasion of privacy is divided into four types:

1. Intrusion on the seclusion or private concerns of another
2. Public disclosure of private facts

A Case in Point

Intrusion on the Seclusion or Private Concerns of Another

The Facts

In *Miller v. National Broadcasting Co.*,[33] an NBC news field producer was preparing a mini-documentary on fire department paramedics and their work. While filming Los Angeles fire department paramedics on their emergency calls, the producer entered the plaintiff's house and filmed the paramedics attempting to save the plaintiff's husband, who had suffered a heart attack. The film was broadcast on NBC's nightly news program. Although the plaintiff was present during the incident, the producer did not attempt to obtain her consent for the intrusion.

The Court Decides

The court ruled that reasonable people could regard the NBC camera crew's intrusion into the bedroom at a time of vulnerability and confusion as "highly offensive" conduct and a violation of the wife's right to privacy.

3. Publicity that places the person in a false light in the public eye
4. Appropriation of a person's name or likeness

Intrusion on the Seclusion or Private Concerns of Another

Intrusion on the seclusion or private concerns of another consists of intentional interference with another's interest in solitude or seclusion, with respect to his or her person or private affairs. Eavesdropping on private conversations, peering into windows, making unwanted telephone calls, illegally searching shopping bags, or otherwise invading a person's home are examples. To put it into context, listening in on hospital telephone calls or searching through a patient's belongings without authorization may also be considered an invasion of the patient's privacy.

In addition, filming or otherwise documenting medical activities without the patient's permission may also be considered an invasion of privacy if it is done for purposes other than treatment of the patient.

On occasion, private individuals may become caught up in publicity as a result of circumstances such as accidents or crimes, which make their condition of interest to the public. This involvement also causes a loss of some of their right of privacy. Publicity surrounding victims of crimes, suicides, accidents, and rare diseases does not usually give rise to liability for invasion of privacy. However, some courts have ruled that the right of privacy should include the right to obtain medical treatment without the publication of this information to the news media.

In *Barber v. Time, Inc.*,[34] a patient was permitted to sue for the publication of her name and picture in a story concerning an eating disorder. Because the use of the patient's name and photograph were not considered necessary to the story, the invasion of privacy could not be justified as newsworthy.

Defenses to Invasion of Privacy

DUTY TO DISCLOSE IMPOSED BY LAW

Much like in defamation, when the nurse has a duty imposed by law to disclose confidential information about a patient and the disclosure is made in compliance with such law, the nurse is protected from liability. For example, according to most state laws, nurses are obligated to report known or suspected incidents of child abuse or elder abuse; the law further provides that nurses shall be immune from lawsuits when they make such a report.

There may be other circumstances in which reporting a patient's condition is mandated by state law, such as the diagnosis of certain communicable diseases. Whenever such reports are required and the report is made with the good faith belief that it is true, the reporting individual should be immune from liability.

RELEASE OF INFORMATION TO THE NEWS MEDIA

Inquiries about patients by news media present serious concerns regarding invasion of patient privacy.

There is no legal obligation to disclose information of any kind about a patient to the news media. Each facility should have a written policy that describes who will respond to media inquiries and what information may be released. This policy should comply with state and federal law and should address when a health care provider may disclose the patient's name, address, age, and sex; a general description of the reason for treatment (whether an injury, burn, poisoning, or some unrelated condition); the general nature of the injury, burn, poisoning, or other condition; the general condition of the patient; or any information that is not medical information.[35] However, this provision of law is ineffective if the patient specifically requests that the information not be released.

Nurses must know the facility's policy and procedure regarding disclosure of patient information.

If the patient is receiving treatment for drug or alcohol abuse, special rules apply regarding the disclosure of information about the patient. No information may be disclosed about the patient, including the fact that the person is or was a patient in the facility, without either the patient's written consent or a court order. Check the federal and state laws.

There is often considerable interest in the medical treatment of a public figure. If the personality and affairs of an individual have already become public, the press has the right to inform the public about legitimate matters of public interest. To some extent that person has lost the right to keep his or her affairs private. This may continue to be true long after the person has ceased to be a celebrity. However, after some time, the individual may have the right to sue for invasion of privacy.

Public Disclosure of Private Facts

Highly objectionable publicity of private information about a patient may be an invasion of privacy. (If the information is false, it may also give rise to a cause of action for defamation.) In some jurisdictions, the public must not have a legitimate interest in having the information available.[36]

A notorious case of public disclosure of private facts is *Bazemore v. Savannah Hospital.*[37] In this case, parents brought an action against a newspaper, its photographer, and the hospital for unauthorized publication of pictures of their malformed child who had been born with his heart outside his body. The hospital had permitted a newspaper to photograph and publish pictures of the child's nude body without the permission or even knowledge of the parents. The Georgia Supreme Court ruled that the hospital had a duty to protect the child from "an invasion of an unauthorized person or persons, whereby its monstrosity and nude condition would likely be exposed to any persons, and particularly to the general public."[38]

In another case, the plaintiff was treated in the hospital for an alcohol-related illness. On admission, she had been assured of privacy by the hospital and its employees. Later, a physician sent a health insurance claim form with the medical diagnosis of "Acute and Chronic Alcoholism Detoxification" to the office of the plaintiff's employer. The employee who opened the mail was not authorized to receive insurance payment forms. The plaintiff alleged that the incident caused severe humiliation, embarrassment, and stress. The court held that the physician could be liable for violating the plaintiff's right to privacy by publishing personal information without the plaintiff's permission.[39]

Information of any kind and in any form pertaining to patients must be protected from improper disclosure. This includes medical records, diagnostic films, photographs, recordings, or tracings. The patient's written permission must be obtained prior to the disclosure of patient-identifiable data or information, unless allowed by state or federal law.

Publicity That Places the Person in a False Light in the Public Eye

Another type of invasion of privacy comes up only rarely in the health care setting. It involves publicity that places a person in a false light in the public eye, such as the unauthorized use of a person's name on a petition or the use of a person's picture to illustrate a book or an article, implying a connection that does not exist.

Appropriation of a Person's Name or Likeness

The nonconsensual use of a person's photograph or image for commercial purposes, such as advertising, is a well-recognized basis for liability based on invasion of privacy.

Invasion of privacy occurred when a plastic surgeon used several "before" and "after" photographs of his patient's cosmetic surgery, without her consent, at a department store presentation and on a television program promoting the presentation.[40]

In another case, the patient had given her physician permission to film her cesarean section on the understanding that the film would be exhibited to medical societies and used to further medical science. The pictures were actually included in a motion picture titled *Birth*, which was shown in commercial theaters. The patient sued both the physician and the camera operator for invasion of her privacy.[41]

KEEP IN MIND

▶ Administering treatment against a patient's will may be considered assault and battery.

▶ When force is used to detain a patient, liability for false imprisonment may also exist.

▶ Performing a medical or surgical procedure without the patient's consent may give rise to allegations of both negligence and medical battery.

▶ The nurse should become familiar with applicable state and federal laws relating to reporting obligations and requirements of confidentiality of patient information.

▶ To successfully prosecute a lawsuit based on the allegations of an intentional tort, a person must prove that the act was committed with the intent to cause an injury, that the act was an invasion of a right, or that it was substantially certain that the injury or invasion would result from the act. It must also be shown that the person was damaged by the action in some way.

▶ To be considered defamatory, publication or communication must be made to some third person that injures the victim's reputation in some way. The statements must not be true or protected by some absolute or qualified privilege, and the disclosure of the information must not have been required by some state or federal law.

▶ Invasion of privacy can occur in a number of contexts in the health care setting. Unreasonably revealing the personal or private affairs of a patient may interfere with the solitude of the person and, if false, may also give rise to a cause of action for defamation.

▶ There is no legal obligation to disclose information of any kind about a patient to the news media.

In a Nutshell

The liability for intentional tortious conduct rests squarely on the person performing the tortious acts. However, there may also be circumstances in which the employer is held liable for the injuries as well. Except in cases of outrageous or malicious conduct, tortious conduct is most likely to result because the nurse is unaware that his or her actions are not protected by applicable laws. To avoid such liability, it is advisable to become familiar with the state and federal laws that apply to the practice of nursing. Such laws include reporting requirements relating to child abuse, elder or dependent-adult abuse, victims of crimes, and communicable diseases. Also, know laws regarding confidentiality of sensitive information. If the nurse is dealing with chemical dependency patients, he or she should also be familiar with federal and state drug and alcohol treatment confidentiality laws. The mental health nurse should be knowledgeable about involuntary and voluntary treatment and confinement laws. The federal and state laws, especially HIPAA, relating to use and disclosure of health information must also be reviewed and followed. Avoiding intentional tort liability involves understanding what intentional conduct is permitted and what is considered improper and tortious in the jurisdiction where the nurse practices.

Afterthoughts

1. Define an intentional tort and distinguish it from negligence.
2. Discuss how quasi-intentional torts differ from intentional torts.
3. Give examples in the health care arena and discuss the following torts:
   a. Defamation
   b. Invasion of privacy
   c. Assault
   d. Battery
   e. False imprisonment
   f. Trespass to land
   g. Intentional infliction of emotional distress
4. Relate how you can prevent invasion of privacy of your patients.
5. Define and give an example of a medical battery.
6. Discuss how informed consent relates to medical battery.
7. Discuss what role the doctrine of informed consent plays in an allegation of intentional tort.
8. What is the policy in your facility regarding disclosure of patient information? How is your facility complying with HIPAA and privacy regulation?
9. Find an intentional or quasi-intentional tort case and discuss (1) the "intent" issue, (2) damages or harm, and (3) how the tort could have been prevented.
10. If a competent patient refuses his medication and you force him to take it by intimidation, have you committed any tort? If yes, which one?

11. Develop and present to the class a case scenario involving an intentional or quasi-intentional tort. Have the class discuss what tort you have selected and the elements of the tort.

ETHICS IN PRACTICE

Three days after his 81st birthday, Mr. E. was admitted to the medical unit with a diagnosis of metastatic cancer of the liver. He had several full-course treatments of chemotherapy and radiation during the previous year with only temporary remissions of the disease. His condition had deteriorated rapidly during the previous month, and his family was no longer able to care for him at home. Dr. K., his physician, expected Mr. E. to die within a few weeks, if not sooner, and admitted him to the hospital primarily for pain control. On admission, Dr. K. ordered morphine sulfate (MS) 5 mg IV to be given every 2 hours around the clock.

Although this was a relatively large dose of a strong narcotic medication to be given this frequently, Mr. E. tolerated the treatment for the first 36 hours and reported a significant reduction in his pain. On the third morning after his admission, Mr. E. was difficult to arouse for his morning vital signs and breakfast. When his nurse, Joan F., RN, finally did get Mr. E. awake, he was confused, and his blood pressure was 82/50 with shallow respirations at 10 per minute. He still complained of severe generalized body pain and asked for "more of that medication that helped so much the day before."

Joan did not give Mr. E. his scheduled 8 AM dose of MS. She phoned Dr. K. and reported her assessment of the patient, expressing her belief that continuing the medication at the previously prescribed dose and frequency would be fatal to this patient. Dr. K., who had been up most of the night with an emergency patient, stated sarcastically, "And Mr. E. has such a productive life to look forward to—give the medication like I ordered it! And don't call me any more about this—I'll be in after lunch!" and slammed down the phone.

What should Joan do? If she continues to give the medication at the prescribed dose and frequency and the patient dies, could she be held civil or criminally liable? What are the ethical principles involved in this case? How could she best resolve the dilemma?

References

1. See Keaton, WP, et al: Prosser and Keaton on the Law of Torts, ed 5. 1984, § 1, at 1 & 2.
2. Legal Dictionary: http://www.law.com, accessed 11/21/02.
3. See Keaton, WP, et al: Prosser and Keaton on the Law of Torts, ed 5. 1984, § 111, at 773.
4. Good Samaritan statutes vary from state to state but generally absolve from liability the health care provider who in good faith provides emergency care at the scene of an accident.
5. Baca v. Velez, 833 P.2d 1194 (N.M.App. 1992).
6. Roberson v. Provident House, 576 So.2d 992 (La. 1991).
7. Canterbury v. Spence, 464 F.2d 772 (D.C. Cir. 1972), quoting Schloendorff v. Society of New York Hospital, 211 N.Y. 125 (1914).
8. Witkin BE: Summary of California Law, Torts, ed 9. 1988, § 358.
9. See discussion of the Berkey case by the California Supreme Court in Cobbs v. Grant, 8 Cal.3d 229, 239 (1972).
10. Gaskin v. Goldwasser, 520 N.E.2d 1085 (Ill. 1988).

11. Patrich v. Menorah Medical Center, 636 S.W.2d 134 (Mo.App. 1982).
12. See Rennie v. Klein, 102 S.Ct. 3506 (1982); and Large v. Superior Court, 714 P.2d 399 (Ariz. 1986).
13. See Calif. Bus & Prof. Code § 2397 (West 1990).
14. Mattocks v. Bell, 194 A.2d 307 (D.C.App. 1963).
15. See Restatement (Second) of Torts § 35 (1965).
16. Cook v. Highland Hospital, 84 S.E. 352 (N.C. 1915).
17. Big Town Nursing Home, Inc. v. Newman, 461 S.W.2d 195 (Tex.Civ.App. 1970).
18. Blackman for Blackman v. Rifkin, 759 P.2d 54 (Colo.App. 1988), cert. den. (1989).
19. Hapgood v. Biloxi Regional Medical Center, 540 So.2d 630 (Miss. 1989).
20. Maben v. Rankin, 55 Cal.2d 139 (1961).
21. Witkin, BE: Summary of California Law, Torts, ed 9. 1988, § 604, at 704.
22. See Restatement (Second) of Torts § 158 (1977).
23. Fardig v. Municipality of Anchorage, 785 P.2d 911 (Alaska App. 1990).
24. Adams v. Murakami, No. C418409 (Los Angeles County Superior Court).
25. O'Keefe, ME: Nursing Practice and the Law. FA Davis, Philadelphia, 2001.
26. See Keaton, WP: Prosser and Keaton on the Law of Torts, ed 5. 1984, § 111, at 773.
27. Schlesser v. Keck, 271 P.2d 588 (Cal. App. 1954).
28. Witkin, BE: Summary of California Law, Torts, ed 9. 1988, § 493 at 580.
29. Mickens v. Davis, 132 Kan. 49 (1931).
30. Bolling v. Baker, 671 S.W.2d 559 (Tex. App. 1984).
31. Murphy v. Herfort, 528 N.Y.S.2d 117 (1988).
32. Fairfield v. American Photocopy Equipment Co., 138 C.A.2d 82, 86 (1955).
33. Miller v. National Broadcasting Co., 187 C.A.3d 1463 (1986).
34. Barber v. Time, Inc., 159 S.W.2d 291 (Mo. 1942).
35. Calif. Civil Code § 56.16 (West 1982).
36. See Restatement (Second) of Torts; § 625D cmts. a-k (1977).
37. Bazemore v. Savannah Hospital, 155 S.E. 194 (Ga. 1930).
38. Idem., 195.
39. Prince v. St. Francis–St. George Hospital, Inc. 484 N.E.2d 265 (Ohio App. 1985).
40. Vassiliades v. Garfinckel's, Brooks Bros., 492 A.2d 580 (D.C. App. 1985).
41. Feeney v. Young, 191 A.D. 501 (1920).

Resources

Association of Trial Lawyers of America
The Leonard M. Ring Law Center
1050 31st Street, NW
Washington, DC 20007
(800) 424-2725
(202) 965-3500

Defense Research Institute
750 W. Lake Shore Drive
Chicago, IL 60611
(312) 944-0575
(312) 944-2003

Common Areas of Negligence and Liability

7

Key Chapter Concepts

Nursing negligence

Liability

Falls

Restraints

Medication errors

Burns

Equipment injuries

Retained foreign objects

Failure to monitor

Communication

Chapter Thoughts

During the course of an average workday, the typical floor nurse carries out numerous treatments, passes out a large number of medications, performs frequent physical assessments, and makes multiple decisions that affect the health and well-being of patients. Nurses rarely have the time to fully investigate and consider all the ethical and legal implications of their actions. They often make critical decisions about patient care while in the midst of high-pressure situations that force them to act quickly. Sometimes nurses make mistakes.

Fortunately, only a small percentage of the mistakes made by nurses actually produce injury to patients. Of this small number of injured patients, an even smaller percentage goes on to seek compensation for damages through legal action. Nevertheless, the number of lawsuits filed against nurses continues to increase. Many of these suits are well publicized in the news media and give the impression that every action a nurse takes can leave that nurse open to a lawsuit. This is a false impression.

The best defenses a nurse can have against being sued by patients are to remain competent in skills and knowledge, practice nursing at the highest standards of care, and document thoroughly. Remaining competent and knowledgeable about nursing skills, techniques, treatments, assessments, and medications is not only a legal imperative but also one of the key requirements for ethical nursing practice. Nurses have the minimal ethical obligation or duty of nonmaleficence, which means doing no harm to patients. If nothing else, remaining competent in one's skills and knowledge helps prevent injury to patients.

Another important factor in preventing lawsuits is to establish a friendly, trusting relationship with the patient and his or her family. As nursing has sought more independence and status as a profession, there has been an unfortunate movement toward less personalized care. Most patients and their families have an inherently positive attitude toward nurses, whom they see as the only individuals in the often impersonal institutional atmosphere who personally care about them.

Nurses teach, counsel, and provide comfort and understanding to patients and families in stressful situations. A little extra time spent talking with patients; allowing them to express anger, fear, or anxiety; or even bending the rules to accommodate visitors often pays big dividends later. In reality, if the nurse has a good relationship with the patient, it is less likely that he or she will be named in a lawsuit if a mistake is made.

OBJECTIVES

Upon completing this chapter, the reader will be able to:

1. Analyze cases and define common areas of nursing negligence and liability
2. Recognize common deviations from the nursing standard of care
3. Identify areas in which nursing risk management can reduce patient injury and resulting exposure to nursing liability
4. Identify appropriate measures to minimize risks and avoid liability
5. Discuss common breaches for different areas of nursing practice

Introduction

The second report of the Committee on Quality of Healthcare in America (Institute of Medicine [IOM]), "Crossing the Quality Chasm: A New Health System for the 21st Century," made several recommendations. The IOM report recommended an overhaul of the United States health care system and established specific directions for leaders, regulators, policymakers, and clinicians to "close" the quality gap and identify current practices that inhibit quality care. The goals of the proposed changes are to make patient care timely, safe, equitable, efficient, and centered.[1] Nurses are instrumental in ensuring quality patient care.

Nurses' Liability

Nursing negligence is conduct that is unreasonable under the circumstances or that fails to meet the appropriate standard of care as discussed earlier. **Liability** means legal responsibility: a nurse is legally responsible for actions that fail to meet the standard of care or for failing to act and thereby causing harm. For example, when a nurse gives the wrong medication to a patient and the patient suffers harm, the nurse may be liable for negligent administration of the drug.

Many cases of nursing negligence also involve other parties. For example, a patient may argue that his injury is the result of negligence on the part of a nurse and a doctor, hospital, or other employer; any combination of defendants may be found responsible for the injury and liable for a deviation from the standard of care (Box 7–1).

BOX 7–1

Defensive Nursing Practice Tips

1. Avoid blaming or criticizing other health care providers in the presence of the patients or family members.
2. Recognize the "problem patient" and troubleshoot.
3. Use thorough documentation for the noncompliant patient or complainer.
4. Maintain thorough and accurate documentation.
5. Send only copies and never the originals of records or radiographs requested.
6. Know the charting policies and procedures of the facility and your unit.
7. Know the accepted abbreviations for the facility.
8. Maintain thorough documentation of telephone calls involving you, patients, family members, physicians, and other health care providers.
9. Maintain good communication and rapport with the patient and family. Many lawsuits are pursued because the patient or family did not like the way they were treated by the facility's staff or physician.

Common Causes of Liability

Nursing negligence cases are found in legal reports, legal journals, or insurance company publications. Northrop[3] reviewed 33 cases reported in 1 year by plaintiffs' attorneys alleging nursing malpractice. For the most part, nursing actions fell into the following categories (Box 7–2):

1. Treatment
2. Communication
3. Medication
4. Monitoring, observing, and supervising

See Appendix A, which divides common nursing actions into nursing areas of practice.

Another study ranked the top 10 most common allegations in nursing malpractice claims in one insurance program over 6 years.[4] The top 10 allegations found were as follows:

1. Patient falls
2. Failure to monitor
3. Failure to ensure patient safety
4. Improper performance of treatment
5. Failure to respond to patient
6. Medication error
7. Wrong dosage administered
8. Failure to follow facility procedure
9. Improper technique
10. Failure to supervise treatment

A CASE IN POINT

A Focus on Patient Care

The Facts

In *Nieto v. State of Colorado,*[2] an inmate at a correctional facility sought treatment at the facility's medical clinic and was given cold and flu medication by the nurse. Three days later he returned to the clinic with increased pain. On the second visit he was seen by another nurse who was the medical coordinator at the facility. The nurse instructed the inmate to continue the medication given to him. Several days later the inmate returned with continued pain and a swollen right eye. The clinic nurse told the inmate to leave and not to return or he would be disciplined.

However, he returned again in a couple of days with worsened symptoms and complained to the nurse that he thought he was suffering a stroke. The nurse briefly examined him and gave him an antibiotic and decongestant with instructions to continue other medications given and return the next day. The inmate failed to return to the clinic but sought assistance from the prison guard, who told him to apply a hot compress to his eye and return to bed. The inmate unsuccessfully sought help from the guard two more times in the next 3 days.

He was found in his cell incontinent and unconscious with his right eye bulging from its socket. He was taken to the emergency department of the local hospital and diagnosed with a severe sinus infection that had spread to his right eye and to the base and frontal lobe of the brain. He also suffered a stroke and was permanently paralyzed on the left side.

He filed a civil suit seeking damages for injuries he sustained as a result of inadequate medical care.

The Court Decides

The individual defendants were dismissed. The claim, based on Respondent Superior, proceeded. The court found that the correctional facility was responsible for failure of the employees to provide adequate medical care

Nurses can best avoid liability for negligence by giving safe, high-quality nursing care. It is also helpful to be aware of potential problem areas, identifying the risk areas in individual practice, and taking measures to minimize exposure to those risks. Such measures include staying current in the field of practice, establishing a good relationship with patients, documenting thoroughly all treatment and communications, and following approved procedures.

The following sections provide an overview of common types of patient incidents. These are not listed in any particular order, but they are fairly representative of the types of lawsuits to which staff nurses in health care facilities might be exposed in the course of their practices.

BOX 7–2

Nursing Negligence Cases

Treatment

1. Enema to a preoperative patient with appendicitis, which resulted in ruptured bowel and appendicitis
2. Improperly used equipment, resulting in air embolisms
3. Failure to administer the correct oxygen level
4. Failure to attach a fetal monitor as ordered
5. Burns to an infant from formula heated in a microwave
6. Failure to attend a patient having an asthma attack, resulting in injuries such as brain damage

Communication

1. Failure to notify the physician of changes in signs and symptoms
2. Failure to chart vital signs for hours in a labor room
3. Failure to advise the physician of jaundice
4. Failure to notify the physician of circulatory compromise in a casted leg

Medication

1. Wrong medication given on discharge (topical eye anesthetic instead of artificial tears)
2. Failure to give diazepam (Valium) as ordered
3. Improper administration of potassium chloride

Monitoring/Observing/Supervising

1. Failure to recognize dehydration and electrolyte imbalance
2. Failure to monitor intravenous therapy
3. Failure to monitor fetal heart rate
4. Negligent supervision of a psychiatric patient who attempted suicide
5. Negligent assignment and supervision of a student nurse who did not take blood pressure for 6 hours

---

Patient Falls

According to the Centers for Disease Control and Prevention (CDC), more adults 65 and older die from fall-related injuries each year than from any other cause. The CDC attributes the high fall rates to a growing number of people age 89 and older.[5]

With respect to patient **falls,** the most important measures for preventing lawsuits are assessing for fall potential (e.g., fall risk assessments) and implementing measures to prevent falls. For instance, health care providers should document that the patient was instructed to remain in bed or that a family member was told that the patient should remain in bed and voiced understanding. They should ensure that the bedside rails are up and that the call light is at the bedside. It is difficult to defend a claim if, at minimum, there has not been frequent documentation of the patient's care. If a patient does fall, information on the chart and in an incident report must include an evaluation of the patient's physical and mental condition (including the integumentary, respiratory, cardiovascular, musculoskeletal, and neurological systems). But most cases involving patient falls that lead to liability for practitioners do so because of the lack of documentation regarding the circumstances prior to the fall, rather than after the incident.

If a "fall warning" mechanical device or alarm is used, record its use on the chart. This gives the appearance to a judge or jury that the nurse is aware of the potential problem and attempted to prevent any injuries and provide a safe environment for the elderly patient.

Patients in hospitals and nursing homes may be medicated, sedated, disoriented, or restricted by a cast or walker. They may not be expecting sudden dizziness upon rising from a recumbent position. They may be confused by unfamiliar surroundings. Injuries often occur when a patient slips on a wet floor or falls trying to climb over a side rail. Many patients fall when trying to walk without needed assistance or getting up from a wheelchair that has not been locked. The nurse has a duty to assess the situation and then provide adequate assistance, supervision, or restraint to ensure patient safety. Failure to do so may result in liability.

Restraints

Restraints are applied to restrict patient movement in cases where the patient may cause personal harm or harm to others. The trend today leans toward a restraint-free environment; however, this is not possible at all times. There are certain situations in which restraints are appropriate and necessary. That said, however, if a patient is restrained or detained inappropriately, it may lead to allegations of false imprisonment. Physical restraints can cause skin breakdown, impaired respiratory status, strangulation, and death. Chemical restraints may cause drowsiness, decrease coherence and judgment, and increase confusion in elderly patients. Therefore, if a patient must be restrained, it is important to chart the following items:

1. Ineffective alternatives that were tried prior to restraints
2. Reason for restraints; describe patient's specific behavior and type of restraint used
3. The time and date when restraints are applied
4. The times when the patient is monitored while restraints are in place
5. Patient's response to restraints
6. How facility policy and procedures are followed with regard to how often a patient in restraints must be checked and released from restraints, as well as the care to be given the patient when out of restraints

7. For every patient check, assessments of skin integrity; circulation; respiratory status; patient's verbal response; reasons, based on patient behavior, for continued restraints; and physician's orders

Most institutions, hospitals, clinics, and nursing homes have policies and procedures addressing restraints and other patient safety measures. It is important to know and follow these guidelines to prevent injuries. Injuries can result in asphyxiation, death, fractures, brain damage, circulatory compromise, and nerve damage.

There is no absolute liability for falls that occur in hospitals. Before the duty to protect the patient (e.g., with restraints) arises, there must be proof that the nurse had reason to foresee that the patient could be harmed by falling. This is illustrated in a New York case[6] in which a plaintiff was denied recovery after a fall in the hospital. The patient was recovering from surgery on his leg. On the ninth postoperative day, he fell from bed and suffered serious injuries. The nurses testified that they had no reason to foresee this fall and that the patient was alert and oriented. The physician testified that the patient's condition did not warrant the use of side rails. The court denied recovery to the patient.

Medication Errors

According to a report by the United States Pharmacopeia that summarized medical error data from 56 facilities nationwide, the most commonly reported types of **medication errors** included the following:

1. Improper dose and quantity errors
2. Unauthorized drug errors (e.g., administration of the wrong medication)
3. Omission errors (medications were not administered)[7]

The key factors contributing to these errors were heavier workloads and distractions.[8] According to the study, however, the majority of errors studied did not cause harm.

Errors in the administration of medications are another common source of liability for nurses. Examples of negligence in medication administration are plentiful. Common errors include administration of the wrong drug; administration of a drug to the wrong patient; administration of the wrong dose or by the wrong route; improper injection technique; administration of a drug that the nurse knows is contraindicated; or the failure to recognize side effects, adverse reactions, or toxic signs and symptoms. The standards of nursing care require that nurses understand the medications they administer and use their judgment in following medication orders. When a physician orders a medication for a particular patient, the dose, route, frequency, and other parameters are specified. Failure to meet any one of these specifications may cause an injury to the patient and result in liability for the nurse. Nursing professionals are constantly reminded of the importance of knowing the reason why a drug is administered and how treatments are to be administered.

A CASE IN POINT

Restraints

The Facts

One Massachusetts case involved an elderly man who fell out of bed following eye surgery.[9] The nurse's notes indicated that the patient returned from surgery "very sleepy" but did not note anything about side rails or instructions to the patient regarding ambulation. In the early morning of the first postoperative day, the patient was found on the floor, disoriented, with a fractured wrist. The patient's family alleged that they had requested that the patient be restrained for his own protection because he "seemed so disoriented" after surgery.

The Court Decides

This case resulted in money damages for the patient.

The Facts

In *Reifschneider v. Nebraska Methodist Hospital*,[10] a patient sued a hospital and others for injuries she sustained when she fell from a hospital cart while in the emergency room. The patient was admitted to the emergency room semiconscious and unstable. She was placed on a cart with the side rails raised but was not strapped in or otherwise restrained. The physician testified that after he examined the patient, he requested that someone remain with her at all times, but he did not recall the person to whom he gave that order. The nurse attending the patient was called from the room on another task by the charge nurse. The charge nurse asked the patient's father to remain in the room with her. However, the father left, and, while attempting to climb off the end, the patient fell from the cart and suffered a severe blow to her face and temporomandibular joint. The patient alleged negligent failure to restrain and negligent failure to provide attendants or supervision.

The Court Decides

At trial, the defendants were granted a summary judgment in their favor due to the absence of expert testimony from the plaintiff on the standard of care. The appeals court reversed in part and remanded (returned the case to the lower court) for further proceedings against the hospital on the question of adequate supervision.

The Facts

In *Ashcraft v. Mobile Infirmary Medical Center*,[11] a 71-year-old patient in a psychiatric ward complained of sore and swollen feet following a day trip. She was given a bucket of warm water to soak her feet while sitting in the recreation room. Afterward, the nurse carried the bucket of water to the patient's room. The patient testified that the nurse pushed the door open with the bucket. As the patient stepped from the carpeted hall to the tile floor, she slipped, fell, and broke her right arm.

The Court Decides

The court decided in favor of the defendants.

The Appellate Court Decides

On appeal, the decision was reversed and the case remanded for resolution of the issue in dispute regarding whether the nurse was negligent in spilling the water or in failing to warn the patient about spilled water. The final outcome of the case is not reported.

The Facts

Brookover v. Mary Hitchcock Memorial Hospital [12] illustrates how charting practices can complicate the question of liability for a fall. A 36-year-old patient underwent brain surgery. Three days postoperatively he pressed his call light for assistance to the bathroom. When no one responded, he got out of bed and fell, breaking his hip. The nurse, who had heard a "thump," wrote in the clinical record: "Found pt. [patient] on floor—Apparently crawled out of bed—trying to get to BR (bathroom)—had called for help but not a quick enough response." This speculation was damaging for the nurse. Further problems for her defense arose when the patient's mother testified that the nurse admitted that she had heard the patient but could not respond because the hospital was shorthanded.

The Court Decides

The court issued a verdict against the hospital.

Drug Patient Safety System

Medication errors dropped by 86 percent after a Boston hospital, in 1993, installed a computer system that alerts physicians when they make potentially dangerous decisions when ordering medications. Brigham and Women's Hospital's system informs physicians of drug allergies and interactions. Fewer than 5 percent of hospitals nationwide have such a patient safety system. [13]

Burns

Patient **burns** are another common source of nursing liability. Burns can be caused by heating pads; hot bath and shower water; hot water treatments, including enemas and sitz baths; electrocautery equipment; heat lamps; and warmer beds. Chemical burns can occur from operative prep solutions. Cigarette-related burns are also common. Nurses must be particularly alert to the risk of burns when the patient has decreased sensitivity to heat or is unable to communicate discomfort. Children, elderly people, and patients who are sedated or anesthetized are often victims of burns (Box 7–3).

A CASE IN POINT

Medication Errors

The Facts

In *Hallinan v. Prindle,*[14] a hospital operating room nurse inadvertently supplied formaldehyde (Formalin) instead of the procaine (Novocain) requested by the surgeon who was preparing to anesthetize the patient. Several drops were injected before the error was discovered. The patient suffered great pain and required excision of an area of tissue.

The Court Decides

In affirming a judgment against the nurse, the court noted that there was no question that the nurse was negligent. In fact, the nurse accounted for her mistake by frankly admitting that she took no pains to read the label on the Formalin bottle before pouring.

The Facts

In *Penaloza v. Baptist Memorial Hospital,*[15] a nurse mistakenly administered a potassium permanganate pill to the patient orally when it was meant for external use only. The patient was receiving daily baths in water in which potassium permanganate had been dissolved for treatment of a rash. The labeled container of potassium permanganate pills was kept in the patient's medication box. One evening the supervisor made a change of nursing personnel on the unit, and the nurse giving medications administered all the pills in the patient's box orally. She testified that the medication was clearly labeled and that she knew that it should not be administered internally.

The Court Decides

In spite of the fact that the nurse admitted knowing how the drug should be administered, the court affirmed a judgment in favor of the hospital, noting that the hospital was not negligent in assigning the nurse to give medications. This nurse was licensed and had 3 years of continuous competent service. The suit did not individually name the nurse as a defendant.

The Facts

In *Holbrooks v. Duke University,*[16] a patient alleged negligent injection technique by a nurse. The patient testified that she was given an intramuscular injection of meperidine (Demerol) and hydroxyzine (Vistaril) approximately 3 to 4 inches above her knee and subsequently suffered nerve injuries. An expert nurse witness testified that the location in question would not be in accordance with the standard of care among members of the nursing profession. A physician testified that the injection could have caused the nerve damage alleged by the patient.

The Court Decides

The court ordered a new trial on the issue of nursing malpractice.

The Facts

Documentation can play an important role in liability determination. In *Briggs v. U.S.,*[17] a patient alleged that he had a psychotic reaction to preoperative medication because he received a double dose. The medications were noted twice on his "PRN and One-Time Medication Records." However, the evidence showed that he in fact received only one dose of medication despite the double notation. Two student nurses were both training on the ward where the patient was hospitalized. One of the student nurses had previously administered injections of preoperative medications. The other student nurse had no experience in this skill, and the nursing supervisor suggested that she administer the preoperative medication to the patient. The student nurses testified that they prepared the injection together, and that the inexperienced nurse gave it. Both documented the medication. Fortunately, the student who administered the injection remembered this incident clearly because it was her first preoperative injection. Also, it was clearly documented in the nurses' written notes that the injection was given by the student nurse with no injection experience.

The Court Decides

The court decided in favor of the defendants.

Equipment Injuries

Another patient safety concern for nurses involves the equipment used in patient care. The nurse's duty to exercise reasonable care includes a duty to select, maintain, and use equipment properly. This can pose quite a challenge in today's highly technological health care environment. The patient is often surrounded by complex and confusing monitors and other machines that require familiarity on the nurse's part. Most hospitals and other health care organizations have policies addressing the need for orientation to new equipment and procedures for identifying items in need of repair or maintenance. Anyone who is expected to use new or modified equipment should be provided with an adequate orientation. Nurses faced with an unfamiliar device to be used in patient care have a duty to seek the necessary orientation and training. Keep in mind that the instruction manuals for the equipment may be used to show the standard of care.

At the same time, many **equipment injuries** result not from unfamiliarity with the equipment but from haste, carelessness, or outright misuse. Nurses should never make their own modifications to patient equipment unless, after careful review of the intended and safe uses of the equipment, such modifications have been recom-

A CASE IN POINT

Burn Cases

The Facts

In *Flower Hospital v. Hart,*[18] two nurses who were hospital employees placed an unshielded lamp globe directly on the naked flesh of an unconscious patient and covered it with a towel while a physician was involved in emergency treatment of the patient. The patient sustained burns.

The Court Decides

The court held the hospital responsible.

The Facts

Nicheter v. Edmiston[19] involved a patient undergoing a breast biopsy and removal of a lesion from her arm. Tincture of benzalkonium chloride (Zephiran) disinfectant was applied to the patient, and fumes from the disinfectant ignited on contact with a heated needle. The patient suffered second-degree burns over a 4-inch area of her arm, resulting in permanent scarring. The nurse involved was not sued.

The Court Decides

The court ruled in favor of the plaintiff.

The Appellate Court Decides

On appeal, the issue of nursing negligence was raised, and the court noted that the patient could have sued the hospital and nurse as codefendants, in addition to the doctor, because of the nurse's actions.

The Facts

In *Smelko v. Brinton,*[20] a 3-month-old child suffered second- and third-degree burns on his buttocks while undergoing surgery. The infant was placed on a heating pad to keep him warm during a hernia repair. At the request of the anesthesiologist, the circulating nurse placed the pad in the operating room. Nothing unusual was noted after surgery. When the parents got home, they discovered blisters draining bloody fluid on the infant's buttocks. The child required skin grafting. Prior to trial, the defendants admitted liability and sought to exclude from evidence the warnings on the heating pad that read, in part, "Burns will result from improper use. Never use pad without cover in place.... Caution: Do not use on an infant, invalid, or a sleeping or unconscious person."

Because the defendants admitted liability before the trial, the case went to trial before a jury on the issue of damages. A verdict in the sum of $400,000 for the minor and $2250 for the parents was rendered.

The Facts

In *Bowers v. Olch,*[21] a paraplegic patient was burned when he was given his pipe to smoke while the nurse was out of the room. He dropped the pipe and set the bed on fire.

The Court Decides

The court wrote that the nurse had a duty to ensure the safety of patients, especially protecting them from known hazards such as fire.

mended by the manufacturer or the institution. Sometimes patient injuries are the result of poorly designed or improperly manufactured devices. In these situations it is especially important for the nurse to use the equipment in the way in which it is meant to be used.

Retained Foreign Objects

Retained foreign objects are a problem primarily for operating room nurses and others who are involved in invasive procedures in which drains, instruments, needles, cotton balls, sponges, hemostats, or monitoring devices are used during the surgery. Facilities generally have very specific instrument and sponge count policies and procedures. Most cases in which a patient alleges that a foreign object was retained involve extensive examination of the facility's count policy and the nurse's compliance with that policy.

BOX 7–3

Common Causes of Patient Burns

- Heating pads
- Hot bath or shower water
- Hot water treatments such as enemas and sitz baths
- Electrocautery equipment
- Heat lamps
- Warmer beds
- Chemical burns from prep solutions
- Cigarette-related burns

A CASE IN POINT

Equipment Injury Cases

The Facts

In *University Community Hospital v. Martin*,[22] the patient was a paraplegic with a gunshot wound to his neck. He was in a special bed that enabled immobilized patients to be rotated to a vertical position. The nurse responsible for checking the position of an essential bolt failed to do so, and as she rotated the bed, the patient fell.

The Jury Decides

A jury awarded $350,000 in damages to the patient.

The Facts

In *Davenport v. Ephraim McDowell Hospital*,[23] a postoperative patient was on a heart monitor. A recovery room nurse observed that the patient was not breathing and was turning blue. The heart monitor showed no heartbeat, but the alarm had not sounded because either it had not been turned on or its volume had been set too low to be audible. The patient was resuscitated, but remained comatose.

The Jury Decides

In a malpractice suit brought against numerous defendants, a jury found in favor of all the defendants.

The Appellate Court Decides

On appeal, however, the court noted that at the time when the patient suffered cardiopulmonary arrest, the heart monitor alarms were either disconnected or inaudible, and evidence was introduced that this was a deviation from the accepted nursing care standards. The nurses testified that the alarms were unreliable and not necessary because the patients were constantly watched in the recovery room. The case was remanded to the trial court for a new trial.

The Facts

A premature infant died 1 week after receiving an excessive amount of hyperalimentation fluid in a short time because of an incorrectly set intravenous infusion pump.[24] A nurse who did not have primary responsibility for the infant, but who was assigned to the unit, made an adjustment to the intravenous (IV) line that resulted in the IV fluid being pumped directly into the infant, bypassing the infusion pump. The infant received 300 mL of solution over 30 minutes, resulting in a severe fluid overload.

The Outcome

The case was settled without trial.

A Case in Point

Retained Foreign Objects

The Facts

In *Tams v. Kotz*,[25] a surgeon was alleged to have failed to remove a laparotomy pad before closing the patient's incision. The patient had undergone surgery for intestinal cancer, and according to the records, more than 400 items, including instruments, needles, sponges, and laparotomy pads, were accounted for using the standard procedure prescribed by the hospital. The nurses testified that they had meticulously conformed to all the procedures set forth in the hospital policy manual.

The Court Decides

Although the hospital settled out of court during the trial, the jury found no negligence on the part of the nurses or the physician. The verdict was affirmed on appeal.

The Facts

In *Truhitte v. French Hospital*,[26] a surgeon was alleged to have failed to remove a large surgical sponge from the patient's abdomen after a hysterectomy. The nurses testified that the particular sponges in question could have been omitted from their handwritten list of sponges prepared at the initial count because they were packaged separately from the usual linen pack used for gynecologic surgery.

The Jury Decides

The jury returned a verdict finding the hospital 55 percent negligent and the physician 45 percent negligent. The jury also specifically found that the operating room nurses were the agents of the hospital and not of the doctor.

The Appellate Court Decides

On appeal, the court found that the jury could reasonably infer from the evidence that the initial inventory of sponges was performed negligently or that the procedure for counting sponges was below the standard of care required of the hospital.

Failure to Monitor Adequately

Although many lawsuits involve a specific act by a nurse, such as administering an incorrect medication, a **failure to monitor adequately** can also result in allegations of nursing negligence. For example, a nurse does not have a duty to continuously watch or provide electronic monitoring of a patient unless some special need makes such observation necessary. Such a circumstance typically arises in clinical areas where the patient's condition changes rapidly, such as in the postanesthesia recovery unit, the intensive care unit, or the labor and delivery unit. The nurse also has a duty to monitor closely those patients who have known self-destructive tendencies or those situations in which a severe drug reaction is possible.

Failure to Take Appropriate Nursing Action

As the profession of nursing has developed over the years, it has become widely recognized that nurses have a much higher duty to patients than merely following physician orders. The nurse is expected to exercise good nursing judgment and to intervene on the patient's behalf when a physician's order seems inappropriate or when a physician does not respond. Nurses are also expected to recognize patient responses that are unusual and to report such responses to the physician. Because nurses have independent responsibilities and a specific level of expected professionalism, there are many examples of situations where a nurse's actions are inappropriate and generally do not meet the expected level of professionalism. These actions result in allegations of nursing negligence. Some cases involve simply failing to recognize that a patient's needs are beyond the nurse's training or expertise; others involve acts of nursing incompetence that appear to be almost intentional mistreatment of the patient.

Communication Problems

Today, avenues of **communication** between patients and health care providers include Web sites, e-mails, faxes, computerized documentation, telephone calls, and face-to-face conversations. Communication of patient care information among members of the health care team is a major area of importance to every hospital, clinic, physician's office, and other health care delivery site. Much time is spent devising and refining documentation systems and forms for patient records. It is important to have thorough and accurate communication and to preserve information learned about patients from interviews, examinations, laboratory studies, phone calls, literature searches, consultations, and conversations with other health care providers. Failures in communication can have serious consequences for a patient and can result in liability for nurses.

However, although communication is important, it is not necessary and would in fact be impossible for a nurse to notify the physician of every single thing that a patient relates. The nurse must exercise good judgment and must advise the physician promptly of significant history, symptoms, reactions, and other observations that the physician relies on the nurse to make.

A Case in Point

Failure to Monitor

The Facts

In *Gillis v. U.S.*,[27] a patient alleged that the late application of a fetal heart monitor and the resulting delay in diagnosis of fetal distress caused severe neurological problems in her infant. The mother testified that she came to the hospital in labor at 7:30 PM and was left unattended in her room until the fetal monitor was applied at 10:30 PM. She denied that any examinations, procedures, or visits from physicians or nurses occurred during that time. When the fetal monitor was applied, fetal distress was noted, and after attempts to relieve the fetal distress by the usual measures, a cesarean section was performed.

The nurse's notes and testimony differed sharply from the mother's testimony. The records and testimony indicated several examinations by physicians and nurses and the administration of an enema. The nurses noted that the patient was assisted to the bathroom to expel the enema. When she returned to her bed, the nurses had their first opportunity to apply the fetal monitor, which had been ordered 40 minutes earlier.

The Court Decides

The court found that the failure to monitor during this period was not outside the standard of care and, because there was no breach of duty, dismissed the plaintiff's claim. This case proves yet another example of how accurate, detailed nursing notes can help in the event of a lawsuit. Although the nurses involved in this case may not have remembered the details of this particular evening, their notes indicated their assessments and interventions and the patient's responses in sufficient detail that they were able to convince the court of the patient's inaccurate recollection of the events that transpired. The court noted, "Too many documents show that Mrs. Gillis did receive attention.... These documents were not falsified."[28]

Failure to Confirm Accuracy of Physician's Orders

Nurses are not protected from liability simply because they follow a physician's order. Nurses are expected to use good nursing judgment; to be familiar with medications, procedures, and anticipated responses to treatments; and to be able to recognize an unusual medication or treatment that might be ordered for a patient. When the nurse is unfamiliar with a medication or uncomfortable with any order, treatment, or procedure, the prudent nurse is expected to investigate further. He or she may consult a textbook, formulary, or pharmacist to check dose ranges for medications or call the physician, supervisor, or head nurse.

A Case in Point

Appropriate Nursing Action

The Facts

In *Austin v. Conway Hospital*,[29] the plaintiff alleged that the nurse came into her husband's room and rapidly began to pour a tube feeding into his nasogastric tube without checking the placement of the tube. The plaintiff claimed that the nurse, who was in a hurry to go home, continued the tube feeding even though fluid was coming out of the patient's mouth and nose and he was gagging and in respiratory distress. Despite the patient's distress, the nurse left. An orderly came in some time later and sought assistance for the patient, who was by then unresponsive. The patient died a short time later.

The Outcome

The lawsuit against the hospital was dismissed because the plaintiff failed to file within the time required by the statute of limitation.

The Facts

In *Schleier v. Kaiser Foundation Health Plan*,[30] a patient who had recently been seen by a physician for possible cardiac problems called a health plan "advice nurse" to report that he had experienced vomiting, weakness, heavy sweating, and exhaustion after mowing his lawn. The nurse allegedly responded that he should "sweat it out." The patient died a short time later in an ambulance en route to a hospital.

The Court Decides

The health plan was held liable for the negligence involved in this case.

The Facts

Cooper v. National Motor Bearing Co.[31] illustrates the nurse's duty to recognize the limits of nursing interventions when a patient is not responding to a treatment. An occupational health nurse failed to refer a patient for medical treatment even though a wound she had treated had not healed over a period of 10 months. The patient eventually discovered that the lesion was cancerous and had to have extensive resection of the area. The nurse testified that she was aware of the warning signs of cancer, yet she continued to treat the wound in spite of its failure to heal as expected.

The Court Decides

The nurse was found liable. The court noted that the nurse should know whether a condition is within her authority or whether it should be referred to a physician.

A Case in Point

Communications Case Studies

The Facts

In *Ramsey v. Physician's Memorial Hospital,*[32] two children were brought to the emergency room with rashes and high fevers. The mother told the nurse that she had removed two ticks from one of the children. The physician was not told about the ticks. In the absence of this history, the physician diagnosed the children with measles. The younger child died 4 days later of Rocky Mountain spotted fever. The older child was subsequently treated and cured, but sustained a limp that resolved within 6 months.

The plaintiffs presented undisputed evidence that the nurse knew that ticks had been removed from one of the children. A medical expert testified that "it is incumbent upon an emergency room staff ... to record significant medical data. I feel that the knowledge by a nurse that ticks were removed from a patient in the spring ... represents significant data. If this were not passed on I would consider that a failure to apply an adequate level of conformance as to standards...."[33]

The Court Decides

The facility was found liable for failure to diagnose Rocky Mountain spotted fever in two children, which resulted in the death of one child. The court wrote that there was ample evidence that the failure of the nurse to communicate this element of the patient's history to the attending physician was a serious violation of her duties as a nurse. Further, there was evidence that this failure to communicate was a contributing proximate cause of the injuries suffered by the children.

The Facts

In *Phillips v. Eastern Maine Medical Center,*[34] a patient died from an infection that resulted from a 6-hour delay in surgery, after a nurse failed to tell the physician that the patient had the signs and symptoms of an esophageal tear. The patient underwent surgery to remove a foreign object lodged in his esophagus. About an hour after surgery, the patient's wife reported to the recovery room nurse that her husband was wheezing and in pain. Although the symptoms indicated a possible tear in the esophagus, the nurse failed to inform the surgeon. Six hours later the surgeon was finally advised of the patient's distress, and corrective surgery was performed. Unfortunately, the patient's condition worsened because of an infection transmitted from the intestinal tract during the 6 hours before the tear was repaired. The patient died, and his wife brought a malpractice action against the hospital, alleging negligence through the actions of the nursing staff.

The Jury Decides

After a jury trial, judgment for more than $1 million was entered for the plaintiff.

The Appellate Court Decides

On appeal, the court wrote that the failure of the hospital staff to promptly notify the surgeon was a departure from the standard of care, but ordered a new trial unless the plaintiff agreed to accept a damage award of $370,000.

The Facts

In *Duplan v. Harper*,[35] a patient learned that she was pregnant. Her job environment put her at risk of becoming infected with a cytomegalovirus (CMV), which causes severe birth defects. The physician examined the patient and tested for CMV. The physician instructed the nurse to notify the patient of her test results, which were positive. The patient called the nurse back because she wanted a clarification. The nurse incorrectly told her that a positive result meant that she did not have an ongoing primary CMV infection. Based on the erroneous information, the patient decided *not* to abort.

The patient brought wrongful birth and medical malpractice claims against the United States under the Federal Tort Claims Act (because the clinic obstetrician/gynecologist was at a United States Air Force base). The child was born with CMV-induced birth defects such as nystagmus, microcephaly, mental retardation, developmental delays, loss of fine and gross motor skills, and hearing loss.

The Court Decides

The court determined that there was improper communication by the nurse and awarded the plaintiff $3,056,100.

AUTHOR TIP: *It is also important that the nurse confirm any order that cannot be understood. Whether the problem is illegible handwriting or an unclear or incomplete order, the standard of care generally requires that the nurse must not carry out any order that is not clearly understood.*

Vital Statistics

According to the IOM report by the Committee on Quality of Health Care, medical error was a leading cause of death and injury in the United States.[36]

According to an article in the *Chicago Tribune*, since 1995 approximately 1720 hospital patients have been accidentally killed. Another 9584 have been injured from acts or omissions of registered nurses nationwide. The newspaper analyzed 3 million state and federal computer records and created a database.[37]

Facilities looking for an improved bottom line often cut staffs to skeleton crews,

? What Would You Do?

A cardiac patient complained to the nurse that he had chest pain and shortness of breath. The nurse, who was on her way to lunch, decided to wait until she got back before calling the patient's physician. She gave the patient the medications that were ordered for him in the event that he should get chest pains. She did not tell the nurse who was covering her patients during lunch. Half an hour later, when she returned from lunch, the nurse had forgotten about the patient's complaints. Later that day the patient was found to have suffered a massive heart attack.

1. What possible deviations from the standards of nursing care occurred in this case?
2. Discuss the ethical issues in this scenario.
3. In what other ways could this situation have been handled?

endangering patient safety and overworking the registered nurse who is already stretched thin.

KEEP IN MIND

▶ Be familiar with and do not deviate from applicable policies and procedures.
▶ Assess patients carefully for foreseeable risks, such as falls and burns.
▶ Document accurately, in a timely manner, and concisely.
▶ Concentrate on what you are doing when preparing or administering medications. Remember that many medication errors can be avoided by using care in reading orders, labels, and patient identification tags.
▶ Be sure you are familiar with the proper uses of equipment before using any machine in patient care.
▶ Never continue to use equipment that is malfunctioning, and never modify equipment yourself.
▶ Carefully assess patients for monitoring needs.
▶ Use good nursing judgment when deciding when to notify the physician of patient status.
▶ Know the limits of your training, expertise, and license, and do not practice beyond those limits.
▶ Do not carry out an order that you do not understand or that is clearly inappropriate.
▶ Remember that excellent communication between health care providers helps to best meet the patient's needs.
▶ Keep up with current trends in your area of specialty. Should it ever come to litigation, your practice will be compared with the standard of care expected from nurses with a similar background and education.

IN A NUTSHELL

Allegations of nursing negligence can arise from almost any act or omission by a nurse that results in injury to a patient. This chapter has reviewed some of common areas of nursing negligence and liability. These cases illustrate the importance of several basic guidelines for protecting yourself from liability exposure: Document thoroughly, follow hospital policies and procedures, conform your professional behavior to the highest standards of nursing care, and develop trusting relationships with your patients.

AFTERTHOUGHTS

1. Identify four common areas of nursing liability and give an example of a deviation from the standard of care for each.

2. Identify two types of patients who are at a high risk of falling and discuss nursing interventions that are appropriate to minimize the risk.

3. If a patient falls and is injured, discuss the liability issues involving the nurse who is assigned to that patient. What should be documented?

4. If a physician writes an order for a medication and mistakenly orders a dangerously high and very unusual dose, is the nurse automatically protected legally? What should the nurse do?

5. Many types of equipment are used in patient care today. Discuss the types of injuries that can result from not knowing how to use the following types of equipment:
   a. Heating pad
   b. Heart monitors
   c. Intravenous (IV) infusion pumps
   d. Electronic beds

6. Operating room instrument and sponge count policies are very important evidence in a trial involving retained foreign objects. Discuss how such a policy can help in the defense of a nurse.

7. If a suicidal patient is ordered to have "10-minute checks" and the nurse does in fact check that patient every 10 minutes, is it necessary that each check be documented? Why or why not?

8. If a nurse administers a medication and the patient suffers an allergic reaction, can the nurse be found negligent? Discuss.

9. How do you determine if an action or inaction is a breach of the standard of patient care?

10. What are the elements of negligence? Apply and discuss the elements of a case you find on the Web or in a law library or journal.

11. List two common breaches for five nursing specialties.

12. Discuss two cases or scenarios involving breaches of the standards in two nursing specialty areas.

13. Obtain a case from any of the areas mentioned and discuss the elements of negligence.

14. Watch a medical television program and discuss the sections of the show involving the following:

    a. Policies and procedures

    b. Breaches of the standards of care

15. Poll your class and determine what they think are the most common areas of nursing liability and why.

ETHICS IN PRACTICE

Sarah T. and Beth W. were two RNs who worked the 3 to 11 PM shift on a busy surgical unit. Over the past 3 weeks, they had run a high census, had received a large number of seriously ill postoperative patients, and had been under a great deal of pressure to work overtime.

A particularly tenacious respiratory virus had been affecting several other members of the staff, causing many "call-ins." One afternoon during shift report, both Beth and Sarah realized that they were showing the initial symptoms of this respiratory virus. Because three very critical postoperative patients were to be admitted to the surgical unit during their shift, Beth and Sarah took some over-the-counter cold medications so that they could remain at work and not contribute to the shortage of nursing staff that already existed. They realized they probably should be at home and wondered if they might be causing more harm to the patients by communicating their illnesses to individuals who were highly susceptible to infections. They also recognized that the cold medications contained antihistamines that might affect their nursing judgment and performance of complicated skills.

What is the ethical dilemma in this situation? Did the nurses make the right decision in staying at work? What ethical principles are involved in making this type of decision? Could an "I was sick and taking medication" defense be used if either of them had made a serious mistake in patient care? What if a patient became ill with the viral infection the nurses had?

References

1. RN Magazine 64(2), 2001.
2. Nieto v. State of Colorado, 954 P.2d 834 (Colo App. 10/1/97); State of Colorado v. Nieto, 993 P.2d 493 (Colo 2/14/2000).
3. Northrop, CE: Nursing actions in litigation. QRB 13(10):343, 1987.
4. O'Keefe, ME: Nursing Practice and the Law—Avoiding Malpractice and Other Legal Risks. FA Davis, Philadelphia, 2001.
5. Hip fractures on the increase. Your Shift, May/June, 2000.
6. Mossman v. Albany Medical Center Hospital, 311 N.Y.S.2d 131 (N.Y. 1970).
7. Study links heavy workloads to medication errors. RN Magazine 64(2):164, 2001.

8. Ibid.
9. Martin, PB: Closed claims abstract. The Risk Management Foundation Forum (Jan–Feb):5, 1988.
10. Reifschneider v. Nebraska Methodist Hospital, 387 N.W.2d 486 (Neb. 1986).
11. Ashcraft v. Mobile Infirmary Medical Center, 570 So.2d 593 (Ala. 1990).
12. Ramsey v. Physician's Memorial Hospital, Inc. 373 A.2d 26 (Ind App. 1977).
13. In touch with Louisiana Trial Lawyers Association. Washington Post, March 18, 2001.
14. Hallinan v. Prindle, 62 P.2d 1075 (Cal. App. 1936).
15. Penaloza v. Baptist Memorial Hospital, 304 S.W.2d 203 (Tex. App. 1957).
16. Holbrooks v. Duke University, Inc., 305 S.E.2d 69 (N.C. App. 1983).
17. Biggs v. U.S., 655 F. Supp. 1093 (W.D. La. 1987).
18. Flower Hospital v. Hart, 62 P.2d 1248 (Ok. S.Ct. 1936).
19. Nichter v. Edmiston, 407 P.2d 721 (Nev. 1965).
20. Smelko v. Brinton, 740 P.2d 591 (Kan. 1987).
21. Bowers v. Olch, 260 P2d. 977 (Cal. 1953).
22. University Community Hospital v. Martin, 328 So.2d 858 (Fla. App. 1976).
23. Davenport v. Ephraim McDowell Hospital, 769 S.W. 2d 56 (Ky. 1988).
24. Martin, PB: Closed claim abstract. The Risk Management Foundation Forum (Jan–Feb):15, 1989.
25. Tams v. Kotz, 530 A.2d 1217 (D.C. Ap. 1987).
26. Truhitte v. French Hospital, 180 Cal. Rptr. 152 (Cal. App. 1982).
27. Gillis v. U.S., 722 F. Supp. 713 (M.D. Fla. 1989).
28. Idem., 715.
29. Austin v. Conway Hospital, 356 S.E.2d 153 (S.C. 1987).
30. Schleier v. Kaiser Foundation Health Plan, 876 F.2d 174 (D.C. App. 1989).
31. Cooper v. National Motor Bearing Co., 288 P.2d 581 (1955 Cal. App.).
32. Ramsey v. Physician's Memorial Hospital, Inc., 373 A2d 26 (Md. App. 1977).
33. Idem., 30.
34. Phillips v. Eastern Maine Medical Center, 565 A2d 306 (Me. 1989).
35. Duplan v. Harper, 188 F.3d 1195 (OK. 1999).
36. Errors in health care: a leading cause of death and injury. In Kohn, LT, Corrigan, JM, and Donaldson, MS (eds), Committee on Quality of Health Care in America, Institute of Medicine: To Err Is Human: Building a Safer Health System. Washington, DC, National Academies Press, 2000, pp 26–48. Available online at http://books.nap.edu/books/0309068371/html/26.html.
37. Berens, MJ: Nursing mistakes kill, injure thousands. Cost cutting exacts toll on role on patients, hospital staffs. Series: Dangerous Care: Nurses' Hidden Role in Medical Error. Chicago Tribune, (Sept 15):20, 2000.

Resources

American Prosecutors Research Institute
99 Canal Center Plaza, Suite 510
Alexandria, VA 22314
(703) 739-0321
http://www.ndaa-apri.org/apri

Appendix A

General Breaches of the Standard of Care

Many breaches may be alleged in the different nursing specialty areas:

1. Failure to access care through the hierarchy or chain of command
2. Failure to clarify orders
3. Failure to provide a safe environment for the patient
4. Medication errors
5. Failure to follow standards of care or facility policy and procedure
6. Failure to recognize or notify the physician of significant changes in the patient's condition
7. Failure to document in a timely and proper manner
8. Failure to monitor properly
9. Failure to give discharge instructions properly to the patient or family
10. Failure to protect patient against harm

Common Medication Errors

1. Wrong medication given to patient
2. Wrong route of administration
3. Wrong site of administration
4. Wrong dosage
5. Wrong time
6. Failure to document administration of drug
7. Transcription errors on the Medication Administration Record (MAR)
8. Omission of a dose
9. Duplication of a dose
10. Administration of a drug not ordered
11. Administration of a drug to a patient who has a known allergy to the drug, as documented in the record
12. Failure to detect and obtain timely treatment of an anaphylactic or severe allergic reaction
13. Failure to detect signs and symptoms of adverse reactions or drug toxicity
14. Failure to properly administer chemotherapy by administering medication outside the therapeutic range
15. Failure to select and administer the proper medications when two bottles of different medications look alike (e.g., potassium chloride and sodium chloride)
16. Failure to clarify the physician's order

Intravenous Lines

1. Failure to properly start an IV, resulting in injury to the patient
2. Failure to change IV dressings in a proper and timely manner, resulting in undetected infection or infiltration

Orthopedic Nursing

1. Failure to properly assess
2. Failure to detect signs and symptoms of compartment syndrome
3. Failure to detect problems or go through the chain of command to get help for extremities in casts that are constricted
4. Failure to detect signs and symptoms of a fat embolism

Long-Term Care

1. Failure to protect the patient from falls
2. Failure to prevent the development of decubitus ulcers
3. Failure to detect decubitus ulcers and treat them in a timely manner, resulting in amputations, gangrene, sepsis, or death
4. Failure to monitor polypharmacy effects, side effects/adverse reactions, and toxic levels of drugs used by patients
5. Failure to provide a safe environment (e.g., prevent wandering off the premises)
6. Failure to prevent abuse, neglect, or injury by other patients or the staff
7. Failure to prevent burns

Pediatrics/Neonatal Intensive Care Unit/Pediatric Intensive Care Unit Nursing

1. Failure to properly monitor
2. Failure to properly check IV sites, resulting in infiltration or infection
3. Failure to prevent falls or injuries from cribs or beds
4. Failure to protect the infant from burns (e.g., by a bottle heated in a microwave)
5. Failure to prevent or detect overhydration or underhydration
6. Failure to report suspected child abuse
7. Equipment injuries (e.g., failure to check Isolette temperatures)
8. Failure to maintain equipment in proper working order (e.g., turning off alarms).
9. Failure to properly administer injections

10. Failure to properly insert tubes, resulting in tissue and organ damage
11. Failure to routinely check IV boards and dressings, resulting in nerve damage and tissue necrosis
12. Failure to properly feed, resulting in aspiration

Emergency Care

1. Failure to properly monitor
2. Failure to provide a safe environment (e.g., patient falls off stretcher because rails are not raised)
3. Failure to give proper discharge instructions
4. Failure to properly administer medication
5. Failure to triage in a timely and proper manner
6. Failure to take an accurate and thorough history
7. Failure to assess the patient in a timely and proper manner
8. Failure to give proper telephone advice
9. Failure to properly report signs and symptoms of the patient to physician on call
10. Failure to properly gather evidence and preserve the chain of custody
11. Failure to perform cardiopulmonary resuscitation (CPR) in a timely and proper manner
12. Failure to honor advance directives
13. Failure to report suspected patient, spousal, child, or elder abuse
14. Failure to discharge patient to the proper facility or via the appropriate means, such as ambulance or relative

Occupational Nursing

1. Failure to detect signs and symptoms of a condition and to refer to a physician or consultant
2. Failure to properly document all treatment and medications given to employees

Case Manager

1. Failure to exercise due care in the discharge of the contractual duties
2. Failure to properly document care activities and outcomes
3. Failure to inform a subscriber of a managed-care company of the contractual right to an impartial review and arbitration of a disputed claim
4. Failure to obtain all the necessary documents and medical records, resulting in the denial of care

5. Failure to properly investigate the qualifications and competencies of the providers and facilities to which patients are referred for treatment
6. Failure to act as patients' advocates

Any type of "kickback" or "incentive" program between a provider/payor and the case manager is considered illegal (conflict of interest). This is also unethical behavior that may result in the patient not receiving the best possible care by the most appropriate provider.

Office Nursing

1. Failure to make a proper nursing diagnosis or use good nursing judgment when a patient calls in with signs and symptoms
2. Failure to properly administer medication (e.g., intramuscular injection causing sciatic nerve injury)
3. Failure to notify the patient of important test results (e.g., Papanicolaou smear, positive cancer or human immunodeficiency virus [HIV] blood test) in a timely and proper manner

Correctional Nursing

1. Failure to refer to a physician or consultant in a timely and proper manner
2. Failure to detect and report signs and symptoms of a medical condition

Perioperative Nursing

1. Failure to prevent falls
2. Failure to properly use or place restraints or tourniquets, resulting in nerve palsies
3. Failure to perform proper sponge and instrument counts, resulting in retained foreign objects
4. Abandonment of the patient
5. Failure to properly administer medication
6. Failure to protect the patient from burns (e.g., from thermal pads or Bovie pads)
7. Failure to properly use monitoring equipment
8. Failure to properly handle specimens (e.g., losing specimens)

Intensive Care Unit/Critical Care Unit Nursing

1. Failure to properly monitor
2. Issues dealing with conflicts among the patient, family, and physician regarding the living will, health care agent, and do not resuscitate (DNR) order

3. Failure to properly monitor or notify physician of change in status
4. Failure to detect life-threatening changes in condition
5. Failure to properly maintain the airway
6. Failure to suction the patient in a proper and timely manner
7. Failure to restock the crash cart

Certified Registered Nurse Anesthetist

1. Failure to properly intubate (e.g., improper placement)
2. Failure to detect equipment failure
3. Failure to properly position the patient, causing nerve injuries
4. Failure to properly monitor
5. Failure to properly administer anesthesia

Oncology Nursing

1. Failure to properly administer chemotherapy, resulting in injury (e.g., extravasation into tissues)
2. Failure to notify patient of important laboratory or diagnostic results

Dialysis Nursing

1. Failure to properly perform dialysis
2. Failure to detect or prevent infection at shunt site
3. Improper use of solutions used in dialysis

Urology Nursing

1. Failure to notify patient of important laboratory or diagnostic results (in an office setting)

Educators

1. Failure to properly delegate duties to a student
2. Failure to properly document students' nursing skills
3. Failure to require students to obtain more education in areas of poor performance
4. Failure to notify students of areas of failure/poor performance: the faculty member fails to discuss or present a plan for improvement to the student outlining areas that need improvement such as behavior, skills, or knowledge base
5. Failure to allow due process

Medical-Surgical Nursing

1. Failure to monitor vital signs
2. Failure to prevent falls
3. Failure to prevent aspiration
4. Failure to properly administer medication (e.g., sciatic nerve injury)
5. Failure to prevent patient injury from:
    a. Enemas
    b. Catheters
    c. Feeding tube misplacement
    d. Transportation
    e. Restraints
    f. IVs

Psychiatric Nursing

1. Failure to assess the risk of suicide
2. Failure to properly monitor
3. Failure to prevent harm
4. Failure to communicate and document observations
5. Failure to detect drug toxicity
6. Failure to protect the patient from other patients
7. Failure to provide a safe environment

School Nursing

1. Failure to report signs and symptoms of child abuse
2. Failure to properly administer medications and treatments
3. Failure to know the school board's policy on "Do Not Resuscitate" (DNR) orders and whether advance directives and DNRs are allowed and upheld in the school setting

Obstetric Nursing

1. Failure to detect signs and symptoms of fetal distress
2. Failure to perform proper nursing functions when fetal distress is detected (e.g., turning patient on side, administering oxygen, calling the physician)
3. Failure to notify the physician in a timely manner of problems or deterioration of the patient's condition

Other allegations may include the physician's failure to perform a cesarean section instead of a vaginal delivery in a timely manner; the infant may suffer from Erb's palsy as a result of vaginal delivery. Also, rectal sphincter injuries from improperly performed episiotomies may be alleged.

Allegations Against the Facility

1. Failure to provide adequate staffing
2. Failure to provide proper working equipment
3. Negligent hiring: failure to make proper background, criminal checks, and credential checks
4. Failure to properly charge for services; Medicare/Medicaid fraud and abuse
5. Failure to provide a safe patient environment
6. Failure to comply with Consolidated Omnibus Budget Reconciliation Act of 1985 (COBRA) and Emergency Medical Treatment and Active Labor Act (EMTALA) regulations

Documentation and the Nurse   8

Key Chapter Concepts

Documentation

Quality assurance

Continuous quality improvement (CQI)

Risk management

Veracity

Health Insurance Portability and
    Accountability Act (HIPAA)

Narrative charting

Problem-oriented charting

PIE charting

Focus charting

Charting by exception

Clinical pathway

Electronic charting

Against medical advice (AMA)

Do not resuscitate order

Abandonment

Incident

Incident, variance, or occurrence
    report

Chapter Thoughts

The universal dislike of paperwork in general, and charting in particular, is the
one issue in health care that probably all nurses agree on. The amount of time
nurses spend completing forms, filling out checklists, and organizing progress
notes has increased in proportion to the amount of government regulation and
the ever-increasing complexity and specialization found in today's health care
system. Although most nurses realize the importance of accurate and timely
documentation of patient care, they also see it as an activity that removes them
from the patient's bedside and that increases their overall work load. Seldom is
documentation included as an element in the nurse's proficiency evaluation, thus
reducing its importance as an activity for nurses. The one aspect of patient care
that is most likely to be abbreviated during a nurse's busy day is charting.

In recent years, the medical record (i.e., the patient's chart) has attained
tremendous stature as a key element in most lawsuits and disciplinary proceedings brought against health care providers, including nurses. Because of this
increased interest in documentation by the legal and administrative systems, the
ethical and legal principles involved in documentation have been welded into one
inseparable issue. Yet the ethical principles that underlie good charting also serve
to form the underpinnings of the legal value of that charting in a court of law.

First and foremost, the ethical principle of veracity serves as the bedrock issue
in documentation. Although veracity (truth telling) is an important element in all
aspects of health care, it loses its ambiguity when it takes on a written form. It is
a generally accepted principle that health care providers should "tell the truth" to

patients concerning their health care. Yet most nurses realize that truth telling is not an absolute principle. Telling the truth to a patient can have a number of meanings, ranging from giving the patient all the information available, to providing the patient with the information he or she "needs," to withholding information that is considered to be harmful to the patient's health or recovery. Perhaps the only activity that is prohibited in relation to truth telling and patient care is outright mistruths or lies.

In documentation, there is no room at all for misinformation involving patient care.

The main purposes of charting are (1) to furnish other health care providers with information about the patient's condition and the care planned and rendered and (2) to protect the health care provider from the legal and administrative systems should something adverse or unexpected happen to that patient or the patient's safety is at issue.

Not only is dishonest charting a violation of the ethical issue of veracity, but it is also a violation of the legal system and the nurse practice acts. Charting activities that are not done, observations that are not made, or vital signs that are not taken constitute fraud in the eyes of the legal system. Depending on the situation and the state where it occurs, fraud may be treated as a crime punishable by either a fine or a jail term.

Another ethical principle that underlies charting is that of beneficence. To do good for the patient is a well-accepted principle in health care. A nurse must believe that accurate, truthful, complete, and timely charting aids in the cure of patients' diseases and hastens their recoveries. The antithesis must also be accepted, namely that inaccurate, untruthful, incomplete, and late charting is harmful to patients' cures and recoveries.

Finally, as a practical issue in charting, it is important to consider what may possibly be done with that chart in the future. The quality of nurses' charting, particularly the nurses' notes, should improve drastically if nurses keep it in the back of their minds that this chart may eventually turn up in a court of law. As nurses chart, they should ask themselves "How will this entry sound if it is read to me while I sit on the witness stand in front of a judge and a jury?"

Professionalism is more than wearing a clean uniform and providing competent patient care. Professionalism is reflected in how nurses speak, how they present themselves to patients and the public, and how they record the activities of patient care in the chart.

OBJECTIVES

Upon completing this chapter, the reader will be able to:
1. Discuss purposes for documentation.
2. Identify appropriate documentation, as required by the current health care system, including the electronic documentation system.
3. Discuss pitfalls that lead to weak documentation and potential problems.
4. Relate the process of continuing quality improvement (CQI) to documentation.

5. Identify the appropriate use of variance, incident, or occurrence reports.
6. Identify the appropriate use of employee health records, including postexposure tests to human immunodeficiency virus (HIV) and hepatitis B virus (HBV).
7. Relate the importance of confidentiality in patient care documentation.
8. Define the different documentation formats.
9. Discuss tips for more effective and thorough documentation.
10. Identify potential areas of legal liability in charting.
11. Discuss case law involving documentation errors and problems.
12. Discuss the Health Insurance Portability and Accountability Act (HIPAA).

Introduction

Documentation is the cornerstone of all health care decision making. The old adage, "If it was not documented, it was not done," is as true today as ever before. The nurse is responsible for the largest part of the patient care record. **Documentation,** the recording of all pertinent information concerning the patient's care in the medical record, is a critical factor from various perspectives: legal-ethical, bioethical, patient outcome, continuous quality improvement, and medical-legal.

Purposes of Documentation

In addition to serving as a confidential record that identifies the patient and health care services provided, the medical record is a business and legal record that has many uses and serves multiple purposes. The primary purposes of the record are to identify the patient's status, to document the need for care, and to plan, deliver, and evaluate that care. Secondary purposes include the following:

1. Provides evidence of the provision of quality nursing care
2. Provides evidence of the nurse's legal responsibilities to the patient
3. Records information for personal health protection
4. Provides evidence of standards, rules, regulations, and laws regarding nursing, medical, and allied health practices
5. Records statistical information for standards and research
6. Provides cost-benefit reduction information
7. Provides risk management information
8. Provides information for student learning experiences

9. Provides evidences of protection of patient rights
10. Records professional and ethical conduct and responsibility
11. Provides data used to determine the type of care needed on discharge
12. Provides data for planning future health care
13. Provides data on nursing and medical history for future admissions
14. Provides data for quality-of-care review
15. Provides data for continuing education and research
16. Provides data for billing and reimbursement
17. Provides data to record nursing care, which forms the basis of evaluation by the Joint Commission on Accreditation for Healthcare Organizations (JCAHO) and other federal or state agencies
18. Provides communication between the responsible nursing professionals and other practitioners contributing to managing patient care

Documenting for Continuous Quality Improvement

Nursing has been concerned with the process of ensuring quality patient care since the time of Florence Nightingale. The initial primary focus on patient care quality began with single events and single settings. Dissatisfaction by consumers with both the cost and the quality of care led to attempts to change health care through intense regulation and reliance on legal decisions to support patients' rights. Health care leaders responded by focusing on entire patient care episodes and recognizing the importance of synergy between the provider and the system in affecting quality outcomes.

In the past, facilities have used quality assurance and risk management to manage and control the quality of care and financial losses. **Quality assurance** is a process used to evaluate the type and level of patient care that is given by the health care provider. Patterns and recurring incidents are evaluated to determine how to change them so that a more optimal level of patient care can be achieved.

Continuous quality improvement (CQI) is a more mature process than quality assurance (QA) or quality control (QC). The origins of CQI lie in the work of Joseph Juran and W. Edward Deming, Americans who developed effective processes for implementing them as consultants to the Japanese manufacturing industries following World War II. Juran and Deming refer to CQI as total quality management (TQM) or quality improvement processes. CQI assumes that work groups are experts about their work and should be the focus for monitoring quality, identifying problems, and devising solutions. Data for improvement purposes is collected from the nurses' documentation and is used to assist in problem verification, analysis of problems, measurement of improvement over time, and conformance to standards of care.

The staff nurse responsible for implementing patient care services actively participates in the actual patient care processes and is in the perfect position to analyze those processes with a view toward system improvement and to document those processes appropriately. Merely to monitor the status quo is inadequate.

Documenting for Risk Management

Risk management is a quality assurance process used by facilities to prevent financial losses before they happen by identifying, analyzing, minimizing, and preventing risks in problem areas that result in claims by injured patients, staff, or visitors.[1] Risk management tools commonly used include incident, variance, or occurrence reports; surveys; committees; training and retraining of staff; communication between patient and staff and among health care providers; patient and staff education; monitoring of risks and injuries; and accurate and comprehensive documentation.[2]

Legal and Ethical Responsibilities

Nurses use various systems or formats to document patient care and status. These systems are crucial in ensuring quality care, managing risks to avoid and decrease exposure to litigation and disciplinary actions, validating why there should be payment for care delivered, meeting state and federal licensure requirements, and meeting accreditation requirements.

The first line of defense for the nurse is factual and thorough documentation. Good documentation can "save" the nurse in medical malpractice claims, disciplinary actions, and conflicts arising from ethical dilemmas. **Veracity,** or telling the truth, is essential in a patient's medical records, because all health care providers caring for a particular patient rely on the records to make decisions about treatment. Therefore factual, concrete, descriptive, and truthful entries must be used when charting.

Failure to Maintain Records

Lack of time to document is the most common reason given by nurses who fail to adequately document a patient's care. In these days of nursing shortages, it is more often than not the truth. However true, it is not an accepted explanation in litigation or disciplinary action. Absence or sparseness of documentation that fails to demonstrate the care and treatment given to the patient in question can negatively implicate a nurse regardless of the quality of care provided. It is imperative that the nurse focus on the crucial line of defense that can protect the nurse, staff, and facility.

Additionally, the facility has the responsibility to safely keep the patient records to ensure that, in the event of legal action, there is a reliable source of information concerning the care the patient received.

Confidentiality of Patient Records

Confidentiality of patient records is essential because of the legal, ethical, employment, and social implications attached to unauthorized disclosure.

A CASE IN POINT

Missing Records

The Facts

A woman alleged res ipsa loquitur regarding the care and treatment rendered for removal of four wisdom teeth. Two weeks later she developed left facial asymmetry, hearing loss, and diparthia. She had no "hard" evidence of any specific act of negligence, but three copies of anesthesia records were missing and never produced.[3]

The Jury Decides

A jury delivered a $2.5 million verdict against the hospital and anesthesiologist.

In 1996 Congress passed the **Health Insurance Portability and Accountability Act (HIPAA)** to address the serious need for a national standard for patient record privacy. The Department of Health and Human Services (DHHS) released HIPAA privacy rules and deadlines for implementation.

Faxing Medical Records and Patient Information

Whenever materials are faxed, there is the potential for breaches of confidentiality if the fax machine is in an area that is not limited to staff access or if the material gets faxed to an incorrect number. To protect the patient's confidentiality, institutions must develop policies and procedures regarding the kind and types of information that can be faxed, especially concerning the information that is confidential, such as human immunodeficiency virus (HIV) and hepatitis B virus (HBV) test results or status reports. Policies and procedures must also address safeguards to ensure that the material is not transmitted to the wrong person or received by the wrong person or facility.

Documentation Standards

Standards governing documentation come from various sources, such as federal and state laws, the American Nurses Association (ANA), JCAHO, institutional policies and procedures, and other health care organizations.[4]

Standards must be "reasonable." If the standard at your facility is set at providing the optimal or highest level of care, nurses may be held to a higher standard of care even though the national standard may be lower. Keep this in mind when writing your policies and procedures.

Types of Documentation

Several effective methods of ensuring accurate documentation exist. The type used is determined by institution policy.[5]

Narrative Charting

Narrative charting is the most common and well known of all the documentation systems. The format is a narrative paragraph that describes the patient's status, treatments, medications, and other pertinent information.

Advantages

- Most familiar method of documentation.
- Can be combined easily with other documentation methods or systems.
- Chronological events can be easily documented (e.g., emergency situations).
- Contains information on patient's status interventions, treatments, and responses to same.
- Most health care providers feel comfortable with this format.

Disadvantages

- Handwriting may be illegible.
- Either too much information or too little information may be charted.
- Can be disorganized.
- Is time consuming.
- May fail to consistently demonstrate that all the nursing process is taking place, especially evaluation and planning.
- At times may fail to show critical thinking, analysis, and decision making by nurse.
- Makes data retrieval difficult.
- Makes tracing the patient's condition and problems difficult.

Problem-Oriented Charting

In **problem-oriented charting,** all members of the health care team can document their information of the patient's problems and their plan of care to address them. This type of charting gives a comprehensive picture of the patient's clinical status and how the patient responds to interventions. Two formats are used.

The SOAP format:

S—Subjective data (what the patient or family tells the nurse)
O—Objective data (the nurse's observations)

A—Assessment (what the nurse believes is occurring based on data)
P—Plan (the nurse's plan of action)

And the SOAPIE format:

S—Subjective data (what the patient or family tells the nurse)
O—Objective data (nurse's observations)
A—Assessment (what the nurse believes is occurring based on data)
P—Plan (the nurse's plan of action)
I—Interventions (specific treatment implemented)
E—Evaluation (of patient's response to interventions)

Advantages

- Well structured in a specific format.
- Easier to monitor problems.
- Can be used with care plans by numbering problems for quick reference in the progress notes.
- Nursing process is reflected.
- Enhances communication and collaboration among health care providers as part of an integrated record.
- Provides discharge summaries of each problem and whether or not it is resolved as written. With unresolved problems, notes are written regarding further treatment or action needed and the manner in which the information will be disseminated to other health care professionals and facilities.

Disadvantages

- Nurses must relearn the documentation process and "fit" the information into the SOAP(IE) format.
- Blanks occur in the format if the nurse does not know or cannot decide which category to place the information when charting.
- Redundant information in the care plan, problem list, and flow sheets.
- Time consuming because each problem requires that the nurse document a separate SOAP(IE) entry.
- May be resistance by other health care professionals of integrated progress notes.

PIE Charting

PIE charting is a problem-oriented documentation method based on the nursing process. The acronym PIE stands for:

P—Problems
I—Intervention
E—Evaluation of nursing care

PIE charting consists of progress notes, assessment, and patient care flow sheets.

Advantages

- Simplifies charting.
- Decreases redundancy.
- Eliminates separate care plan.
- Ensures ongoing care is documented because nurses record their evaluation of identified problems every shift.
- Improves quality of progress notes.
- Works well in primary nursing and psychiatric settings.

Disadvantages

- Can result in lengthy documentation due to charting requirements every 8 and 24 hours.
- Staffing mix may be a problem because the care planning is the registered nurse's (RN's) responsibility.
- May not be suited for patients with unchanging problems.
- Inconsistency may result due to no practice guidelines, care plans, or clinical paths.
- Fails to address patient outcomes.

Focus Charting

Focus charting is a documentation system that organizes narrative documentation to include the following for each concern identified:

D—Diagnosis
A—Action
R—Response
T—Teaching

The term *focus* refers to the patient's concerns and is used instead of *problem*.

Advantages

- Creates structured progress notes.
- Nursing process is promoted and includes patient's response.

- Nursing judgment and analytical thinking are used to determine patient's status from the data.
- Patient's concerns and needs are identified.
- Focus column makes patient information easy to read.

Disadvantages

- May be difficult to integrate and document notes on content and focus.
- Must sort data into categories of data, action, and patient's response.
- May evolve into just narrative charting without patient responses noted.

Charting by Exception

Charting by exception (CBE), another type of documentation system, requires only the documentation of abnormal findings and adherence to the standards of practice. This method was created to decrease charting and end-of-shift change reports time and to make the patient's most current information easily accessible, so patient trends or patterns are more obvious.

Advantages

- Consists of flow sheets, SOAP progress notes, protocols, incidental orders, standards of practice–based documentation, and nursing diagnosis–based care plans.
- Readily accessible current patient data.
- Flow sheets eliminate jot sheets, scratch paper, and so on.
- Form guidelines on the back are helpful to nurses.
- Normal patient findings are identified.
- Most repetitive narrative charting is eliminated.
- Easily adapted to clinical pathways documentation.

Disadvantages

- Creates redundancy in charting.
- Developed for use with an all-RN nursing staff. Institutions that do not have all-RN staff would need to change the nursing care delivery system used.
- Requires changing numerous documentation tools.
- Requires re-education of the staff experienced with other more extensive documentation methods.
- Reimbursement may be affected because of the lack of documentation of routine activities.[6]
- Legally CBE can be difficult to defend because it sometimes appears that conditions, signs, or symptoms are not detected by the nurse because there are gaps in charting or intermittent charting.

Clinical Pathway

A **clinical pathway** is an abbreviated plan of care that is event oriented and provides a multidisciplinary mechanism for predicting specific disease outcomes, problems, and interventions.

Electronic Charting

Electronic charting, or charting by computer, is the trend in all aspects of health care. Using either computer terminals on the facility units or handheld computers, electronic documentations systems have revolutionized the way the nurses document patient care and treatments, allowing quicker and greater accessibility to patient information.

Advantages

- More accurate and timely charting.
- Easier access to patient information.
- More efficient method of communicating.
- Assists in providing patient confidentiality.
- Allows more legible patient information.

Disadvantages

- Risk of breaches in confidentiality may be increased.
- Downtime is increased.
- Difficult for health care providers to transfer to a "paperless" chart.
- Cost of equipment and education. Training is a must and takes time and resources.
- Insufficient number or terminals can delay inputting of data.
- Can promote a false sense of security that the computer information is always correct.
- Software issues are possible. It may take awhile for facilities to find the best program to meet their needs. Once they do, there are often "bugs" to be worked out.

Legal and Ethical Issues in Electronic Charting

Confidentiality.   Institutions must develop policies and procedures to ensure that breaches in confidentiality do not occur when patient records are kept electronically. Those policies and procedures should cover the following:

- Limiting the time that information is left on a screen if the nurse has to leave the station or laptop for some reason.

- Placement of computer terminals, so they are in an area where there is limited access by other individuals.
- A mechanism to determine which individuals are requesting sensitive information such as HIV results so that leaks of confidential information can be traced.
- Creating passwords that are used and routinely changed to prevent use and access.
- Creating levels of access so that only those who have a need to know get access to patient records.

Employee Access.   Policies and procedures must be developed to designate the process of accessibility; how employees can obtain accessibility; why (for what reasons) they wish to access information; what information can be accessed; and what information is confidential and has limited access. To ensure system integrity, the access codes for the nurse-employees or health care providers should not be alphabetical or in numerical order, which can be deciphered by someone. Access codes should be a random choice of numbers and letters.

Patient Privacy.   Privacy of information obtained from the patient and family members must be protected from those who may "abuse" such information.

Accuracy of Data Input.   Policies and procedures must be developed so that health care providers have guidelines for making sure that the information obtained is entered into computerized records accurately and in a timely manner. Orientation and training programs must be developed so that employees' computer skills can be checked and policies and procedures can be instituted for charting.

Patient's Right to a Copy of the Medical Record.   Patizents also have a right to a copy of the medical records. However, with computerized charting, policies and procedures must be developed regarding when a patient or patient's attorney can actively obtain a copy of the computerized chart. Because the computerized chart can be printed out immediately, decisions such as whether a partial chart can be released or whether the patient must be discharged before he or she can obtain a copy of the chart must be made.

On December 28, 2000, the HIPAA Rules for Standards for Privacy of Individually Identifiable Health Information were published. The final rule must be complied with by the majority of affected, covered entities by April 14, 2003, or by April 14, 2004, for small health plans. The final rule applies to the following:

1. Any health care provider who transmits any health information in electronic form in connection with a standard transaction
2. Any health plan
3. Any health care clearinghouse

The purpose of the privacy rule is as follows:

1. To enhance and protect the rights of the patient consumer by controlling the inappropriate use of health care information
2. To provide patients with access to their health information
3. To improve health care quality and restore trust among patient consumers
4. To create a national framework for health care privacy protection

Effective Documentation

Documentation forms the framework for all nursing activities, and documentation standards establish specific regulatory guidelines and policies. Effective written documentation ensures that all health care providers caring for the patient receive the most accurate description of their patients' problems and interventions and provides evidence that standards were followed in providing patient care. Effective documentation includes *f*actual, *a*ccurate, *c*omplete, and *t*imely record entries (Box 8–1).

Documentation that is not fact is considered falsified and can lead to serious problems if a patient sues for medical negligence and it is discovered that records are altered or falsified, if there are accusations of Medicare and Medicaid fraud and abuse, or in nursing disciplinary actions. Inaccurate documentation can lead to mistakes. For instance, if an order is given for Meperidine 25 mg and is written on the medication record as Meperidine 125 mg, the patient could potentially receive five times the amount of drug ordered. Documentation such as "Demerol 25 mg PRN" is incomplete because both the route and frequency with which the drug can be given is missing. Although it may be difficult to do with 10 seriously ill patients and no aide or licensed practical nurse (LPN), timely documentation can be critical for patient care. For example, if a dose of insulin is given but not documented and a supervisor or a medication nurse tries to "help out" and does not talk to the nurse who actually gave the insulin, the patient could be overdosed and suffer severe consequences.

Effective documentation includes the following:

1. Written communication of essential facts to maintain a continuous record of events over time

---

BOX 8–1

Fact

When documenting, keep in mind the following acronym:

F   Factual
A   Accurate
C   Complete, and
T   Timely

2. Preparation and maintenance of accounts of events through charts, records, or documents
3. Entries into patient records to give evidence of the need for care, to identify patient problems, and to plan, deliver, and evaluate that care
4. Professional monitoring and evaluation of the patient, nursing judgments, and actions, the patient's progress with regard to health or illness, and the outcomes
5. Entries of nursing activities performed on behalf of the patient
6. Entries discussing or evaluating the care and treatment rendered (e.g., documentation that the pain medicine given alleviated the patient's back pain)

Tips for Effective Documentation

Remember these important points when documenting in a patient's medical record.

Factual

- Use concise, factual, concrete, and specific terminology; for example, "The reddened area on the left lower calf is 2 cm long" or "Sharp, intermittent abdominal pain."
- Do not write relative statements such as "wound is healing." Describe the wound.
- Use the patient's words in describing symptoms whenever these words are helpful. Examples: "My back feels great today."
"I am not having any pain in my stomach."
"I am depressed about being here."
- Avoid using such words as "apparently," "appears to be," or "in no acute distress." For example, on the 11-to-7 shift the nurse documented that the patient "appears to be sleeping." There are no objective facts documented regarding the patient's status. When the nurse on the 7-to-3 shift arrives, make rounds, and finds that the patient is dead, there is no specific information to indicate when the death may have occurred.

Accurate

- Be sure the patient's name is on each sheet of the medical record. Many times charting may take place on the wrong chart because the nurse has not checked the actual patient's name on the chart.
- Do not chart until you have checked the patient's name to make sure that you are charting on the proper record.
- Describe only what you actually observe or assess.
- Do not use medical terms unless you know their meaning.

- Do not spell words incorrectly, because this can cast doubt on your credibility.
- Stay current with terminology and pathophysiology, new diseases, and new assessment concerning ongoing illnesses, and chart only information about which you are certain.

Complete

- Document specific information communicated to other health care providers.
- Clarify orders that are not complete.

Timely

- Write the complete date and time of each entry. This is important because if there is a medical negligence case involving a patient, a chronology of events will be developed to pinpoint the exact times when events occurred. Military time is the "norm" and is more effective because you do not have to determine if treatment was done in the AM or PM.
- Make entries in order of consecutive shifts and dates. Remember, it is acceptable to document late entries if you have forgotten to put something in your records. The farther away from the actual time that you document, the more suspicious it becomes to a judge or jury that you are trying to add information to protect yourself from potential exposure.
- Do not chart in advance. Medical records have been discovered that state, for example, "Patient tolerated procedure well," when in fact the patient died during the procedure. Finding a point like this in the medical record lessens the credibility of the health care provider regarding what else might not have been properly done. Also, state boards of nursing have rules regarding "precharting."
- Do not backdate, tamper with, or add to notes previously written. Use the appropriate charting procedure for late entries.
- Do not allow long periods to elapse between entries, because it may appear that the patient is abandoned.

Follow Institutional Policies and Procedures

- Document according to your institution's method of charting.
- Document only on approved institution forms.
- Use acceptable institution abbreviations. Refer to the institution's approved abbreviation list. Be sure that you know what the abbreviations mean in your institution. For example, do not use "h/a" for both "headache" and "heart attack."

- Sign each entry with your name or initials and title. (Know your facility's policy on how your signature must be documented in the record.)
- Do not leave any space between your last entry and your signature. Do not give others the opportunity to access additional or false information and expose you to legal liability.
- If a section or line on a chart is not applicable, mark "NA." Do not leave blank.
- Do not use slang.
- Do not erase.
- Do not use liquid correction fluid.
- Chart only in black or blue ink, according to your institution's policy. Green or red ink may not reproduce well if your chart is copied.
- Do not use sticky notes or clipped-on pieces of paper as part of the patient's records. They get removed and can get lost.
- Avoid block charting or charting everything that you did for the patient and the patient's care, treatment, and status for the entire shift in one note with no specific times indicated.
- Use graphic records to record the patient's vital signs
- Know the facility's policy and procedure for documenting highly sensitive information (e.g., HIV status).
- Do not rewrite notes.
- Document according to the standards of care.

Patient Status

- Read the prior nurses' notes for a patient before charting your care. It is important that you know the status of your patient prior to charting to determine whether or not there has actually been any deterioration of the patient's status.
- Document allergies.
- Report and document notification of abnormal laboratory or other tests ordered and response by physician or other health care provider.
- Thoroughly document intravenous (IV) therapy, peripherally inserted central catheter (PICC) lines, and blood administration—site, dressing change, drainage, vital signs, reactions, and other pertinent findings.

Legal

- If you have made an error in your charting, draw a line and follow the procedure noted in your facility's policy and procedure manual. Many facilities are eliminating the use of "error" or "mistaken entry"—it implies that something was done wrong and again it becomes a credibility issue that an attorney can use to attack a nurse during a trial. Attorneys sometimes play word games.

- Remember that the record will be used in a court of law in any type of medical negligence claim, personal injury case, workers' compensation claim, custody matter, social security claim, child or elder abuse claims, or other legal proceedings.
- The record contains confidential information and must not be placed where unauthorized persons, facility personnel, family members, or strangers can access it.
- Avoid bias, sarcasm, and prejudicial reports or comments about the patient.
- In your charting, do not blame others for acts or omissions that occur in patient care and treatment.
- Do not state personal feelings about patients. For example, "Mrs. Stacey is bullheaded and obnoxious and won't take her medicines." Although the statement may be true, if insulting or derogatory remarks are made by the staff and the patient is unhappy with the care rendered, a lawsuit is more likely to result.
- Document the patient's or family's noncompliance.
- Document inability or refusal to give needed information.
- Document unauthorized materials or items found in the patient's room.
- Do not chart for anyone else, especially nursing actions performed by another nurse. Remember, it may be crucial to you if a lawsuit ensues and several years later the only documentation that can protect you from exposure is the charting by another nurse who didn't accurately chart your care and treatment. You may not remember that patient and what exactly happened.
- Avoid any admission of liability involving patient care when charting. In a New Hampshire case, a hospital was held liable when a nurse documented in her chart that the patient was found on the floor and had apparently crawled out of bed while trying to get to the bathroom. She wrote that the patient had called for help, but "there was not a quick enough response."[7]
- Document the chain of custody and preservation of evidence in domestic violence, abuse, and rape cases.
- Document that you have made the necessary reports according to state laws, such as in cases of child or elder abuse.
- Do not document incidents in your diary. Any personal notes that are used to prepare for a deposition or trial may be requested by the plaintiff's attorney. When there is the possibility of a lawsuit, write factual and concrete statements with dates and times. Sign and date your notes. Some nurses mail their notes to themselves to actually show the postmark and the date when the notes were written. Be cautious in writing facts or assumptions about an incident in personal notes. Always show any such material to your attorney prior to your trial or deposition.
- If you are aware of a lawsuit or anticipate a lawsuit regarding a particular patient, do not rewrite your nurse's notes. Attorneys and handwriting experts review charts and can detect when and what records have been rewritten. Handwriting analysis can be done on each chart to determine the date and type of ink, indicating when the actual recordings were made.

▨ Documenting in Special Situations

Telephone and Verbal Orders

Telephone and verbal orders must be written and cosigned according to the facility policy and procedure. Accepting by telephone a do not resuscitate (DNR) order on a patient is not recommended. If there is any type of controversy regarding the death of a patient with a DNR order, the nurse may be exposed if the physician states that he or she did not give the order and refuses to cosign. If a DNR order must be obtained over the telephone, it is imperative that the nurse and another witness receive the telephone order. The nurse must document the fact that she or he and the witness heard the DNR order given by the physician.

Medications

When administering a medication, document the name of the medication, route, site, time, reason for giving medication, your name or initials, and patient's response. It is extremely important to document the site, because if a lawsuit claims sciatic nerve damage as a result of an injection, the attorney will focus on which nurses administered injections in the gluteus maximus during the crucial period.

Also, thoroughly read any affidavits regarding your nursing care before signing. In a sciatic nerve injury case that was settled out of court, a statement was prepared by an attorney to aid in proving that the hospital's nurses were not negligent in their method of administration. However, neither the attorney nor the nurse who signed the affidavit read it. Unfortunately, it stated that the nurse always gave her injections in the right lower inner quadrant of the gluteus maximus—a damaging statement resulting in immediate settlement of the case.

Controlled Substances

Controlled substances must be documented properly or there could be legal disciplinary or criminal implications. Discarding drugs or removing drugs from the pharmacy machines requires following policies and procedures to detect and prevent diversion of drugs. When controlled substances are administered, it is essential to document the reason for administering the drug, the administration site, the time given, and the patient's response to the drug.

Medication Error Reporting

When using or developing a form for medication error reporting, the following information should be documented:

1. Type of event (e.g., wrong medication given, adverse drug reaction)
2. Facts surrounding the event
3. Witnesses—names and addresses
4. Date, time, and location of event
5. Name of staff person notified or who discovered event
6. Status of patient—effect of event on patient
7. Names and time of persons notified of event (e.g., physician)
8. Name and title of person completing the form
9. Date of report[8]
10. Names of persons receiving a copy of the report

Against Medical Advice Documentation

When a patient leaves **against medical advice (AMA),** proper documentation must be made to decrease the potential liability exposure for the health care providers.

The physician or other appropriate health care provider should inform the patient of the risks of leaving without proper treatment. For example, if a patient is having chest pains radiating down the left arm, the patient should be warned that he could suffer damage to the heart and death if not treated. A form devised by your facility attorney should be given to the patient to sign stating that he has been advised of the risks and dangers of leaving the facility AMA. Also, discuss with the patient and document what tests have been ordered and completed and those tests that have not been done. If the patient refuses to sign, document what was told to the patient and that he or she refused to sign the form.

If the physician is not available to discuss the dangers of leaving AMA, the nurse should discuss them with the patient. Documentation of the conversation should be made in the nurse's notes.

Document the mental status of the patient and the patient's reason for leaving in his or her own words. Document that other family members or friends are present and have been informed of the dangers of leaving and given instructions about what to do. Instructions on follow-up care and drugs or prescriptions given to the patient must also be documented. If relatives who are not with the patient are notified, document the name, time notified, and what information was relayed. Finally, document the destination of the patient, how the patient is being transported, who is accompanying the patient, the time that the patient left the facility, and the patient's mental and physical condition.

Do Not Resuscitate Orders

Do not resuscitate orders must be written to protect the health care provider in situations where there is a potential for a medical malpractice suit. There should be policies regarding DNR orders, and a time limit should be placed on the orders so that they are renewed periodically. A patient's status may change, and the DNR orders may no longer be required. Also, any discussions with the patient or family regarding DNR orders should be documented. Institutions may also have a form for DNR cases that explains what happens if the patient is not resuscitated. This form should be signed and dated by the patient and the family member who consents to such an order. A copy should be given to the patient, and a copy can remain in the chart.

Also, facilities must have plans in place to determine what patients have DNRs. For example, some facilities use specific color designations in the form of wristbands or colored stickers on the door or charts.

A word of caution: If your facility has no method of designating patients with DNRs, what are the potential legal implications if a patient is outside his or her room and arrests or another nurse discovers the patient and is not familiar with the patient's wishes? The facility and staff should have methods to determine what patients have DNRs, so that their wishes can be honored. Lawsuits have occurred because staff have resuscitated patients that had DNRs.

Discharge Planning and Discontinuation of Home Health Services

When planning for a discharge, it is of the utmost importance that there be documentation that the patient or the patient's family is aware of the fact that treatment and care will be discontinued on a specific date and the consequences; alternative resources; and specific plans that must be put into action after the effective date. A specific form should be used that can be signed and dated documenting the information that is discussed with the patient. Both the patient and the family member should sign and date the form. Both should be given a copy and a copy should remain in the patient's chart. This may decrease the possibility for exposure if there is a claim of medical malpractice and abandonment. **Abandonment** is the unilateral termination of care and treatment by the health care provider without the patient's consent.

Documentation Weaknesses

In documentation, every word counts. Legally speaking, your documentation is just as important as the care you provide. It must indicate assessments noted and the interventions performed in response to those assessments. Furthermore, a summary of actions that are taken but lack of a record of follow-up presents a legally damaging document. A nurse attorney, legal nurse consultant, risk manager, or another health care provider should be able to review the patient record and reconstruct the care the patient received, even if months or years have passed. If key facts or notes on follow-up are not documented, it is difficult to defend the nurse.

To be certain that your documentation is complete, address these three vital aspects of care: assessment, intervention, and patient response (Box 8–2). Be particularly alert in the following instances, where documentation weaknesses commonly occur.

When Vital Signs Are Abnormal

Any significant deviation from normal—whether it is elevated or decreased temperature, elevated or decreased blood pressure, or accelerated or slowed respiratory rate—demands a notation showing what is being done about it. When notifying a physician or other provider, record the time, the provider's response, and what you did. Note also when you are unable to reach the provider, as well as when you reattempted to contact the provider or contacted someone else. Document every time you called or paged.

If your response to abnormal findings is to monitor the patient more closely (and frequently), specify that in your documentation, and note whether the patient's condition improves or deteriorates, and your response to that change in condition.

When a Patient Codes

An unexpected bad outcome can result in legal action. Documenting what happened during a code or other emergency is especially crucial, because it is often argued that monitoring was inadequate and intervention occurred too late.

Emergency situations are precisely when documentation is apt to fall short. To avoid documentation gaps, many facilities keep code sheets on crash carts and documentation is assigned to one member of the team who does only the documentation.

BOX 8–2

Prevention of Documentation Errors

When documenting, remember the following tips:

- Take your time when documenting.
- Double-check your work.
- Use computerized/electronic charting when available. It has many "prompters" to ensure that you don't forget to document important information.
- The Institute of Medicine (IOM) estimated that medical errors cause 98,000 deaths yearly. Approximately 7000 are attributable to drug errors. One immediate source of errors is sloppy handwriting.
- Handheld electronic prescribing devices have been developed that use a printed order that can reduce risk of errors from transcription mistakes or sloppy handwriting.[9]

A Case in Point

Inadequate Documentation

The Facts

A 62-year-old stroke patient was admitted to the hospital. The doctor ordered that she wear a restraining jacket and that the bedrails be raised at all times. One month after the patient's admission, a nursing assistant found her on the floor, where she apparently had fallen from the bed and fractured her right hip. The family of the patient sued the hospital for malpractice.

What did the nursing notes document? The nurses' notes documented that the patient had "escaped from her restraining jacket and left the bed on several occasions." On the morning that she fractured her hip, it was documented that at 6:30 AM she was resting quietly in bed and the restraint was on and the side rails were up. At 7:15 AM a nursing assistant found the patient on the floor still wearing the restraints, and the side rails were up. However, the nurse's notes actually contradicted the nurse's contention that she actually saw the patient at 6:30 AM. In fact, she actually did not check on the patient until 9:30 AM.

The head nurse spoke to the patient's husband about the problem and voiced her concern that he was unfastening her jacket and forgetting to retie it, which he denied, and asked that his wife be checked on almost constantly. This was documented in the notes. The head nurse informed him that she would require private duty nurses. The problem with the documentation was that there was no notation about the conversation showing that the husband was informed of the problem of his wife getting out of bed. The documentation on the chart showed that the hospital took no special steps to protect the patient. The court ruled that the conversations of the head nurse with the patient's husband did not relieve the hospital of the duty to take extra precautions and that the damage award was not excessive.[10]

The Jury Decides

The jury returned a verdict in favor of the hospital. The plaintiffs moved for a new trial. The trial judge granted the motion and awarded $225,000 for general damages and $60,897.37 for medical expenses.

The facility appealed the award.

Once a crisis is over, check the documentation to be sure it is complete and review the chart to see that nothing crucial was omitted.

When a Patient Is Transferred

Any patient moved—from the emergency department to intensive care unit or other department, even from one medical-surgical unit to another—calls for a patient assessment. Document the condition of the patient soon after the patient arrives on your unit, and again right before the patient leaves. The chart should also contain a record of the patient's condition on admission to your institution and assessments at the beginning and end of each shift or change of staffing according to policy and procedure.

Failure to Document Vital Information

Failure to document vital information that can be used by other health care providers in rendering treatment can result in a malpractice action. In a Louisiana case, the hospital was held liable because a hospital employee was told by the family and patient that a knife used in the stabbing of the patient had a broken blade. Because this information was not charted on the patient's history and not communicated to the emergency room physician, no radiographs were taken. Two months later, x-ray examinations were done because of continued pain and swelling in the shoulder, and knife blade fragments were found.[11]

Who Owns the Medical Records?

Medical records are owned by the facility, but the facility must provide copies to patients on request. States have carefully created laws outlining such things involving time limits for providing the records after they are requested and the amount that can be charged for duplication.

Use in Legal Disputes

Medical records are not only used to follow the course of the patient's treatment but are also used in legal matters. For example, records may be used in claims involving medical malpractice, personal injury, domestic or custody battles, workers' compensation cases, toxic torts, social security hearings, Americans with Disabilities Act disputes, sexual abuse, rape, kidnapping, psychiatric hearings for institutional commitment, guardianship hearings, ethical dilemmas, or disputes in which the patient's medical or physical status, care, and treatment must be analyzed.

Review of Medical Records: An Analysis by the Plaintiff's Attorney or Expert

When a plaintiff feels that there has been medical negligence in care and treatment, he or she seeks an attorney who specializes in the area of medical negligence. The attorney or an expert reviews the records to determine whether there has been a breach of the standard of care that has caused damage to the plaintiff. Records that may be reviewed include home health records; doctor's office records; insurance forms; history and physical examination forms; admittance fact sheets; physician orders and progress notes; nurses' notes; flow sheets; narrative notes; medication records; nursing care plan; vital signs sheets; surgery documents (including the record of the operation, anesthesia record, operating room nurses' notes, and postanesthesia records); emergency room record; consultations; ambulance run sheets; consents for treatment or surgery; discharge teaching; x-ray reports; discharge summary; autopsy reports; records of treatments and care given by physical therapists, occupational therapists, respiratory therapists, dietitians, and social services; hospital, clinic, and physician records; and medical bills (itemized statements).

Medical records can be obtained by the patient from the medical records department of the facility or the doctor's office. Medical records can also be obtained after a lawsuit has been filed by a subpoena duces tecum (SDT), which means "to appear and to bring with you." After a lawsuit has been filed, the plaintiff may also obtain medical records through a discovery tool called request for production of documents and things.

Employee Health Records

Employee health records are essential to care for the staff of any institution. Those records may be reviewed by outside agencies and generally should be carefully constructed to provide adequate information without divulging privileged or confidential information. Of particular concern, following implementation of the Occupational Safety and Health Administration's (OSHA) *Standard for Prevention of Transmission of Bloodborne Pathogens in the Workplace*, are test results following occupational exposure to HBV or HIV. These records should be separated from the balance of the employee's personnel record and maintained in a separate medical file so that the results are not provided to attorneys who subpoena a nurse's personnel or health file.

Incident/Occurrence/Variance Reports

An **incident** is an occurrence, accident, or event that is not consistent with the facility or routine care of a patient in the facility.

Common types of reportable incidents include the following:

- Falls from bed, wheelchair, or commode
- Medication errors or unusual reactions
- Treatment errors (e.g., skin tears)
- Incidents caused by patients (e.g., burns, self-mutilation)
- Wandering
- Drinking or eating substances

■ Abusive actions toward staff/family or abusive actions of family/friends toward patient
■ Patient or family complaints regarding care and treatment
■ Stolen or missing personal property
■ Visitors injured (e.g., fall)

An **incident, variance, or occurrence report** is a written report or form made when a patient or visitor problem or "incident" has occurred. The report is a formal document and depending on the state law may or may not be discoverable by attorney.

Documenting the pertinent information is important. Some incident reports are set up as "check-off sheets," with very little narrative space. Others are largely narrative. Because state laws vary, incident reports may be obtained by the plaintiff's attorney in some states.

Purposes of Incident Reports

Joint Commission standards dictate the establishment of an incident reporting system. Incident reports are useful tools that are used by nurses, physicians, attorneys, risk managers, health care administrators, other facility committee members, and insurance carriers. Incident reports are a source for the following:

■ Assessing problem areas
■ Assessing subjects for in-service teaching
■ Minimizing patient/family risks
■ Evaluating individual health care providers
■ Assessing needs for policy and procedure revisions

This form is also assessed and appropriate interventions are discussed by the risk management department to determine if there is the potential for a lawsuit or a patient care issue that requires changes in policy or procedure. Also, it may be determined that the nurse requires additional training or counseling on the issue at hand.

Legal and Ethical Issues

Only complete an incident report on incidents of which you have firsthand knowledge. All incidents must be reported. Failure to report could result in termination of your job. Personal liability could result if your failure to report if an incident causes harm to a patient or other person. You have a responsibility, both professionally and ethically, to follow the institution's policy for reporting incidents.

The incident report is not part of the medical record. It is an administrative record. The medical records should include only factual observations. The incident report does not replace proper documentation in the record. In some sates, the incident report is protected and confidential. Be aware of the laws in your state.

What to Include in an Incident Report

Incident reports are made up of statements and general facts, along with the specific information sought. Most incident reports should include the following:

- Names and information about persons involved in the incidents
- Patient: Name and name of attending physician
- Visitor: Name and reason for presence at facility
- Date of occurrence
- Environment (e.g., lighting, position of bed, position of side rails)
- Time of occurrence
- The date of the report of the incident
- Patient or visitor
- Room number
- Age
- Marital status
- Gender
- Facility
- City, state
- Diagnosis prior to incident/surgery; date and type of surgery
- Location of incident (e.g., patient's room, operating room, lobby)
- Type of incident (e.g., fall, medicine relating, missing/lost property)
- Service (e.g., emergency, surgery, obstetric)
- Administrative code section for falls and other patient incidents
- Person who discovered the incident
- Specific facts related to the incident
  Incident-related cause (e.g., wet or foreign material on floor, side rails not used, defective equipment)
  Fall/accident involved (e.g., bed, bedrails were (1) up, (2) down, (3) absent; tub or shower)
  Restraints used prior to accident (yes/no, type)
  Physician's orders prior to occurrence (e.g., restraints, up with assistance, no orders)
  Nature of incident relating to medication procedures, treatment, or disease (e.g., wrong patient, infiltration, suspected reaction, wrong treatment/medicine)
  Incident-related cause (e.g., transcription error, wrong medication from pharmacy, patient identification not checked, physician's orders not clear)

In reportable incidents—those that are dictated as reportable by state and federal laws, the JCAHO, and facility policies and procedures—the following information should be documented:

- Brief factual description (area for brief narrative)
- Witnesses—names, addresses, and phone numbers

- Result of occurrence or injury (e.g., death, no apparent injury)
- Patient condition prior to occurrence (e.g., alert/oriented, confused/disoriented, senile)
- Last time patient seen and by whom
- Patient/visitor's attitude after occurrence (e.g., cooperative, unaware of the occurrence, angry (see comments)
- Name/title/department of person most closely associated with incident
- Department head/head nurse review
- Signature/title of person preparing the report; date
- Signature/title of person reviewing report; date
- Comments section
- Was there injury? Yes/No
- Treatment refused? Yes/No
- Was physician notified? Yes/No
- X-ray ordered? Yes/No
- Results:_____
- Clinical findings:_____
- Follow-up:_____
- Person reported to:_____
- Follow-up:_____
- Copy to:_____

Who Should Write the Incident Report?

Incident reports are written by the nurse who has experienced the problem firsthand or someone who has secondhand knowledge of the incident. The supervisor or nurse manager may also write information on the form. It is extremely dangerous to allow someone else to write the report if you witnessed the incident. Inaccurate or incorrect information may be documented that could be a problem if the matter ends up in court.

What Should Be Excluded from an Incident Report?

It is critical that information that could "hurt" the institution be omitted from the incident report. Some of these "danger zones" include the following:

- Physician comments
- Physician orders (Some argue that if an order is written by a physician, it becomes part of the medical record and loses its confidentiality privilege.)
- Opinions/assumptions
- Conclusions (e.g., what caused the incident)

- Suggestions regarding who is the responsible party
- Recommendations on how things can be improved
- Recommendations on what you would do differently
- Recommendations on how you can prevent that incident from happening again[12]
- Details from witnesses
- Descriptions of actions taken to correct the problem
- Accusations
- Staff evaluations on incident reports
- Multiple copies of the report disseminated to numerous parties

A single report should not be made from a compilation of witness reports (that have been obtained by nursing supervisor) and added or attached to the incident report. Be careful not to state information inaccurately (e.g., "Patient fell out of bed," if you did not witness the incident; "Patient found lying on floor" is the correct form). Also, do not make admissions in the record, such as "Patient fell out of bed because the call light was out of reach and the staff didn't check on him quick enough."

Who Will See the Incident Report?

After the incident, several people or committees may evaluate and investigate the incident reported. The following are some who may read the report:

- Nurse who witnessed the incident
- Nursing supervisor/department head
- Attending physician
- Administration
- Quality Assurance
- Risk Management
- Institution's attorney
- Institution's insurance company
- Plaintiff's attorney (if allowed by law).

What Happens to the Report?

After the incident, several events or procedures take place as part of the facility's quality assurance process:

- Patient/visitor incident occurs.
- Nurse documents factual information about incident in the medical record.
- Nurse fills out an incident report during the shift.
- Incident report given to nursing supervisor/department head.
- Incident report is sent to appropriate administrator, who reviews the report.

- Administrator sends the important information to appropriate person/department for follow-up.
- Trend data is reviewed so that problems/problem areas can be determined and changes can be recommended through:
Education
Policy changes
Personnel changes
Personnel reprimands/terminations

What to Do After the Incident

No one likes to see someone get hurt or the wrong medication given. It is, or can be, upsetting. However, some tips on what to do after the fact include the following:

- Remain calm.
- Continue patient/staff rapport.
- Do not act "guilty."
- Do not blame anyone.
- Follow procedures if family or patient requests information about the incident.
- Do not speak to patient's attorney.
- Ombudsman, patient advocate, and patient relations department should be called if necessary.

KEEP IN MIND

- ▶ The primary purposes of documentation are to identify the patient's status to document the need for care and to plan, deliver, and evaluate that care.
- ▶ Continuous quality improvement (CQI) is a process that assumes that work groups are experts about their work and should be the locus for monitoring quality, identifying problems, and devising solutions.
- ▶ Types of documentation are contemporaneous, accurate, and fraudulent.
- ▶ Electronic charting policies and procedures must be especially sensitive to the potential risk of liability based on breach of a patient's privacy and confidentiality.
- ▶ The common systems of documentation are narrative, problem oriented, PIE, focus, and charting by exception.
- ▶ Documentation policies and procedures must be created and used in situations involving telephone and verbal orders, medications, do not resuscitate orders, discharge planning and discontinuation of home health services, patient cardiac or respiratory arrest events, patient transfers, documentation of vital signs and patient status, and employee health records.

▶ Incident, variance, or occurrence reports should be used as a toll to change behaviors, policies, procedures, equipment, or rules that can cause harm or damage.

In a Nutshell

Documentation is your first and best line of defense. Regardless of the type of system used, keep in mind that your documentation must be factual, accurate, complete, and timely (FACT). By documenting in this manner, you not only legally protect yourself and your facility, you also provide a good solid record for use in other possible legal or ethical matters. Along with documenting appropriately, you must maintain health information privacy. Under HIPAA, federal privacy standards are mandated and must be followed by health care providers and facilities.[13]

Afterthoughts

1. List five reasons for documentation.
2. What is "effective" documentation?
3. Discuss the continuous quality improvement (CQI) method.
4. Discuss important aspects of the incident, variance, or occurrence report and what should be included in a report.
5. Outline and discuss 10 charting tips.
6. Discuss current charting systems available to the nurse.
7. Discuss the advantages and disadvantages of each charting system.
8. Outline important points that should be remembered when dealing with a DNR order.
9. Relate ethical and legal issues involved with electronic charting.
10. Discuss what must be documented with a patient who leaves a facility against medical advice (AMA).
11. Relate three areas in nursing of potential danger and legal exposure when documenting.
12. Discuss an ethical issue involving documentation.
13. Discuss the possible legal, ethical, and disciplinary implications of false documentation.
14. Outline the documentation/charting policies in your institution.
15. Discuss if precharting is allowed in your state. Why or why not? Define your state board's position on precharting.

Ethics in Practice

It was an extremely busy 3 to 11 PM shift on the surgical unit of a large city hospital. Because it was a Wednesday evening, the unit was not only receiving new postoperative patients from surgery but was also in the process of discharging patients and admitting new patients for the next day's surgery schedule.

Melinda L., RN, charge nurse for the 3-to-11 shift, had worked on the surgical unit for 2 years. She had a reputation as being a well-organized, competent, and hard-working nurse who seemed to be able to bring order out of chaos. On this particular shift, even her considerable skills in organization were failing to settle the unit to a point where she felt in control.

Mrs. Star J., a 66-year-old patient with diabetes, was being admitted at 4:00 PM to the surgical unit because of poor circulation in her legs and possible infection of her right foot. One of her admission orders was to culture the drainage from the sore on her great right toe. In checking the orders after the unit secretary had noted them, Melinda decided to do the culture herself because the staff was already tied up in other activities. Melinda explained the procedure to Mrs. J. and then proceeded to culture a draining sore on her left toe. The culture was taken to the lab with the appropriate slips by the unit secretary.

During supper, a patient aspirated and coded. Later that evening, a patient fell while attempting to climb out of bed with the bedrails up. It was almost 11:45 PM when Melinda finally got to sit down and do her charting. After all that had happened that evening, she was having some trouble remembering what she had done earlier in the shift.

When she came to Mrs. J.'s chart, she remembered that she had gotten a culture and checked back on the orders to make sure it was actually ordered. The order said "C&S right great toe," so Melinda charted, "1630—Culture of right great toe obtained and sent to lab. Procedure explained to patient" and signed it.

On her way home that night, Melinda was thinking about how busy the shift was and all that had happened. She wondered if she had done everything that was supposed to be done, and charted everything that needed to be charted. She also began thinking about Mrs. J. and the culture. By the time she reached home, she felt pretty sure that she had cultured the wrong toe. She would correct the chart in 2 days when she worked again.

When Melinda returned after her 2 days off, she discovered that Mrs. J. had had a below-the-knee amputation of her right leg. The physician had decided to do the amputation because the culture that was sent to the lab had grown *Clostridium perfringens* (gas gangrene). Melinda feels that she is responsible for this mistake. What should she do? If she "tells" or tries to correct the chart, could she be open to a lawsuit?

References

1. Fishbach, F: Documenting Care Communication, the Nursing Process, and Documentation Standards. FA Davis, Philadelphia, 1991.
2. Northrop, C, and Kelly, M: Legal Issues in Nursing. CV Mosby, St. Louis, 1987.
3. Weintaub, Michael I: "Mistake May Represent Negligence." M.D. Consult, accessed online 1/2/01.
4. Iyer, P, and Camp, N: Nursing Documentation—A Nursing Process Approach. Mosby, St. Louis, 1999.
5. Ibid.

6. Ibid.
7. Brookover v. Mary Hitchcock Memorial Hospital, 893 F.2d 411 NH (1990).
8. Cohen, MI: "Mistake May Represent Negligence." M.D. Consult, Jones and Bartlett Publishers, Boston, 2000.
9. Weintaub, MI. "Mistake May Represent Negligence." M.D. Consult, accessed online 1/2/01.
10. Keyworth v. Southern Baptist Hospital, 524 So.2d 56. La. App., 5th Cir. 1998.
11. Brown v. Conway Memorial Hospital, 588 So.2d 295 (La. 1991). Tammelleo, AD: The Regan Report on Nursing Law 32:9, 1992.
12. Weintaub.
13. Kumekawa, JK: Health Information Privacy Protection: Crisis or Common Sense? Online Journal of Issues in Nursing, American Nurses Association, accessed online 12/12/02.

Resources

Arikian, VL: Total quality management: Application to nursing service. Journal of Nursing Administration 21(6):46, 1991.
Deming, WE: Out of Crisis. Massachusetts Institute of Technology, Cambridge, Mass, 1982.
JCAHO Transition: From QA to CQI—Using CQI Approaches to Monitor, Evaluate, and Improve Quality. Oakbrook Terrace, Ill, 1991.
Juran, J: Juran on Leadership for Quality. Free Press, New York, 1989.
Jech, AO. "The Next Step in Preventing Medical Errors." RN Web ® Archive, April 1, 2001.
Showers, J: Safeguarding Against Nursing Negligence. Springhouse Corp. and Gale Group, 2000. (web article)

The Georgetown University Health Privacy Project
http://www.healthprivacy.org

Electronic Privacy Information Center
http://www.epic.org

Office for the Advancement of Telehealth, DHHS
http://telehealth.hrsa.gov

Centers for Medicare and Medicaid Services (formerly Health Care Finance Administration [HCFA])
http://cms.hhs.gov

Federal Trade Commission
http://www.ftc.gov

Food and Drug Administration
http://www.fda.gov

National Telecommunications Information Administration, Department of Commerce
http://www. ntia.doc.gov/

HIPAA Privacy Final Rules
http://www.hhs.gov/ocr/part3.html

Electronic Documentation 9

Nancy M. Matulich, RN,C, MSN

Key Chapter Concepts

Health information

Computer-based patient record
 (CPR)

Electronic documentation system

Computer hardware

Computer software

Physical security

Personnel security

Password

System security

Encryption

Audit trail

Authentic

Chapter Thoughts

The benefits of electronic charting include reducing work and time-intensive tasks, eliminating lost or misplaced files, improving access to authorized users, providing a quicker turn-around time or production time, and increasing security measures through audit trails. Some even advocate a "health card" that contains the patient's medical history in a credit card format that will be carried by the patient and used when needed.

In any format, ethical issues face health care providers when dealing with such sensitive and confidential information. These issues include being truthful in what is recorded and actually done with the record. The duty to warn, required disclosure of specific types of information on a need-to-know basis, privacy issues, and the duty to do no harm all come into play.

Therefore it is critical that guidelines, policies, and procedures are clear and cover all the situations in which medical information may be requested, used, or reported, whether it is in a hospital or clinic, business (insurance companies, employers, or health maintenance organization), or school setting.

OBJECTIVES

Upon completing this chapter, the reader will be able to:
1. Describe the need for electronic documentation in health care.
2. List the basic elements of an electronic documentation system.
3. Discuss the confidentiality and security of information documented electronically.

4. List the advantages of electronic documentation.
5. Describe the problems associated with electronic documentation.
6. Discuss the future of electronic documentation of patient care information.

Introduction

Health information, which is any information that is created or received by a health care provider, health plan, public health authority, employer, life insurer, school, or university or health care clearinghouse, must be protected to ensure patient confidentiality and privacy. Today there is rapid expansion in health care information and multiple demands for ways to use it. Managers, payers, regulator agencies, quality improvement initiatives and insurance companies, schools, and health maintenance organizations (HMOs), to name a few, want this information. To manage this explosion of information in patient care, health care organizations are rapidly implementing electronic documentation systems, including using a **computer-based patient record (CPR),** which allows the gathering of data in a format that can be stored, retrieved, and analyzed.

Electronic documentation systems attempt to meet these needs in a variety of approaches. Systems can be designed to address the electronic documentation needs of a single department or a single type of caregiver, such as a freestanding laboratory or small physician's office, or the needs of all the caregivers and various departments within one institution.

Regardless of the approach, electronic documentation must be more than simply converting paper forms and requisitions into a computerized format. The system must be able to collect, store, retrieve, and share information generated during patient care. Electronic documentation systems must also permit analysis of clinical information within the institution and across multiple health care sites so that health care outcomes and processes can be evaluated and improved. For instance, a facility's utilization review process, which determines whether medical care is appropriately and properly performed, will use information collected from the system to assist in its review.

What Is Electronic Documentation?

Electronic documentation is a system that uses computer hardware and specialized software to collect, process, sort, store, print, and display the information generated as a result of the delivery of health care to patients. This information includes information to identify the patient (name, address, age, next of kin, marital status), financial or payer information, and clinical information (Box 9–1).

BOX 9–1

Clinical Information

Diagnosis

Surgical procedures

Medical and nursing assessments and examinations

Physician's instructions for care (nursing care plan, nursing interventions, treatments)

Results of diagnostic tests

Physician's notes outlining the plan of care and the patient's responses

Assessments and care provided by physical therapists, occupational therapists, respiratory therapists, and other contributors

Patient and family teaching

Social worker's assessment and plans for posthospital support

---

Computer Hardware

The **computer hardware** forms the interface that allows the caregiver to enter and retrieve information. The hardware may be a single personal computer used to document and report a single type of information, such as the results of diagnostic testing. Or it can be multiple personal computers connected to create a network. The network may link several areas within one department or among all departments in the institution. The data entered into the system is then transferred to a mainframe computer, where it is processed and stored.

Computer Software

Computer software is the instruction that tells the hardware what, when, and how to do something. A set of software instructions can be relatively simple, such as instructions to verify that a patient's identifying information is included with a request for a diagnostic test, or it can be more complex, such as when a physician enters an order for an intravenous pyelogram (an x-ray examination of the kidney) and the software automatically instructs the computer to do each of the following activities:

- Notify the radiology department that the test has been ordered.
- Inform the supply department to send supplies for pretest treatments.
- Notify the food service department to modify the patient's diet.
- Notify the pharmacy to send pretest medications to the nursing unit.
- Instruct the nurse to perform the treatments and administer the medications.
- Track the time required to do each of the tasks associated with patient preparation for the x-ray examination and the test itself.
- Provide an electronic checklist for each caregiver to document completion of each of the activities associated with the patient preparation for the test.

- File the completed electronic checklist so that each caregiver can see what has been completed.
- Alert caregivers if part of the pretest preparation has not been completed.
- Record the charges for the test and the pretest preparation.
- Document the results of the x-ray examination.

Ensuring Confidentiality

The Health Insurance Portability and Accountability Act (HIPAA) requires compliance by health care providers and all others who gain access to health information to protect the privacy, confidentiality, and security of the patient's information. In addition, most professional and regulatory agencies, including the American Medical Association, the American Nurses Association, and the Joint Commission on Accreditation of Healthcare Organizations, also stress the importance of maintaining the confidentiality of patient information (Box 9–2).

Although confidentiality of patients' health care information is very important, it is not absolute. Some information may be shared with others in specific situations. These situations may vary by state but usually include the following:

- Information given to other health care providers for the diagnosis and treatment of the patient.
- Information used in medical education, but only as necessary for the educational activities.
- Information used by qualified personnel for the purpose of conducting audits, program evaluations, peer review, and similar activities, as long as the patient's identity is not disclosed.

All health care providers have an ethical and legal responsibility to maintain the confidentiality of patient information, and yet the ease with which information stored in an electronic documentation system can be accessed and disseminated can increase the potential for a breach of security and confidentiality by increasing the user's abil-

---

BOX 9–2

Security and Confidentiality of Electronic Documentation

"The patient has the right to expect that all communication and records pertaining to his/her care will be treated as confidential by the hospital except in cases such as suspected abuse and public health hazards when reports are permitted or required by law. The patient has the right to expect that the hospital will emphasize the confidentiality of this information when it releases it to any other parties entitled to review information in these records."[1]

A CASE IN POINT

Protection of Patient Confidentiality

The Facts

A hospital retained a law firm to screen for the records of patients who qualify for social security income reimbursement for their medical expenses. For those patients who did qualify, the hospital could file for the payment of services for which they would otherwise not be paid. A portion of the payments received would be paid to the law firm based on contingency fee contract.

The hospital provided the following information to the law firm: the patient's name, age, telephone number, and medical diagnosis and the patient registration forms.

For $2^{1}/_{2}$ years, the hospital routinely released the records to the law firm without obtaining patient consent or authorization.

A class action suit was filed against the hospital law firm and the administrators, chief executive officer, and executive director of the hospital alleging invasion of privacy, intentional infliction of emotional distress, negligence, breach of implied contract, statutory violations, and improper solicitation claims against the law firm.

The Court Decides

The court held that an independent tort exists for unauthorized, unprivileged disclosure to a third party of nonpublic patient medical information obtained via a physician-patient relationship. Disclosure to the law firm required consent of the patient.[2]

ity to access, transmit, and copy information quickly. As more individuals access computer-based patient information, the risk for abuse increases. As this risk increases, supervisors and software developers work to develop security systems that will decrease the risk of a breach of confidentiality.

However, any attempt to increase the security and confidentiality of health care information must balance the patient's right to privacy and confidentiality with the caregiver's need for information to safely and effectively provide care. To help endure the confidentiality and security of patient information, three approaches are generally used:

- Physical security
- Personnel security
- Security of the system

Physical Security

The **physical security** of electronic documentation systems is the need to protect information from being accessed by unauthorized persons. Some threats to the physical security of data include the following:

- *Poor placement of video displays and personal computers,* which may allow individuals to view confidential information. Video displays and other hardware must be placed so that caregivers can easily view and enter data without others being able to read information that may be confidential.
- *Theft of data storage devices,* such as a hard drive or other media containing data. Physical security measures must also consider the location of the stored data. The confidentiality of data stored in a personal computer can be breached simply by transferring the information to a diskette or CD-ROM or by picking up the computer and walking away. These risks can be minimized by utilizing the following methods:
  1. Transferring or storing data in a secure, remote location
  2. Disabling disk drives so that information cannot be copied
  3. Securing personal computers used for data storage to an immovable object to prevent theft
- *Damage to hardware or storage devices* by power surges, floods, fire, or even a spilled cup of coffee.

Personnel Security

Any security system is no better than the personnel who operate it. Effective **personnel security** procedures, including careful selection of employees who will have access to confidential information, can minimize the risk of breach of confidentiality. Once selected, employees who are authorized access to the electronic documentation system must be thoroughly trained. The training must include the following:

1. Description of procedures used to maintain confidentiality
2. Proper use of the system
3. Institutional policies mandating confidentiality of patient information
4. Disciplinary actions that are taken if a breach of patient confidentiality occurs

Completion of this training should be documented and usually includes a statement signed by the employee agreeing to maintain confidentiality of patient information and adhere to the institutional policies regarding the electronic documentation system.

Another method of increasing personnel security is the use of **passwords** or sign-on codes to prevent unauthorized individuals from accessing information contained in the electronic documentation system. Employees who do not have a valid password cannot enter or retrieve information in the electronic documentation system. Employees who do not have a need to use the system are not issued a password. Passwords also serve several other security functions. The password identifies users to the system and limits users to sections of the system that apply to their job functions. For example, a clerk's password will not allow him or her to document nursing care; a nurse's password will allow him or her to document the results of an x-ray examination. To further ensure that users do not jeopardize the confidentiality of data, software can be instructed to terminate the user's access to the system after a specified period of inactivity.

System Security

System security ties physical security and personnel security together to create a multilevel system that helps ensure that the information in the system is confidential and secure. System security measures typically include institutional policies that protect the system. The policies usually describe the following:

1. The type and amount of information that may be collected
2. The job classes of employees that may be given access to the system
3. Use of the password system, including issuing, tracking, and deletion of passwords

System security should also include protection from computer viruses, a reliable mechanism for backing up data, and routine monitoring of activities at high risk for a breach of security.

Encryption, the manipulation of data to prevent anyone but the intended recipient from reading that data, also helps prevent unauthorized individuals to access confidential information. To help detect unauthorized users who access a patient's record, most systems include an **audit trail** function that maintains a log of who accesses each record and when.

Integrity of Electronic Documentation

Maintaining the security and confidentiality of patient data and information is meaningless if the integrity of the electronic documentation is questioned. Is the information in the system what the users intended it to be? Has the data been altered? Who changed the information? Why? When? Being able to answer these questions will help determine if the information contained in the electronic documentation system is accurate.

The first consideration in maintaining the integrity of the data is ensuring that the

? | What Would You Do?

Student Confidentiality

As a school nurse, you have an ethical and professional responsibility regarding confidentiality of student information. You have recently been assigned a school in District A whose health records are computerized. You have discovered that a list of student health problems is circulated monthly to all the teachers in the school. You know that this list should be directed only to those staff members who have a need to know.

You have also learned that student information is transferred over the Internet and is not encrypted or encoded to prevent access by outside parties.

What should you do?

1. What are the potential legal liabilities?
2. What are the potential problems that may arise from these practices?

data is **authentic.** Electronic data is considered to be authentic when the data is the same as the individual originally entered into the system. This commonly means that the software provides an opportunity for the user to read the data before it is added to the patient's electronic documentation. Most systems achieve this by displaying the information for review before the information is accepted by the electronic documentation system. If the user is not satisfied with the data, changes and corrections can be made before the information is added to the patient's electronic patient record. In addition to the user's review of data, most systems also compare the data with a set of input requirements before accepting the data. This helps to ensure that those basic elements, such as the patient's identification, the date of a diagnostic procedure, required charting elements, and similar data, are included in entry. If the user identifies an error after the information is added to the record, an error removal mechanism with its resulting audit trail allows corrections to be made. Another element of data integrity is positive identification of the individual making the entry or retrieving data. On-line this is achieved by the user's password, which identifies the user to the system and attaches the user's name or initials to each of his or her activities in the system. Printouts identify the user with full name and license or initials based on the user's password. If initials are used to identify a user, the initials must be unique to one individual and a record kept of the individual identified by the initials.

Advantages of Electronic Documentation

There are numerous advantages of a well-designed, comprehensive electronic documentation system. It can:

- Save time and money.
- Improve the quality of care.
- Promote interdisciplinary care.

Increasing demands for detailed documentation have resulted in a significant increase in the time devoted to documentation. Caregivers are told, "If it is not charted, it was not done." This has resulted in some caregivers devoting approximately 30 to 50 percent of their time to documentation activities. Preformatted electronic documentation and standardized documentation has been reported to eliminate nurse overtime due to charting.[3] Time can also be saved when the input of a single piece of information initiates multiple activities. For example, documentation of the completion of a diagnostic test might result in the following:

- Charges for supplies or equipment used in the test are entered in the patient's bill.
- The type and number of activities completed are recorded for evaluation by management.
- The patient transport service is notified that the patient is ready to return to his or her room.

Prompt notification of the caregiver of abnormal test results by automatic printout can also save time by expediting alterations to the plan of care and reducing the time needed for a patient to respond to changes in care. On-line retrieval of diagnostic information can also save time by reducing the time used to place and answer phone calls to the various diagnostic departments.

Electronic documentation systems can also improve the quality of documentation. Software can prompt the user to include each of the items necessary for acceptable documentation of each aspect of care. Poor or illegible handwriting is not a concern with electronic documentation. Information contained in printouts and on-line retrievals are legible and organized by the software.

The quality of care the patient receives can also be improved when data are entered and stored in electronic documentation systems. The computerized format of the data allows analysis of the data to identify trends and identify the most effective approaches to care. Software that is instructed to remind users about potential problems can also improve the quality of care the patient receives when caregivers are notified of special aspects of the patient's care, such as a risk for falls, allergies, or handicaps that might not be obvious.

Electronic documentation systems can also promote interdisciplinary care and documentation when all caregivers use the same system for electronic documentation, discipline-specific forms are eliminated, and related data are grouped together regardless of discipline. For example, information obtained during discharge planning conferences can be documented by nurses, social workers, and physical or occupational therapists. However, all information will be automatically grouped together and printed under one heading, "Discharge Planning," regardless of the individual making the entry (Box 9–3).

BOX 9–3

Electronic Charting

Advantages

- Legibility is increased.
- Improves nursing productivity and decreases paperwork time.
- Reduces record tampering.
- Provides a graphical display of data.
- Supports the use of nursing process and individualization of patient assessment. Nursing diagnosis can be suggested by software, depending on findings.
- Decreases redundant documentation.
- Categorizes nursing notes according to nursing diagnosis.
- Automatically prints reports.
- Documentation is created according to standards of care.
- Knowledge of patient outcomes is improved by analyzing data in records.
- Recruitment and retention of nurses are improved.
- Availability of data for nursing research projects and aggregate information about patient outcomes or problem areas are increased.
- Allows basing charges on care delivered.
- Simultaneous use of patient's records is possible.

Disadvantages

Computerized patient records increase the potential for legal problems through:
- Accidental or intentional disclosure of private data to unauthorized individuals.
- Modification or destruction of patient records.
- Entering inaccurate information into the computer.
- Making clinical decisions based on the inaccurate information.[4]

Problems Associated with Electronic Documentation

One of the most common problems with electronic documentation is lack of commitment by the institution to the concept of electronic documentation. Without this commitment, documentation of care is fragmented. Some information is available on-line, other information might be found on a paper form used by one type of caregiver, and related information might be found on a different paper form used by a different type of caregiver. It becomes difficult, if not impossible, to determine exactly what care patients have received and how they responded to it. Lack of a consistent computer-based system makes it impossible to evaluate aggregate data and patient outcomes. Access to the system hardware is often a problem. There may not be enough terminals to meet the caregivers' needs. Hardware may not be located near the point of care or may be located in high-traffic areas, where it becomes difficult to concentrate on complete and accurate data entry. Any of these problems discourages use of the system and results in a loss of data. Access to data can be another problem. If today's data are only available when a printout is generated, users will not be able to make decisions and deliver care based on the most current information.

Once users have become accustomed to using the system, loss of the system through planned or unplanned computer downtime can result in a disruption of care and loss of information usually documented in the electronic documentation system. Well-designed backup procedures can help minimize, but not eliminate, users' responses to the loss of the system even for a relatively short period.

Implementation and use of an electronic documentation system can also be a problem. Successful system development and use require planning, cooperation, and communication among the multiple disciplines and multiple types of caregivers who document patient care and information. Many times these caregivers have never truly worked together. They are now faced with having to establish a common vocabulary, create working relationships, and learn how to understand the information (e.g., fall risk scores, types of allergic responses, different types of impairments) generated by different types of caregivers. This problem may be further complicated by failure of the institution's administration to provide adequate time and resources for these tasks.

Orientation time is usually increased in an electronic documentation system. Most caregivers are familiar with the use of paper forms and can usually decipher the use of the form after a brief review. This is not possible with an electronic documentation system. Documentation displays are not stacked on a shelf. They are hidden in the computer, available only to those who know how and where to find them. For some it is like searching for an invisible needle in an electronic haystack.

Although most systems provide at least one mechanism for review and verification of data before it is added to the patient record, errors occur in the electronic record. These errors may never be discovered and corrected. Failure to trust the electronic documentation system, either on the part of administration or on the part of the bedside caregiver, can result in duplicate charting—once in the computer and once on paper. When questioned about the reason for this time-consuming pattern, the usual response is "just in case something happens to the computer."

The Future of Electronic Documentation

To reach the potential that electronic documentation offers to health care professionals, standards for electronic documentation of health care information have to be developed and implemented. The federal government and private enterprise have

---

BOX 9–4

Proposed Data Sets

Uniform clinical data set
Nursing minimum data set
Uniform hospital discharge data set
Ambulatory medical care minimum data set
Health professional minimum data set
Uniform data set for home care and hospice

---

proposed a number of standards (Box 9–4). None of the proposed standards has gained widespread acceptance, and none meets the diverse needs of all types of care-givers. Data standards, common definitions of terms, and computer languages and software that permit the transfer of aggregate data to others, such as health care payers, governmental agencies and regulatory bodies, will help electronic documenta-tion move toward a unified computer-based patient record (Box 9–5). This will allow large bodies of data to be analyzed to identify clinically effective approaches to care, care based on research, not based on habit or intuition.

A computer-based patient record also benefits the individual patient. A single record contains information about each contact with a health care provider, including the patient's past and present health problems, and may minimize the risks that one caregiver may overlook a significant problem not usually associated with his or her specialty. The CPR will also minimize or eliminate duplicate requests for the same information from the patient, a problem that can cause the patient to question the information available to the caregiver and the decisions he or she makes.

BOX 9–5

Elements of the Computer-Based Patient Record

Multidisciplinary problem list
Measures of health status
Documentation of clinical reasoning
Linkages to other health care providers
Protection from unauthorized access
Support for continuous access
Support for surveillance and multiuser views
Support for other clinical resources
Facilitation of clinical problem-solving supports direct data input by the physi-cian
Support management of patient care
Flexibility and expandability

KEEP IN MIND

▶ Electronic documentation uses computer hardware and software.
▶ Security and confidentiality are the biggest problems that electronic documentation presents to the user.
▶ Three approaches used to ensure security and confidentiality are physical security, personnel security, and system security.
▶ The advantages of electronic documentation outweigh the disadvantages.
▶ The advantages of electronic documentation include reduced paperwork, elimination of lost or misplaced files, improved access to authorized users, quicker turn-around time for providing records, increased security measures, improved cost efficiency, enhanced quality of care, and promotion of interdisciplinary care.
▶ The disadvantages of electronic documentation include potential claims of security breaches or breaches of confidentiality; lack of total commitment by an institution to the concept of electronic documentation, leading to fragmented patient documentation (some on paper and some in electronic format); difficulty in accessing system hardware; difficulty in evaluating aggregate data and patient outcomes; and problematic implementation and use if not properly planned and staff not adequately trained.

IN A NUTSHELL

The wave of the future is electronic documentation. Although this format has many advantages, one of the greatest concerns is a breach of confidentiality. Therefore, to avoid ethical breaches and litigation based on breaches of confidentiality by providing unauthorized access to a patient's records, clear and specific policies and procedures must be created and used by health care providers.

AFTERTHOUGHTS

1. Discuss the advantages of electronic charting.
2. Discuss the disadvantages of electronic charting.
3. What are three ways to protect patient confidentiality when using electronic charting?
4. Describe a scenario showing how a health care provider can breach patient or student confidentiality when using electronic charting.
5. What are the necessary components needed to use electronic charting?
6. Find a case involving confidentiality and electronic charting. Discuss the case with the class.
7. What are some things that you feel should be changed in your current system of charting to provide a more thorough, efficient, and confidential way of charting?

ETHICS IN PRACTICE

You are working an 11:00 PM to 7:00 AM shift on a unit that you have been floated to because of short staffing. Tonight is unusually slow, and you notice that the other nurse appears to be on the computer for a long time. You ask her what is she doing as you walk over to the computer. You see that the screen the nurse is viewing has the human immunodeficiency virus (HIV) test results of a surgeon who is on staff at your hospital. She quickly shuts the computer down and wanders off "to check on patients." A month later the rumors that Dr. Smith has acquired immunodeficiency syndrome (AIDS) has circulated throughout the hospital and community because of a "leak" about test results from a recent hospitalization.

What would you do?

1. Do you report what you saw?
2. What legal implications can occur because of a breach of confidentiality?
3. What ethical principles are involved?
4. Should you have reported the nurse a month ago?
5. What are the policies and procedures in your institution regarding this type of scenario?

References

1. American Hospital Association, Patient's Bill of Rights, http://www.hospitalconnect.com/.
2. Biddle et al. v. Warren General Hospital et al., 86 Ohio St. 3d 395 715 N.E. 2d 518 (9/15/1999).
3. Eclipsys: Real-World Examples from our Customers, http://www.eclipsnet.com.
4. Gobis, LJ et al: Bedside computers and confidentiality. Am J Nursing 95(10):75–76, 1995.

Resources

Dick, RS, Steen, EB, and Detmer, DE, Committee on Improving the Patient Record, Institute of Medicine: The Computer-based Patient Record: An Essential Technology for Health Care. National Academy Press, Washington, DC, 1997.

Schwab, NC, Panettieri, MJ, and Berfen, MD: Guidelines for School Nurse Documentation: Standards, Issues and Models, ed 2. National Association of School Nurses, Scarborough, Maine, 1998.

Tomes, JP: Confidentiality of Electronic Medical Records. Heritage Professional Education, Nashville, 1998.

Associations:

The Centers for Medicare & Medicaid Services (CMS)
http://cms.hhs.gov

American School Health Association
Guidelines for Protecting Confidential Student Health Information
http://www.ashaweb.org.

Risk Management 10

Tamela Esham, RN, JD

Key Chapter Concepts

Quality assurance

Risk

Risk management

Risk control

Loss control

Loss prevention

Transfer of risk

"Hold harmless" clause

Subrogation clause

Risk financing

Risk retention

Self-insurance

Going bare

Compliance

Utilization review (UR) process

Peer review

Immunity

Chapter Thoughts

The health care professions in general and nursing in particular focus on curing disease, prolonging or increasing quality of life, and helping patients reach their highest level of functioning. In recent years, this mindset has become formalized into what is called quality assurance. **Quality assurance** evaluates the role of the health care provider with the purpose of reaching as high a standard of care as possible. From the quality assurance viewpoint, the health care institution looks for patterns of care that are less than optimal, or recurring events that diminish the level of care, and then tries to correct them to increase the standard of care.

The idea of quality assurance is built squarely on the ethical principle of benef-icence—that is, doing good for the patient. Although the term *good* has a number of meanings, in the health care setting it is understood to mean provid-ing the best quality and highest standard of care possible. This level of care goes beyond the minimal standard of care that the law generally requires in a defense against a lawsuit.

The legal parallel to quality assurance is risk management. From the ethical viewpoint, risk management is a much narrower and more limited concept. The primary goal of risk management is to identify areas where lawsuits can occur and keep financial losses to a minimum. Risk management usually focuses on individual incidents. Whereas insurance companies use the concept of risk management to reduce their financial losses, facilities apply the same concept to prevent injury, disability, or death to patients and employees by anticipating and preventing accidents. Again, the primary goal is to reduce monetary losses rather than increase the quality of the care being provided.

Quality assurance and risk management overlap in the health care setting. Both involve the general safety aspects of the institution. Many health care providers have both safety committees (risk management) and quality control committees (quality assurance). Whereas the safety committee is usually chaired by an engineer and the quality control committee by a registered nurse, the information developed by both committees is often similar. Sharing this information with each other goes a long way to improving the overall safety of the institution.

OBJECTIVES

Upon completing this chapter, the reader will be able to:
1. Describe risk management.
2. Describe types of risks.
3. Distinguish among risk, injury, and loss.
4. Identify six examples of reportable incidents.
5. Discuss loss prevention.
6. Describe three loss prevention techniques.
7. Describe loss reduction.
8. Describe techniques for accomplishing loss reduction.

Introduction

Risk is the possibility of suffering harm or loss. In health care settings over the years, managing risk has evolved from simply purchasing insurance for financial coverage of losses to a complex, coordinated effort of preventing and controlling loss.[1]

The primary focus of many risk management programs is the risk of a patient suffering an injury in the health care setting and making a claim against the health care organization. The costs associated with the patient's claim are regarded as losses to the health care organization. Many other risks exist as well, including the risks of injury to staff, visitors, and vendors and the risk of property damage.

Risk management refers to a comprehensive plan that identifies, evaluates, analyzes, eliminates, reduces, and monitors risks that may lead to patient or employee injuries or that could result in financial losses or legal liability. The primary goal of risk management is to decrease the incidence of adverse outcomes, legal liability, and financial loss and to minimize loss from malpractice and other civil claims.[2]

Techniques of Risk Management

Risk management techniques fall into two categories: risk control and risk financing. **Risk control** consists of risk avoidance, loss control, and transfer of risk.

Risk Avoidance

Because most health care activities carry some element of risk, risk avoidance could require as drastic a solution as simply ceasing an activity. For example, the only way to completely avoid the risks associated with obstetric deliveries is to eliminate the services.

Loss Control

Loss control includes loss prevention, or controlling the frequency of loss, such as requiring and monitoring the use of side rails on the beds of frail patients. Loss reduction, or minimizing the magnitude of the loss, is another type of loss control. Early intervention and communication with a patient and a patient's family following an incident such as a fall is one way of attempting to reduce losses by minimizing the likelihood of a lawsuit.

Loss Prevention

Loss prevention techniques should serve two purposes—to decrease the incidence of injury to patients and to reduce financial loss for the health care organization.

The real challenge of risk management is not insuring against losses but preventing them in the first place. Risk management must be a continuous process that is not possible without the cooperation of all disciplines within the health care institutions.[3]

Even when an avoidable injury occurs in the course of treatment (an iatrogenic injury), there is no loss to the health care provider if the injured patient does not make a claim for compensation.[4] As an American Hospital Association official said, "Happy patients don't sue."

Studies have shown that most injured patients do not file malpractice claims. Conversely, many patients who file malpractice claims have not suffered an injury.[5] There are important lessons in these facts. Patients may sue a health care provider simply because they feel they had a bad experience in health care. The perception of a bad experience may be well founded when an avoidable injury has occurred, but it may also be based on anger at the physicians or nurses for failing to communicate or for seeming too rushed and uncaring.

J. E. Orlikoff, who has written extensively on risk management, points out that communication difficulties or perceived difficulties can stem from time constraints (i.e., too many patients and not enough time to really "talk") and from the different expectations of patients and professionals regarding the same interaction in a health care setting.

Expanding on this theory, Orlikoff emphasizes that, in addition to the patient's social expectations, there are specific patient needs that health care providers may fail to meet. First is the patient's need to "retain a sense of control over such personal variables as time, body, food, and hygiene, as well as the management of the medical problem."[6] Second is the patient's need to retain a sense of self-worth or dignity while interacting with health care providers. This need is not met if the health care provider views the patient in terms of a diagnosis (e.g., as the gallbladder case in Room 203), instead of in terms compatible with the patient's view of self (e.g., the professor, the parent, the artist).[7]

Nurses can dignify patients by learning how they define themselves and by finding out what their lives are like. Unless the patient has a unique identity to the health care provider, it will be difficult for the patient's dignity to be fully respected.

One obvious method of preserving a sense of dignity and of control is permitting the patient to have privacy, which is another patient need often not met in a health care setting. "An individual needs to maintain a discreet distance from others in matters he or she regards as personal or confidential."[8] Privacy may be difficult to maintain in a health care setting with large numbers of patients and staff. However, simply acknowledging that privacy is important and that the staff will do its best to protect it may prevent a patient from feeling "violated" by the constant intrusions.

Communication can be improved and patients' needs met by recognizing and overcoming these barriers:

1. Health care settings can be frightening and intimidating.
2. Patient independence is often sacrificed.
3. Patients can be confused, frightened, and isolated by the medical jargon used in a health care setting.
4. "Closed" questions asked by a health care provider (i.e., those that demand a limited response) may leave the patient feeling controlled or manipulated.
5. Health care providers "tend not to use 'social cement' [greetings, introductions, laughter, use of patient's name, social touching] when interacting with patients."[9]

Communication skills must be learned and applied by professional nurses in their patient interaction. In addition, the professional nurse will be called on to play a role in educating other staff about appropriate and positive communication with patients.

Transfer of Risk

Transfer of risk is an agreement that specifies that someone else is responsible for paying for a particular loss for the health care organization. Transfer of risk by contract is achieved by **"hold harmless" clauses,** which indicate that one party to the contract agrees to hold the other "harmless" in the event of injury or loss. A **subrogation clause** in the agreement states that one party promises to substitute in the place of the other if a legal claim is brought. Often, contractual clauses require that the contracting individuals have insurance to cover a particular loss or type of loss.[10] For example, when a facility contracts with a physician to provide services, the physician may agree to hold the facility harmless for injuries caused by the physician's care. A subrogation clause may designate that the physician will substitute in the event the physician's assistant is sued.

Risk Financing

Risk financing is another method of transferring risk that involves insurance contracts. For a stipulated amount of money (premium), one party agrees to compensate the other for loss in a specified area of risk. However, an insurance policy is "merely a private contract transferring financial responsibility; it cannot transfer legal responsibility. If the insurer fails to pay, the insured retains its responsibility to the claimant."[11]

Risk is financed either through the purchase of insurance or by risk retention. **Risk retention** is a decision to fund a risk internally—that is, to pay claims out of a business's assets or proceeds. Partial risk retention results from a decision to fund a portion of a loss internally—for example, to pay deductibles out of the business proceeds or assets and to insure the remainder of the loss.

Self-insurance is a formalized risk retention plan, which sets aside specific amounts of money to fund certain risks. For example, many facilities are self-insured to cover liability and risks of potential lawsuits.

Going bare is a decision to retain the risk but without identifying funding to pay potential claims.[12] For instance, a nurse practitioner who fails to renew professional liability insurance policy has no coverage if sued for negligence and is "going bare." Historically the attitude of many nurses was, "If I don't have malpractice insurance I am less likely to get sued. And if I am sued the claimant won't get anything." Fortunately, nurses have become aware of the fallacy behind this "going bare" philosophy. The claimant can be awarded money from the facility if the nurse is employed by it. The facility can then sue for indemnification. Also, although it rarely happens, the nurse's wages might be garnisheed, and personal assets can be at risk.

The nurse is essentially the front line of risk management in any health care setting. The nurse's primary contribution to risk management is in loss prevention and loss reduction. The techniques and principles discussed are applicable in all health care settings, including hospitals, nursing homes, ambulatory care centers, home health agencies, hospices, dialysis units, and so on. These entities are referred to collectively as health care organizations or health care providers.

Quality Patient Care: A Priority and a Challenge

The greatest challenge facing nurses in managed care organizations is their ability to meet the organizational demands of managed care, of providing quality care in a cost-contained environment while providing quality patient care that meets the applicable standard of care. Nurses must stay focused on their primary roles in the health care system, that of patient advocate and patient caregiver. If they fail to do so, they will contribute to the current trend of allowing patient and quality care issues to become lost in the chaotic health care environment, thereby increasing their own liability risks. As such, nurses must take a tough collective stance to ensure that the primary focus of health care remains quality patient care by taking leadership roles in committees and organizations that emphasize patient care issues.

The Nurse's Role in Risk Management

Nurses play a key role in the success of risk management programs because they have unique skills that allow them the opportunity to identify potential risk areas and determine which situations may be detrimental to patients. Nurses can use their expertise, knowledge, and skills to develop programs designed to reduce liability for nurses. Nurses can use their research and administrative skills to gather pertinent data and develop policies, procedures, and practice guidelines that would substantially decrease the risks in known high-risk practice areas. Nurses' assessments, investigative, and practice skills are invaluable in reviewing safety procedures, incident reports, and patient care to develop programs to reduce liability for nurses.

As a result, nurses can develop and implement policies and procedures that ensure that the goals of a risk management program are successfully met and that patients receive safe, quality care.

Compliance with Policies and Procedures

Compliance with a health care organization's policies and procedures can (1) prevent loss, (2) reduce loss from legal claims, and (3) reduce loss from costs related to noncompliance with regulatory requirements.

Other Benefits of Compliance

Besides reducing loss, policies and procedures in health care settings are developed for several purposes, including to provide structure and control to the organization's operation and to give guidance to employees about workplace expectations and about standards of practice in caring for patients. Compliance with policies and procedures ensures a safe environment, enhances appropriate employee and public interaction, and promotes quality patient care. As an added benefit, compliance also reduces incidents and injuries and successful claims against the health care organization.

Policies and procedures also help to ensure compliance with statutory and regulatory mandates. For instance, they may be developed to parallel and thereby ensure compliance with federal requirements such as the Environmental Protection Agency's protocol for disposal of hazardous medical waste or the Occupational Safety and Health Administration's requirements for preventing or managing exposure to hepatitis and human immunodeficiency virus (HIV). In addition, in a health care setting, policies and procedures are developed to meet state licensure requirements, for participation in the Medicare and Medicaid programs, and for accreditation by organizations such as the Joint Commission on Accreditation of Healthcare Organizations (JCAHO).

The underlying purpose of regulatory standards and policies and procedures implemented pursuant to them is maintaining quality care for health care patients. In addition, these standards are imposed to protect the health and safety of employees. Compliance with the standard in infection control policies and procedures, for instance, protects patients from nosocomial infections (infections acquired in a health care facility) and protects employees from occupational exposure to infections such as hepatitis B and HIV. A patient who contracts an infection from another patient or from an employee because the employee failed to follow proper infection control procedures may file a civil claim for negligence, incurring substantial loss for the employer. Likewise, if an employee is infected through occupational exposure, the employee may make a workman's compensation claim, also resulting in substantial loss to the employer.

Consequences of Noncompliance

Policies and procedures responsive to these regulatory requirements, as well as those developed independently of regulations, set standards against which a health care organization is judged. As discussed in previous chapters, breach of a standard of care can lead to liability for the organization or for the individual professional. Breaches of an organization's policies and procedures can lead to loss from liability claims made by patients, employees, contractors providing services for the organization, or members of the public, such as hospital visitors, because the policies help define the standard of care.

In addition to liability, noncompliance with policies and procedures can lead to losses because of actions taken by regulators, reimbursers, and accreditors. Health care entities are continuously surveyed (or inspected) by state health departments for compliance with licensure and Medicaid reimbursement standards, by the Health Care Financing Administration (HCFA) for compliance with conditions of participation in the Medicare program, and by JCAHO for compliance with its accreditation standards. Noncompliance with requirements can lead to the revocation of a provider's license or termination of reimbursement and may pose a risk to a provider's financing.

Many health care providers are largely dependent on revenues from Medicare and Medicaid. Termination of participation in those programs for noncompliance with program standards can threaten the very existence of the provider. As a condition for issuance of loans or bonds, banks may also require that a health care organization be licensed, accredited, and Medicare certified. In addition to the direct loss of income and risk to financing, the increased regulatory scrutiny and legal appeals are costly and can result in dramatic losses to a health care entity.

Ensuring Compliance

Monitoring compliance with policies and procedures becomes the responsibility of all employees. The professional nurse must not only learn and follow policies and procedures, but must also assist in enforcement of these standards. Every nurse should be responsible for making sure that infractions are corrected and compliance is observed.

When it is apparent that a policy and procedure is obsolete and is not being followed, the professional nurse should see that it is updated. Risk is increased when policies and procedures do not accurately reflect current and appropriate practice. When the standard of care set forth in writing is not followed in practice, a potential plaintiff can make a claim based on a provider's deviation from its own standard, even if the "deviant" practice is more appropriate to current technology and knowledge.

Statutory Reporting Duties

Along with regulatory requirements, which set forth standards of practice, are statutory and regulatory reporting requirements. Nurses are expected to report to regulatory agencies when standards are not followed. For instance, many state agencies require reporting suspected patient abuse or neglect, and most state licensure boards require that licensed nurses report professional breaches of the standard of practice that could result in action by the licensure board (for example, giving patient care while intoxicated or performing a task beyond the scope of the nurse's license). Failure to make such a report not only increases the risk of injury to a patient or fellow employee but may also jeopardize the license of the observing nurse. The observation of reportable incidents first should be reported within the hierarchy of the nursing administration. Then a determination can be made regarding who will make the report of the incident to the regulating agency. Also, federal laws such as the Health Care Insurance Portability and Accountability Act of 1996 (HIPAA) establish privacy and security standards to protect and promote standardized electronic transmission of health care, financial, and administrative transactions. The federal regulations establish a uniform minimum standard of privacy and confidentiality protection. The main purpose is to provide accessible health information but protect unauthorized use and disclosure for non–health-related reasons.

Incident Reporting

Another goal of risk management, aside from prevention of injuries, is to reduce loss once an incident has occurred. Losses can be reduced by quick and careful response. Because communication with the people involved is essential, all health care staff must be alert and report information from patients, family members, visitors, and employees whenever a problem or potential for a claim is indicated. Complete and accurate information is vital for those responsible for managing an investigation and response to an incident.

A CASE IN POINT

The Hospital's Duty to Protect the Patient

The Facts

A physician carved his initials in a patient's abdomen after performing a caesarean section on her. Another surgeon mistakenly removed a healthy kidney instead of a cancerous one, resulting in death of the patient. Is the hospital responsible for these physicians' actions?

The Decision

In each case the state Department of Health concluded that the hospitals involved violated legal requirements for reporting such incidences to the Health Department, in addition to having serious lapses in medical care for the patients.[13]

The variance, incident, or occurrence report is a tool used by almost every health care organization to alert the administration to situations that are out of the ordinary in the facility's operation. Although a reportable incident is often concerned with the care of a patient, incidents may also involve employees or visitors.

Each organization has guidelines that define a reportable incident. All employees should know and follow these guidelines. Examples of reportable patient care incidents include patient falls, errors in medication administration (wrong medication, wrong dosage, wrong patient), and complaints by family members that their loved one is not receiving adequate care. (See Box 10–1 for examples of reportable incidents.) Other examples of reportable incidents include injury or potential injury related to equipment failure, treatment-related incidents such as reactions to radio-opaque dyes injected for x-ray examinations, reactions or errors related to transfusions or intravenous therapy, and missed or incorrect diagnoses. An example of a reportable

---

BOX 10–1

Examples of Reportable Patient Care Incidents

1. Patient falls
2. Medication errors
3. Family complaints about inadequate patient care
4. Injury related to equipment failure
5. Treatment-related incidents, such as reactions
6. Missed or incorrect diagnoses

? What Would You Do?

You are a new nurse on a unit. Several reportable incidents have occurred involving patient injury, including a patient fall and medication errors.

Although they were not your patients, you notice that no reports were made to the physician, nor were incident reports written by Betty Moiswitz, RN.

Betty, who is a "friend" of the supervisor, Fred, just ignores you when you ask if she called the doctor to report the incidences.

What should you do?

1. What are the legal implications for Betty, Fred, and you?
2. What are the ethical implications for Betty, Fred, and you?
3. What are the potential reasons for disciplinary action?

incident related to an employee is exposure to blood or body fluids resulting in the potential transmission of infection (e.g., HIV or hepatitis).

Employees should be familiar with report procedures and forms. In some settings the initial report may be oral. The risk manager may then conduct an investigation of the incident and develop a report addressed to, or with the assistance of, the health care organization's legal counsel.

AUTHOR TIP: *Reports should document only facts describing the circumstances around the incident. For example, if the nurse finds the patient on the floor, the chart should read "Pt. found on floor," not "Pt. fell out of bed," which is an assumption, not a fact, because the nurse was not a witness to the incident. The staff should not draw conclusions about cause or fault, such as "The nurse failed to check the patient's identification band and administered the dosage to the wrong patient." The nurse should not document impressions, such as "The patient was stubborn and uncooperative, and the nurse became angry."*

Health care organizations also have guidelines regarding the timing and routing of an incident report. The report may be made first to a department head or unit coordinator, who then reports to the risk management team. Generally it is important that the information reach the risk manager soon after the incident; often this is required to be within 24 hours. See Box 10-2 for advice on reducing damage after an incident.

Finally, the risk manager should identify causes contributing to the incident and develop mechanisms to prevent future incidents. New policies and procedures may be developed and in-service education provided. Most importantly, once change has been implemented, facilities should create systems to monitor compliance with the new procedures.

Confidentiality of Incident Reports

Accurate information about an incident must be documented for internal use. However, protecting information from discovery by a plaintiff in a lawsuit is a universal concern.

BOX 10–2

Damage Control

When an incident is reported to the risk management department, the responsible individual is likely to undertake some, or all, of the following activities to investigate and "manage" the risk related to the incident:

1. Review the medical records for possible deviations from acceptable standards of care.
2. Request and review records from other facilities where the patient has received care.
3. Obtain an "expert" review of the care provided to the patient.
4. Secure any equipment involved in the incident, so that its condition can be evaluated and maintained for evidence.
5. Assess whether an incident actually led to injury or whether the complaint has any merit.
6. Assess damage resulting from the injury and evaluate whether a prolonged stay or additional treatment was required as a result of an injury and whether the injury is temporary or permanent.
7. Conduct interviews of individuals involved in the incident and of any witnesses to the incident.
8. Advise and counsel the patient and family about the incident.
9. Evaluate the patient's and the family's responses to the incident and their general responses to the staff and the care received.
10. Identify the need for and obtain, where appropriate, consultants to serve as support for the patient and family.
11. Notify administrators, attorneys, and insurers.
12. Assist in planning any public response in the event of potential adverse publicity surrounding the incident.
13. Assist administration in deciding whether to forgive outstanding amounts owed to the facility by the patient.
14. Conduct or participate in settlement discussions.
15. Monitor litigation.[14]

In some states, incident reports may be protected from discovery as attorney work product. Under the attorney-client privilege of confidentiality, any type of document created during an attorney-client relationship is considered to be attorney work product. For example, in a lawsuit, reports or memos created to prepare for litigation are attorney work product.

In other states, courts may allow a plaintiff to have access to the incident report if it was not created in a format that would afford it protection.

To protect it from discovery, the report may be addressed to the attorney or may include the attorney's legal impression of the incident.

Health care organizations usually take into account the state laws when developing guidelines, so that the confidentiality of incident reports is protected. Some typical protective strategies include not referring to the incident report in the medical record and not including it as part of the medical record, because plaintiffs always have access to their own medical records.

Maintaining confidentiality of information in the report is of paramount importance. During the investigation of any incident, risk managers and staff involved in an incident obtain confidential information about the patient and perhaps the staff. Discussions about the incident should be limited to the few designated individuals with a need to know. In conducting investigatory interviews, the interviewer should seek information, not share it. The temptation to share the dramatic facts with friends or family must be resisted. In fact, inappropriate sharing of confidential information could become an incident that causes a lawsuit in and of itself. Successful claims for breach of patient (or staff) confidentiality are increasing, as are invasion of privacy claims (mentioned in Chapter 6).

Utilization Review Process: Peer Review

Utilization review (UR) process is a process whereby personnel trained in specialty disciplines evaluate appropriateness, quality, and medical necessity for services recommended.

In most UR processes, nonphysicians (e.g., nurses and social workers) evaluate the case and refer to a physician reviewer if they believe there is no medical necessity for the recommended treatment.

If the physician still believes that there is no medical necessity after discussions with the treatment provider, the care provider is notified of the denial.

The provider can then appeal the denial. Areas that are reviewed and considered during the appeals process include the following:

1. Consultation: Was a consultation held with the treating physician by the UR committee prior to denial?
2. Medical records: Were all necessary records obtained?
3. Independent examination (IME) by a physician: Was an IME arranged if the reviewing party disagreed with the treating provider's recommendation?
4. Review: Were the records reviewed by the appropriate UR specialist?[15]

Liability

Liability exposure due to an oversight may occur if a credentialing program fails to ensure the use of qualified providers or if the UR process affects the treating physician's medical judgment.

Other areas of liability include direct liability of managed care organizations (MCOs), by using cost containment measures, such as improper denial of care or treatment or provider financial incentives that affect patient outcome; failure to properly credential plan providers (e.g., evaluating education, experience, training, and so on); and fraud, breach of contract, bad faith, or misrepresentation by MCOs.

Enterprise liability (strict liability) against MCOs is a recent theory based on the fact that the MCOs have more power than consumer patients, the risk to the MCO is spread by insurance, and the cost of safety is a production cost to the MCO.

Peer Review

Peer review is a method of monitoring and evaluating patient care by the facility's practicing health care providers. Peer review services by the Health Care Financing Administration (HCFA) are medical necessities, reasonable, and within appropriate standards.[16] In addition to evaluating the group of health care providers, individuals' performances may also be scrutinized and assessed, which can result in restriction of privileges or termination. Also, upon completion of the evaluation, the health care providers may be reported to the National Practitioner Data Bank or other entities such as the National Council of State Boards of Nursing Data Bank.

Immunity

In many states, **immunity** from civil suits is provided to individuals who participate in the peer review process because the goal of the process is to improve quality, improve patient outcomes, and reduce patient morbidity and mortality.

Quality Assurance

Quality assurance is a sequential process that involves setting standards of care, measuring patient care according to those standards, gathering data from chart review, observing patient care, interviewing patient caregivers, and then making recommendations for improvement.

To ensure quality patient care, nursing care must be assessed in terms of efficiency, content, resources, and outcomes. Quality assurance programs serve as a tool for the following:

1. Identifying areas of improvement in patient care
2. Reducing liability risks for the nurse
3. Advancing the goals of nursing practice

The Nurse's Role in Quality Assurance Programs

The nurse's role in quality assurance programs focuses on the evaluation of patient care. Nurses must implement programs in their individual areas of practice to monitor patient care and the outcomes of that care to determine if patients are receiving quality nursing. This is essential to reduce the liability risks for nursing.

In today's litigious society, it is imperative that nurses make a collaborative effort to monitor and assess nursing care to ascertain that it is within the applicable standard of care. Quality assurance programs allow nurses to monitor nursing care in a nonthreatening environment. It allows nurses to utilize their assessment and problem-solving skills to identify and solve quality or production problems. In turn, an efficient plan of care can be implemented that ensures quality patient care and decreases liability risks for the professional nurse.

KEEP IN MIND

▶ Risk management involves identifying areas of potential liability and developing techniques to prevent and reduce loss.
▶ Nurses in health care organizations are uniquely situated to contribute to loss prevention and loss reduction.
▶ Loss prevention includes decreasing the incidence of injury, as well as preventing claims resulting from injury.
▶ Loss prevention techniques include optimal patient communication, compliance with policies and procedures, and contemporaneous, accurate documentation of care.
▶ Loss reduction includes careful incident identification, investigation, reporting, and follow-up.
▶ Confidentiality of patient and incident information is essential to an effective risk management program.

IN A NUTSHELL

Quality assurance and risk management are important tools used in the health care setting to reduce risks and improve the health care provided to patients.

Different techniques, such as risk control, loss avoidance, loss control, and loss prevention, are used in risk management in various settings depending on the circumstances. As a health care provider, the nurse plays an instrumental role in proposing, creating, implementing, and improving quality assurance and risk management techniques that affect the patient.

AFTERTHOUGHTS

1. Describe three types of risk in a health care setting.
2. Discuss the elements of risk control.
3. Discuss and compare loss prevention and loss control.
4. Discuss the relationship between documentation and loss prevention.

5. Give examples of how risk is transferred.

6. What is the law in your state with regard to incident or occurrence reports? Are the reports discoverable by plaintiffs?

7. Discuss damage control techniques that can be used by you in a facility setting.

8. Discuss the guidelines for reporting an incident at a local facility.

9. Discuss the goals of risk management.

10. Discuss the goals of risk management in contrast to those of quality assurance.

11. Name some of the consequences of noncompliance with facility policies and procedures.

12. What is the utilization review process?

13. Discuss how the UR process works in your facility. List the good and bad points. How can the process be made better?

14. Discuss how the peer review process can be a risk management tool.

15. What is the mechanism for determining "medical necessity" of a treatment or procedure? Contact providers and discuss with managed care organizations.

16. Discuss areas of liability involving managed care organizations.

ETHICS IN PRACTICE

Mrs. Debbie D., 24 years old, was finally in the delivery room of a large city hospital. She had been in labor for almost 10 hours with her first pregnancy. The labor had been long and difficult to this point, but Debbie felt excited that she was about to deliver.

Dr. P., an obstetrician, noted that Debbie had a constrictive band of muscle tissue in her cervix that was making the delivery difficult. He made an incision through the muscle tissue to relieve the constriction. A short time later, she delivered a 7-pound baby girl. After the delivery, Dr. P. forgot to suture the incision he had made in the cervical muscle tissue.

Debbie was sent to the postpartum unit for recovery care and observation. Trudi F., registered nurse (RN), who was caring for Debbie, noted that there was a larger than normal amount of vaginal bleeding. She called Dr. P. three times, but he assured Trudi each time that the bleeding was normal with such a difficult labor and delivery and that she should not worry about it.

Debbie's blood pressure continued to drop, her pulse rate increased, and she began to show signs of hypovolemic shock. Trudi wanted to call Dr. P. again but was afraid to because of what he had said the last three times she called him.

What would be the best course of action in this situation? What are the legal and ethical implications? Where does risk management come into play here?

References

1. Dellinger, AM (ed): Legal Issues in Facility Management. Diosegy, A: Risk Management. Little Brown, Boston, §5.1, p 390, citing Orlikoff, J, Fifer, W, and Greeley, H: Malpractice Prevention and Liability Control for Hospitals, 1981, pp 28–29.
2. Taber's Cyclopedic Medical Dictionary, ed 19. FA Davis, Philadelphia, 2001.
3. O'Keefe, ME: Nursing Practice and the Law: Avoiding Malpractice and Other Legal Risks. FA Davis, Philadelphia, 2001, p 500.
4. Ibid.
5. See, for example, Collins, L: 20 years of growth: professional risk management emerges. Business Insurance, October 26, 1987, p 4.
6. Sielicki, AP, Jr: Current philosophy of risk management. Topics Health Care Financing (Spring): 4, 1983.
7. Ibid., 5.
8. Dellinger, 396.
9. Orlikoff, JE, with Vanagunas, AM: Malpractice Prevention and Liability Control for Hospitals, ed 2. American Hospital Association, Chicago, 1988, p 32.
10. Sielicki, 4.
11. Ibid., 4–5.
12. Ibid., 5.
13. Serbakoli, F: Hospitals' Duty to Report Patient Harm, http://consumer.pub.findlaw.com/, March 2000.
14. Youngberg, EJ: Quality risk & management in health care. Aspen Publishing, Gaithersburg Md, 1991. In Youngberg, EJ, and Kuhn, MA: Introduction to Risk Management, vol 1, p 3.
15. Brent, N: Nurses and the Law: A Guide to Principles and Applications, ed 2. WB Saunders, Philadelphia, 2001.
16. Ibid.

Informed Consent 11

Key Chapter Concepts

Informed consent

Consent to treatment forms

Capacity

Decision-making capacity

Durable power of attorney statutes

Minor

Emancipated minor

Mature minor

Expressed consent

Implied consent

Duty to disclose

Medical community standard

Prudent patient or material risk standard

Medical disclosure panel

Subjective standard

Objective standard

Advance directive

Living will

Durable power of attorney for health care

Patient Self-Determination Act of 1990

Chapter Thoughts

The term *informed consent* has become a buzzword for the legal system in relation to the provision of today's high-tech, lifesaving, and life-prolonging health care. Simply defined, **informed consent** is the voluntary permission that a patient or patient's legal representative (who know the risks involved) gives to the health care provider to do something to or for that patient.

The legal intricacies of determining the presence of informed consent have led to a number of successful civil suits against health care practitioners and institutions. The underlying ethical principles on which informed consent are based are often lost in the legal maneuvering that surrounds these civil suits.

Informed consent is based on two key ethical principles: autonomy and beneficence. As defined earlier, autonomy is the right of patients to determine how much and what type of health care they want to receive. It is directly opposed to the practice of paternalism, which is the general attitude that health care providers know what the best treatments are for the patient, with or without the patient's approval. From the ethical viewpoint of autonomy, informed consent becomes a process of giving the power of choice to patients by respecting their decisions and providing them with the information they need to make decisions about their own health care.

The ethical principle of beneficence should underlie all aspects of health care and should be an elemental part of the health provider's philosophy of health care. The principle of beneficence demands that the health care provider do good for patients. The principle focuses on the patient's physical and mental well-being. A secondary "good" that arises from informed consent is that the patient is more likely to cooperate with the treatment plan, communicate better with the health care providers, and, if possible, recover more quickly. If recovery is not possible, then perhaps the patient is allowed to die with some level of dignity.

OBJECTIVES

Upon completing this chapter, the reader will be able to:

1. Define and explain the basic elements of informed consent.
2. Define capacity as it relates to a patient's right to accept or refuse medical treatment.
3. In relation to informed consent, explain the difference between (a) an objective standard and (b) a subjective standard.
4. Describe situations in which consent to treat would be implied.
5. Describe procedures that require informed consent.
6. State exceptions to the duty to disclose risks of treatment.
7. Discuss the basic standards relied on by courts for determining what information must be disclosed to the patient to obtain informed consent to treatment.
8. Describe the duty imposed on health care facilities by the 1990 Patient Self-Determination Act.
9. Define advance directive and explain the types of advance directives.
10. Explain the prerequisites for a do not resuscitate or "no code" order.

Introduction

Patients have evolved into consumers who want to play a greater role in understanding and making decisions about their medical care. No longer are they just passive in their receipt of medical care and treatment. This attitude of awareness has increased the potential claims against health care providers because demands for disclosure have risen.

Before the formal creation of the informed consent doctrine in the late 1950s, the courts applied the doctrine of consent and focused on the right to self-determination.

To make an informed decision and consent, President Clinton's commission identified certain attributes for the study of ethical problems in medicine and biomedical and behavioral research. The attributes identified were as follows:

1. Ability to communicate and understand information
2. Ability to communicate values and goals
3. Ability to reason and deliberate about choices[1]

The major aspects of informed consent were formed with the 1957 *Salgo* decision. This decision essentially held that a physician was liable for withholding information that would be necessary to make an intelligent decision about consenting for a proposed procedure. When a patient's legs became paralyzed after an aortography, a court held that the physician failed to provide sufficient information to the patient before performing the procedure. Also, the court recognized the exception of therapeutic privilege, which allowed physicians to provide only material facts deemed appropriate by the physician. The physician should take into consideration the patient's emotional and psychological condition and welfare.[2] Currently, the state of consent law requires consent to treatment to be "informed consent." This means that the physician or health care practitioner has given the patient enough information regarding the risks and benefits of the proposed treatment and its alternatives for the patient to make an intelligent or "informed" decision. It is generally accepted that a competent adult has the right to consent to or refuse any medical or surgical treatment. If the patient is not a legally competent adult, the patient's parents, legal guardian, health care agent, or, in some states, next of kin or friend can make the health care decisions. Health care decisions can also be made by a surrogate decision maker, someone the patient designated before becoming incompetent.

However, this right to consent is not absolute; courts have not allowed patients in certain cases involving minor children, mental illness, and substance abuse to refuse lifesaving treatments. For example, the court authorized a hospital and its medical staff to provide all reasonable medical care, including blood transfusions, to save the life of an 8-year-old child, even though such treatment violated the parents' religious beliefs.[3]

This chapter discusses the law of informed consent generally. The court decisions and statutes cited in this chapter are used as examples to illustrate specific points of law. The law, including the law of informed consent, varies from state to state. Therefore it is necessary to consult each state's statute for specific information on a particular state's mandates. Most state legislatures have enacted specific statutes dealing with the issue of informed consent.

Along with state case law and statutory law, health care providers should also comply with the rules of the appropriate regulatory and accrediting agencies, such as the Joint Commission on Accreditation of Healthcare Organizations (JCAHO).

What Is Consent and When Do You Need It?

When Do You Need Consent?

At the most universal level, consent in caring for a patient is required any time you intend to touch the patient. It is required if, for example, you:

1. Bathe a patient.
2. Administer medication.
3. Obtain blood glucose levels.
4. Take vital signs.
5. Perform a treatment.
6. Perform a surgical procedure.

When a patient is admitted to a facility, **consent to treatment forms** are usually signed, giving the facility general consent to routine types of procedures or treatments, such as taking vital signs. *Routine* is not defined but implies procedures that are typically noninvasive and have a low risk for injury. Surgical procedures require informed consent and documentation that the consent was properly obtained. Routine consent aside, any treatment or procedure that has material risks, complications, or side effects that can impact the patient requires informed consent. Patients must be given information so that they can decide if they will assume the risk of having, for example, a stroke or infection, in the course of medical treatment.

Some examples of types of procedures that require specific informed consent include the following:

1. Major invasive surgery
2. Minor invasive surgical procedures
3. All procedures using anesthesia
4. Electroconvulsive therapy
5. Experimental treatment procedures
6. Blood and blood product transfusion
7. Radiological therapy
8. Procedures and treatments that may cause injury or damage, such as
   a. Chemotherapy
   b. Medications
   c. Arteriograms
   d. Myelograms
   e. Procedures requiring injection of dyes to visualize body structure or organs

Capacity to Consent

To be effective legally, a patient consenting or refusing medical treatment must possess the legal capacity to make his or her own health care decisions. **Capacity** is defined as the "ability to understand the nature and effects of one's acts."[4] Often capacity is a matter of interpretation for the courts. Courts often favor a presumption that a person is competent unless a court has proven him or her incompetent.

Decision-making capacity is the ability to participate in your care decision based on your ability to:

1. Understand your condition and surrounding situation (mandated treatment overrides the patient's autonomy and right to choose treatment or no treatment).
2. Use relevant information presented.
3. Communicate your preference and give a reason for your choice.[5]

For a patient who does not possess the legal capacity to consent, health care decisions may sometimes be made by the patient's legal representative—a parent, a guardian, a surrogate decision maker, or an agent appointed under a state statute that allows for surrogate health care decision makers (Boxes 11–1 and 11–2). Most states have **durable power of attorney statutes** that allow individuals, while they are still competent, to appoint an agent to make health care decisions for them if and when they become incompetent or unable to do so. A few states allow the next of kin or a friend to make health care decisions. As a practical matter, families of incompetent patients most often consent to the patients' treatment. Such consent is not effective legally unless the state has a law that specifically allows the spouse or next of kin to make health care decisions for incompetent persons. If an incompetent patient has no legal representative, the probate court, upon application, may appoint a guardian or advocate making health care decisions for the patient.

Types of Consent

The patient's consent to be treated may be expressed or implied. Although **expressed consent** can be oral or written, written consent is preferable because of the difficulty of proving oral consent. **Implied consent** may be presumed in emergency situations or inferred from the patient's actions. For example, it is expected that a person presenting at a physician's office for a physical examination has consented to whatever touching is reasonably necessary to conduct the examination. Similarly, implied

---

BOX 11–1

Minors and Consent

A **minor** is a person who is below the age of majority according to state law. An **emancipated minor** is one who:

1. Is financially independent,
2. Lives apart from his or her parents,
3. Is married,
4. Is in the United States military, or
5. Is considered to have the same legal capacity as an adult.

A **mature minor** is one who the courts have determined to have sufficient understanding of the nature and consequences of the treatment proposed despite his or her chronological age.

BOX 11–2

Exceptions to Parental Consent

Some states allow minors to:

1. Consent to medical treatment for sexually transmitted diseases, pregnancy-related medical care, physical abuse, and substance abuse.
2. Consent in an emergency medical situation.
3. Consent if they are considered a mature or emancipated minor.

You should know:

1. Your state laws and policies and procedures for consent and minors.
2. What instances you are allowed to notify the parents or guardians according to your state laws.
3. If the person giving consent is the legal guardian (e.g., when dealing with divorced parents).[6]

---

consent applies in an emergency situation where a surgeon encounters a complication during an operation, such as hemorrhaging, that requires additional emergency procedures to correct.

If consent is not implied or waived, it is the responsibility of the health care provider performing the procedure, such as the physician, surgeon, nurse practitioner, or physician's assistant, to obtain the patient's informed consent.

In most states, health care facilities that ask patients to sign informed consent forms are not held liable if the health care provider fails to obtain informed consent, unless the health care provider is an employee of the health care facility.[7]

Ideally the health care provider has the patient sign the consent-to-treatment form at the time the proposed treatment is discussed. As a practical matter, however, this often does not happen. Typically the patient is seen in the physician's office, where treatment is discussed. Subsequently the patient is admitted to a facility where a nurse asks the patient to sign a preprinted consent form stating that he or she has been thoroughly informed and consents to the proposed treatment.

If the health care provider has not informed the patient, or refuses to answer the patient's questions, the nurse should take steps, through the chain of command, to ensure that the appropriate person has the health care provider fulfill the responsibility to obtain consent. The health care provider owes a legal duty to the patient and must act within the acceptable standards to give the information to the patient to meet that legal duty. This duty should not be delegated to the nurse or any other third party. If the nurse feels that an ethical dilemma is at hand, then it should be presented to the ethics committee.

Keep in mind that the law makes an exception to the informed consent rule for medical emergencies. It recognizes that, in some emergency situations, obtaining informed consent is not possible. In those situations, the law presumes that the patient would consent to treatment and allows his or her treatment under the doctrine of implied consent.

Consent may also be implied in situations where a patient voluntarily goes to a clinic or a physician's office and accepts treatment. In the case of *O'Brien v. Cunard S.S. Co.*, for example, the court found that, by extending her arm and not objecting to the administration of a vaccination, a woman gave her implied consent to be vaccinated.[8]

Documenting Consent

Nurses who sign as witnesses are not obtaining informed consent; they are only witnessing the person signing the informed consent form. The nurse does not verify the information given to the patient and should not do so on a form unless actually present when the health care provider talks to the patient. The responsibility for ensuring informed consent remains with the health care provider, provided that the nurse does not attempt to answer additional questions asked by the patient that should be answered by the health care provider. If the patient has additional questions, the nurse should refer the questions to the treating health care provider. The nurse may reinforce the information provided by the physician but may not assume the health care provider's legal duty to inform the patient.

In the event of a lawsuit, proper documentation supports the health care provider's testimony regarding informed consent. Documentation includes both a written consent signed by the patient and the health care provider's notation of the discussion and consent in the patient's medical record. The type and amount of documentation required depend on the law of the state in which the patient is being treated. Some states have statutes that spell out requirements for written consent forms. Consent is considered valid unless the patient can prove that the consent was obtained in bad faith, by fraud, or from a patient who cannot understand English. Some consent forms used by facilities are translated in other languages. Also, facilities use translators to assist in explaining the elements of disclosure of informed consent.

If a lawsuit is filed, a consent form that is not specific, but merely states that the elements of informed consent have been discussed with the patient, may not be sufficient to prove that the patient actually gave informed consent. If it is not clear that the patient received the required information before consenting to treatment, additional documentation must be included in the medical record. Such documentation includes a summary of the information given to the patient, a statement dictating that all the patient's questions were answered, and any response by the patient acknowledging his or her understanding of the information provided.

Duty to Disclose

To obtain informed consent, the health care provider has a **duty to disclose** the following:

1. Name of person or persons providing treatment or procedure
2. Diagnosis or suspected diagnosis of the patient
3. Conflicts of interest

4. Nature and purpose of the proposed treatment or procedure
5. Material risks, complications, side effects, and consequences of the proposed treatment or procedure
6. Benefits and anticipated outcome of the proposed treatment or procedure
7. Available alternatives, if any
8. Consequences if the proposed treatment or procedure is refused[9]

Duty to Disclose: Case Allegations

In recent cases, plaintiffs alleged that physicians failed to disclose the following:

1. Health maintenance organization (HMO) financial incentives seeking increased disclosure to limit patient tests and referrals
2. Physician substance abuse and committed fraud
3. Availability of more qualified and experienced physicians
4. Lack of experience and training
5. Existence of alternative treatments or procedures that were not as risky
6. Failure to truthfully disclose qualifications
7. Failure to inform patients of the facility and staff limitations:
   a. Little or no equipment
   b. Staff and surgical suites not equipped to handle emergencies
   c. No anesthesiologist present when patient was anesthetized
8. Failure to inform patients about the role of nurse practitioners or physician assistants who assist
9. Failure to inform of available alternatives for invasive and noninvasive procedures
10. Failure to disclose that the physician received incentive payments from the patient's HMO for limiting referrals and tests[10]

In another example, in a Wisconsin case the state supreme court upheld the verdict against a neurosurgeon who had misrepresented or failed to disclose his experience and the complication rate, underestimated the procedural risks, and failed to refer to more experienced surgeons who dealt with brain aneurysms. The patient, who suffered brain damage, settled for $6.2 million.[11]

The law imposes a duty on the health care provider to disclose certain risks of treatment to the patient. Exceptions to this duty to disclose include situations in which:

1. Disclosure is precluded by an emergency situation.
2. The patient has waived the right to receive the information.
3. The health care provider believes the information would be harmful to the patient and invokes therapeutic privilege.
4. The risk is obvious.
5. Public health requirements preclude disclosure.[12]

Exceptions are rare and vary from state to state (Box 11–3). If the patient is not informed, the reasons must be thoroughly documented. There are two basic rules

---
BOX 11-3

Exceptions to Duty to Disclose

1. Emergency
2. Waiver of right to receive information
3. Medical judgment that information would be harmful to the patient (the therapeutic privilege)
4. Obvious risk
5. Public health requirement

---

regarding the physician's duty to disclose. The traditional or majority rule requires the physician to disclose the same information that others in the medical community would reveal under the same or similar circumstances.[13] The rule adopted by other courts is patient-oriented and focuses on what information a reasonable patient would need to make an informed decision.[14]

Standards of Disclosure

In deciding informed consent cases, courts have relied on two basic standards (or a combination of the two) for determining what information the physician must disclose for the patient to make an intelligent and informed decision. These two basic standards are (1) the medical community standard and (2) the material risk or prudent patient standard.

Medical Community Standard

Under the **medical community standard,** the health care provider's duty to inform the patient depends on the circumstances of the case and the general practice of the medical profession in such cases. To prevail, the patient must prove, by the testimony of an expert witness, that the defendant health care provider did not disclose what a reasonable health care provider, under the same or similar circumstances, would have disclosed, and that such nondisclosure caused the patient's injury.

Prudent Patient Standard

The second standard of disclosure, the **prudent patient or material risk standard,** is based on the concept of patient self-determination. A Pennsylvania court explained that a prudent patient standard is one that focuses on the risks a reasonable person considers when making a decision regarding whether to undergo treatment. The court further noted that it is the jury, not the expert, who must decide how material the risk is and whether the probability of that type of harm is a risk a reasonable patient would consider.[15] The courts that follow this patient-oriented standard must focus on what a "prudent person in the patient's position would have decided if adequately informed of all significant perils."[16] This standard does not require the testimony of an expert witness. Under the material risk standard, the court does not consider what a reasonable physician would have done, but what a reasonable patient needs to know to make an informed decision. This standard is based on the premise that each individual has a right to make his or her own health care decisions.

This standard raises the question of the definition of a significant or material risk. Some courts specify that the risk must be a known significant risk of the treatment. One defense to a claim of failure to obtain informed consent is that the risk is either too commonly known or too remote to require disclosure.

The "material risk" issue is addressed in the case of a child who died following a lumbar puncture. The parents sued the hospital and the child's treating physician, claiming that the lumbar puncture was performed negligently and without the actual or informed consent of the mother.[17] The child, who was born with anachondroplasia and hydrocephalus, was experiencing symptoms that suggested meningitis. After several unsuccessful attempts, a lumbar puncture was performed and the child went into cardiac arrest. The court, finding no evidence that negligence caused the child's injuries, held that the physician could not be liable for failure to obtain informed consent because there was no evidence that cardiac arrest was a significant risk of a lumbar puncture. The judge in this case noted that to prevail, the parents had to prove that they would have considered the undisclosed risk significant in making their decision to consent to the lumbar puncture and that they would have chosen not to permit it.

In another reported case, the patient-plaintiff, who suffered from severe pelvic inflammatory disease (PID), was hospitalized and treated with intravenous antibiotics for 2 weeks. Two years later, she had an intrauterine device (IUD) inserted by the defendant physician. She subsequently delivered a baby, after which the IUD was removed, not from her uterus but from her rectum. The plaintiff's expert witness testified that, because of the patient's history of PID, the physician should have explained to the patient the purpose and possible complications of the IUD and the alternative methods of contraception. The jury, however, found that the physician was not required to advise the plaintiff of the risks involved in the insertion of an IUD. The court concluded that the duty to disclose only applies to "reasonably foreseeable material risks" and not to the remote possibility that an inserted IUD would perforate the uterus, migrate, and protrude from the rectum.

In *Hondroulis v. Schumacher*, the Louisiana Supreme Court used the objective standard. The patient had a myelogram and laminectomy performed. The consent form signed listed the risks stated in the informed consent stature.[18] After surgery, the patient experienced numbness in the leg, incontinence, and constipation. She filed suit based on lack of informed consent of material risks. The trial court granted summary judgment in favor of the physician. The court held that she was bound by the consent form unless the facts were misrepresented.

On rehearing, the Supreme Court reversed the summary judgment in favor of the plaintiff.

In Louisiana, to recover in informed consent, the plaintiff must show that the physician failed to disclose a material risk, that the undisclosed risk actually occurred, and that if the material risk had been disclosed by the physician, a reasonable person would have avoided the treatment and unwanted consequences.[19] States such as Louisiana have also established a **medical disclosure panel,** which determines what material risks for each treatment or procedure must, by law, be disclosed to the patient. This was done to protect the health care provider from claims based on failure to disclose certain material risks.

In another case, before surgery the plaintiff signed a consent form that listed some of the material risks associated with the procedure and the anesthesia:

1. Death
2. Brain damage
3. Quadriplegia
4. Loss of organ
5. Loss of use or function of the arm or leg
6. Loss of function of organ
7. Disfiguring scars
8. Infection

After surgery, the patient experienced drop foot. The plaintiff stated the "infection" was not written in as a risk when he signed the document. Also, he testified that the surgeon failed to inform him of the risks of surgery. His wife confirmed his story. The court affirmed that trial court's findings that the plaintiff was not adequately informed of all material risks inherent in surgery. Judgment was affirmed against defendant physician.[20]

Some states do not specify which standard of disclosure must be followed. Whatever the standard, it seems likely that the health care practitioner who properly informs the patient of the major risks of a procedure and the feasible alternative treatment should be protected. It would not be credible to a jury that a patient would have refused a particular procedure because of a minor risk if he or she consented to the procedure after being informed of more serious risks.

Additional information is required if the patient requests it. Most consent forms indicate that all the patient's questions have been answered.

Tips for informed consent for the nurse practitioner, physician, and physician's assistant:

1. Have a policy on informed consent.
2. Be honest if asked about your qualifications.
3. Physicians should check with the Board of Licensure and professional sources to determine the laws relating to informed consent.
4. Educate the patient through discussion, videotapes, literature, and questions and answers.
5. Use plain language; eliminate medical jargon.
6. Know the informed consent requirements related to office and surgery procedures.

7. Discuss and educate the patient on the risks of prescription drugs and their side effects, adverse reactions, effects when combining them with other drugs or alcohol, and contraindications.

Treatment Without Consent

Treatment or attempts to treat without informed consent may result in a lawsuit (Box 11–4). An injured plaintiff may claim that the defendant (the physician or health care practitioner) is liable for any of three things: assault and/or battery, lack of informed consent, or negligently obtaining informed consent. If the defendant is found to be liable, he or she may have to pay damages.

Assault and Battery

Any unauthorized touching or threat of touching of another person may precipitate a civil action for assault or battery. An assault is an intentional act by one person that causes another person to fear that he or she will be touched in an offensive or injurious manner, even if no touching actually takes place. Battery occurs if the act results in actual physical contact or touching. Assault and battery can occur when medical examination or treatment is provided without first obtaining the patient's informed consent. A classic example is the surgeon who has the patient's consent to amputate the left leg but actually amputates the right leg. Certainly the plaintiff can file a lawsuit based on a claim for medical malpractice, but that plaintiff can also allege the intentional tort claim of medical battery. After all, cutting off the right leg was an impermissible touching when the patient only gave informed consent to operate on the left.

If health care providers examine patients, conduct diagnostic tests, or treat patients without first obtaining the proper consent, they can be held liable for assault or battery,[21] even if the patient is not harmed by the procedure or the procedure is actually beneficial to the patient.[22] To prove that assault and battery has occurred, the patient has to convince the jury either that no consent was given or that the practitioner exceeded the scope of consent given.

BOX 11–4

Treatment Without Consent

Treatment or attempts to treat without consent may result in a lawsuit based on the following claims:

1. Assault or battery
2. Lack of informed consent
3. Negligently obtaining informed consent

Negligently Obtained Informed Consent

Lawsuits alleging lack of consent are likely to be based on principles of professional negligence rather than claims of assault and battery. In a professional negligence case, testimony by an expert witness is required to prove or disprove the patient's case. The question experts are asked is: What would a reasonable health care provider with the same knowledge, experience, and expertise do under similar circumstances? In a case founded on lack of informed consent, the plaintiff has to prove that the health care provider, by failing to provide the appropriate information, breached a duty, and that the breach of duty caused the plaintiff to make a different decision than he or she would have made with more complete knowledge.[23] Plaintiff would argue that it is the breach of duty that caused the injury.[24] For example, one court held that a physician could be sued for a patient's death when the physician did not inform the patient of the risk of refusing a routine test such as a Papanicolaou (Pap) smear.[25] In this case, the physician had a duty to inform the patient but breached this duty, and as a result of the breach of duty, the patient made a decision not to have a Pap smear, a decision ultimately leading to her death.

Proving Lack of Consent Cases

Consent to medical treatment is informed when the patient has been provided with sufficient information to make an intelligent decision to accept or reject treatment based on a full disclosure of the facts.[26] This information should be provided by the person who is responsible for performing the procedure or providing the treatment, generally the physician. Proving lack of informed consent varies from state to state.

Standards of Proof

Subjective Standard

Although the elements of informed consent are similar from state to state, the courts differ in what the plaintiff must prove to establish the absence of informed consent. For example, some courts require evidence that the individual plaintiff would not have consented to the treatment if he or she had been provided with adequate information. One such court stated:

> A physician's negligent failure to disclose the risks of harm prior to treatment involves the following five material elements: (1) the physician owed a duty to disclose to the patient prior to treatment the risk of the harm suffered by the patient; (2) the physician negligently performed, or failed to perform, his or her duty of disclosure; (3) the patient suffered the harm; (4) the physician's negligent performance, or nonperformance, of duty was a cause of the patient's harm in that (a) the physician's treatment was a substantial factor in bringing about the patient's harm,

and (b) the patient, acting rationally and reasonably, would not have undergone the treatment had he or she been properly informed of the risk of the harm that, in fact, occurred; and (5) no other cause is a superseding cause.[27]

When the court uses a **subjective standard,** it considers what this patient would or would not do under the circumstances. But the majority of courts do not look at the decision of a particular patient involved. Rather, they look at an **objective standard,** or what a "reasonable" patient would do under the same or similar circumstances.

In a Pennsylvania case, the jury awarded a plaintiff $150,000. The jury found that the surgeon failed to obtain the patient's informed consent before his surgery by failing to disclose the Food and Drug Administration (FDA) status of the pedicle screws used in the surgery. Pennsylvania adopted the prudent patient standard for informed consent, an objective standard. Under this standard, a patient must be informed by the physician of the "material facts, risks, complications and alternatives to surgery, which a reasonable [person] in the patient's position would have considered significant in deciding whether to have the operation."[28]

The pedicle screws implanted in the plaintiff's spine were class III medical devices that were not FDA approved as safe and effective. The court thought that a prudent person would deem the FDA status of screws to be significant or material to a patient's decision to consent to the surgical procedure and ruled for the plaintiff.

Objective Standard

Another court relied on an objective standard in a case in which the patient-plaintiff underwent a decompressive central laminectomy by an orthopedic surgeon. The patient immediately lost bowel and bladder control and remained incontinent until his death from an unrelated cause 6 years later. The patient and his wife filed a medical malpractice lawsuit, alleging that the doctor was negligent in performing the surgery and in failing to adequately warn the patient of the risks involved in the surgery. The case was tried before a judge who found that the doctor failed to obtain the patient's informed consent.

The doctor appealed to a higher court. The appeals court sent the case back to the lower court for a new trial in which the plaintiff would have to prove the following essential elements of an informed consent case:

1. The existence of a material risk unknown to the patient
2. A failure to disclose the risk on the part of the physician
3. That a disclosure of the risk would have led a reasonable patient in the plaintiff's position to reject the medical procedure or choose a different course of treatment and
4. Injury[29]

Subjective Versus Objective

Although worded differently, both the explanations of the elements of informed consent given previously establish that the physician has a duty to disclose certain information and that it can be shown that breaching that duty caused injury to the patient. What these courts require the plaintiff to prove, however, is very different. For example, under the subjective standard, the plaintiff must only prove that he would have refused the proposed treatment if properly informed. Under the objective standard, the plaintiff must prove that a hypothetical "reasonable person" in the plaintiff's position would have refused the treatment if the physician had properly explained the risks, benefits, alternatives of the proposed treatment, type of procedure or treatment to be performed, and consequences of not receiving the treatment.

Theory Behind Informed Consent: Patient's Right to Self-Determination

Self-Determination Versus State's Interest

Although it is generally accepted that a competent patient may refuse medical or surgical treatment, there are circumstances when an interested party petitions the court to intervene and require the patient to consent to treatment. In such cases, the courts balance certain state interests against the patient's rights.

In a Georgia case, a pregnant patient refused a cesarean section on religious grounds. Her physician testified that because of placenta previa, there was a 99-percent chance that the infant would not survive a natural delivery. The court's order that the mother undergo the cesarean section was upheld by the Georgia Supreme Court on the grounds that the state's interest in protecting the potential life of an unborn child outweighed the mother's constitutional right to privacy.[30]

A more difficult question arises when the patient is incompetent to make his or her own health care decisions. The courts may also balance the incompetent patient's rights to refuse treatment against certain interests of the state.

A typical case is *Leach v. Akron General Medical Center*.[31] In the *Leach* case, an Ohio appeals court found that an incompetent patient has a right to forego treatment based on the right to privacy. This court balanced the patient's right to privacy and the state's interests in keeping the patient alive (the preservation of life, the protection of third parties, the maintenance of the ethical integrity of the medical profession, and the prevention of suicide), and concluded that the patient's right to privacy, guaranteed by the United States Constitution, outweighed the state's interests. The court, however, required the highest possible standard of proof for a civil case—that is, clear and convincing evidence of what the patient would have wanted if she had been competent to decide for herself.[32]

Many courts have found that the patient's right to privacy outweighs the state's interests. In 1985 a New Jersey court decided the well-known Karen Quinlan case, the first major case on the right to refuse or discontinue treatment. The court permitted the guardian to consent to the removal of Quinlan's respirator. The court held that the constitutional right to privacy found in the 14th Amendment protects an individual's right, exercised through his or her guardian, to forego or terminate life-prolonging treatment.[33]

Likewise, in 1990 the United States Supreme Court decided the *Cruzan* case, which involved a guardian's decision that Nancy Cruzan, an incompetent person, would want to exercise her "right to die."[34] The Supreme Court acknowledged that a competent adult has a constitutionally protected right to refuse unwanted medical treatment. However, it found that for an incompetent patient, in order to protect the state's interests, the court may require "clear and convincing" evidence of what the patient, if competent, would want. The court did not define "clear and convincing," but it did acknowledge that a proper living will, a legal document stating what health care a patient will accept or refuse, would have satisfied this higher standard. Nancy Cruzan never executed a living will, but there was evidence that she once told a roommate that she would not want to be kept alive on machines. This evidence, according to the court, was sufficient to meet the "clear and convincing" test and overcome the state's interests in the preservation of life, and so she was allowed to be taken off feeding tubes so that she could die.

Other courts have upheld patients' decisions to refuse medical treatment because of religious beliefs. For example, one court found that the right of an adult Jehovah's Witness to refuse blood transfusions outweighed the state's interest in preserving the life of the only witness to a murder.[35]

The Patient Self-Determination Act

Many state legislatures have enacted statutes that allow competent persons to execute documents to exercise control over their future health care. These documents, called advance directives, include living wills and durable powers of attorney for health care.

An **advance directive** is a document by which a competent person (1) makes a declaration regarding future health care he or she will accept or refuse (a **living will;** Figure 11–1), (2) designates another person to make health care decisions if he or she becomes incompetent in the future (a **durable power of attorney for health care** or proxy decision maker), or both.[36]

In general, a living will must be executed with the same formality as a last will and testament. A durable power of attorney for health care (DPAHC) or medical durable power of attorney permits a competent adult (the principal) to appoint a surrogate or proxy (the attorney-in-fact) to make health care decisions in the event he or she becomes incompetent to make such decisions. The various state statutes outline the requirements for executing and revoking a DPAHC. DPAHC statutes provide that the surrogate will receive the same information as an aid to informed decision making that the principal, if competent, would be provided. (See Box 11–5 for a list of the legal documents used to designate health care agents.)

Every state has enacted legislation that allows individuals to execute living wills or DPAHC (Figure 11–2). These directives are binding on health care providers. Historically, there were problems between states that had no such legislation and

INSTRUCTIONS	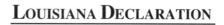 **LOUISIANA DECLARATION**

PRINT THE DATE

PRINT YOUR NAME

Declaration made this _____ day of _____.
                              (day)   *(month, year)*

I _____,
                              (name)

being of sound mind, willfully and voluntarily make known my desire that my dying shall not be artificially prolonged under the circumstances set forth below and do hereby declare:

If at any time I should have an incurable injury, disease, or illness, or be in a continual profound comatose state with no reasonable chance of recovery, certified to be a terminal and irreversible condition by two physicians who have personally examined me, one of whom shall be my attending physician, and the physicians have determined that my death will occur whether or not life-sustaining procedures are utilized and where the application of life-sustaining procedures would serve only to prolong artificially the dying process, I direct that such procedures be withheld or withdrawn and that I be permitted to die naturally with only the administration of medication or the performance of any medical procedure deemed necessary to provide me with comfort care.

ADD PERSONAL INSTRUCTIONS (IF ANY)

Other directions:

Figure 11–1. An example of an advance directive. (Reprinted by permission of Partnership for Caring, 1620 Eye Street, NW, Suite 202, Washington, DC 20006, 800-989-9544.)

BOX 11–5

Health Care Agents

Legal documents used to designate health care agents may be called any of the following, depending on state laws:

1. Durable power of attorney for health care
2. Health care representative form
3. Medical durable power of attorney
4. Medical power of attorney
5. Proxy appointment[37]

---

states that did because some states would not accept advance directives from other states.[38]

To remedy these problems, Congress passed legislation that requires hospitals and other health care facilities, including managed care organizations that receive Medicare or Medicaid funds, to advise all patients of their rights to refuse treatment and of any relevant state law dealing with advance directives. The **Patient Self-Determination Act of 1990** was sponsored by Senator John Danforth, who introduced it with the following words:

> Advance directives encourage people to discuss and document their views of life-sustaining treatment in advance. They uphold the right of people to make their own decisions. And they enhance communication between patients, their families, and doctors, easing the burden on families and providers when it comes time to decide whether or not to pursue all possible treatment options.
>
> Advance directives will not solve all problems related to end-of-life decision…they do not take the pain away from someone we love, but they do ensure that a person's voice continues to be heard, and they do ease the burden, pain, and guilt that families often feel when making decision(s) for their dying loved one.[39]

Do Not Resuscitate Orders

On admission to a health care facility, a competent adult may also exercise control over future medical or surgical treatment by asking the physician for an order not to resuscitate. Per the patient's decision, the physician writes "no code," or a do not resuscitate (DNR) order, on the patient's chart. Such an order instructs the nurses and medical staff to refrain from resuscitating the patient in the event of cardiovascular or respiratory arrest. Such orders do not indicate that other treatment, to which the patient has consented, must be withheld or terminated. Often dilemmas result when nurses caring for the patient attempt to addresses the patient's and the family's wishes. See Box 11–6 for examples of some common dilemmas.

Each health care facility should have its own DNR policy. These policies generally only permit terminally ill patients to have DNR orders. They also should require the

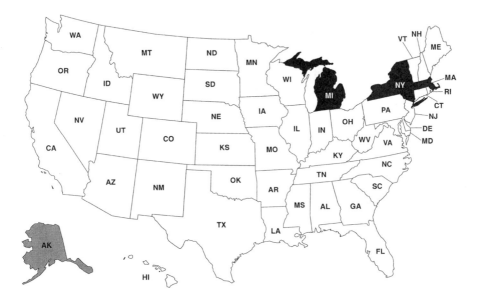

Key

☐ Jurisdictions with legislation that authorizes both living wills and the appointment of a health care agent (the District of Columbia and 46 states: Alabama, Arizona, Arkansas, California, Colorado, Connecticut, Delaware, Florida, Georgia, Hawaii, Idaho, Illinois, Indiana, Iowa, Kansas, Kentucky, Louisiana, Maine, Maryland, Minnesota, Mississippi, Missouri, Montana, Nebraska, Nevada, New Hampshire, New Jersey, New Mexico, North Carolina, North Dakota, Ohio, Oklahoma, Oregon, Pennsylvania, Rhode Island, South Carolina, South Dakota, Tennessee, Texas, Utah, Vermont, Virginia, Washington, West Virginia, Wisconsin, and Wyoming).

▨ Alaska's Power of Attorney Act precludes health care agent authority to terminate life-sustaining medical procedures. The Act does allow the health care agent to enforce a Declaration.

■ States with legislation that authorize the appointment of a health care agent (3 states: Massachusetts, Michigan, and New York).

Note: The specifics of living will and health care agent legislation vary greatly from state to state. In addition, many states also have court-made law that affects residents' rights. For information about specific state laws, contact Partnership for Caring.

Figure 11–2. States with statutes governing living wills and appointment of a health care agent. (Reprinted by permission of Partnership for Caring, 1620 Eye Street, NW, Suite 202, Washington, DC 20006, 800-989-9544.)

BOX 11–6

Common Dilemmas Nurses Face Regarding DNR Orders

1. Lack of documentation in the medical records, especially the progress notes, indicating how the DNR decision was made.
2. No DNR form on the chart.
3. Interpreting DNR orders when a no code order has been qualified as a "chemical code only" or "resuscitate but do not intubate."
4. Performing a "slow code" or "show code" for the benefit of family members.
5. Transfer of residents: Is a DNR order accompanying a resident when he is transferred from one facility to another acceptable? Should a new one be obtained?
6. Abandonment of care by health care personnel of patients designated as DNRs.
7. Family conflicts over DNR orders.
8. Physicians who will not honor the DNR.
9. Family does not understand the difference between a DNR order and a do not treat order.

---

physician to note in the medical record that the patient's decision was made after consultation with the physician regarding his or her medical condition and prognosis. Do not resuscitate or no code orders should always be written in the patient's medical record and periodically reviewed and updated.

In 1990 an Indiana court was the first to consider whether a doctor was liable for issuing a DNR order without the patient's informed consent.[40]

The Incompetent Patient's Right to Self-Determination

If a patient is unconscious or otherwise unable to make health care decisions, someone else may have to make those decisions. If the patient, like Nancy Cruzan, has never discussed his or her wishes with the family and has never executed an advance directive, any assumption made by a surrogate decision maker may not be the decision the patient would have made if competent. Because of this possibility of error, the courts are very protective of the rights of incompetent patients and may, as in the Cruzan case, require a very high standard of proof before allowing the physician to terminate any life-sustaining treatment. In Cruzan the court held that, because of the obvious and overwhelming finality of such life-and-death decisions, the state had the right to err on the side of life.[41] The United States Supreme Court, however, recognized that a living will would have been sufficient evidence of Cruzan's wishes to sustain an order removing her feeding tube.

As a practical matter, physicians face such decisions daily. See Box 11–7 for some commonly asked questions about advance directives and DNR orders. Generally, physicians have been able to rely on close family members to make decisions for the incompetent patient, because it is the family who usually cares about the patient and has knowledge of the patient's wishes. This does not mean that a family member has a legal right to accept or refuse treatment for an incompetent patient. In most states, only a legal guardian (or parent in the case of a minor) can make health care decisions for another, unless the patient has executed an advance directive appointing another person to make health care decisions in the event of incompetence.

However, even if a patient is conscious, there may still be a question of whether he or she is competent to consent to or refuse treatment.

A woman with cancer was admitted to a hospital under a mental illness/mental health statute. The patient believed that she would be spiritually cured and refused treatment on religious grounds. The patient's physician requested that the court order treatment for the cancer, claiming that the patient's belief was a delusion that affected her ability to give informed consent. He also claimed that she was incompetent, because she was hospitalized pursuant to the mental illness statute. The court disagreed, finding that the patient was not legally incompetent and that she had a constitutional right to refuse treatment.[42]

Informed Consent and the Living Will

The concept of a living will is based on the doctrine of informed consent.[43] Some believe that, by voluntarily executing a binding directive, the individual indicates that he or she has weighed all of the factors and has chosen to remove the decision to prolong his or her life from the physician's discretion.[44] Nonetheless, many critics of living wills contend that they cannot be based on informed consent because the patient cannot know what treatment options will be available many years later. Either way, even where there is no state law legalizing living wills, a living will is strong evidence in court of the patient's wishes if a court must make health care decisions for an incompetent patient.[45]

BOX 11–7

Facts on DNRs (and Other Advance Directives)

1. *What types of care should be discussed regarding end-of-life medical needs?*
   a. Cardiopulmonary resuscitation (CPR)
   b. Hydration
   c. Artificial nutrition
   d. Mechanical ventilation
   e. Kidney dialysis[46]
2. *Who should receive a copy of the patient's advance directives?*
   a. Spouse
   b. Health care agent
   c. Family
   d. Primary care provider
   e. Attorney
   (Warn the patient not to keep the only copy in a safe deposit box that only he or she can access.)
3. *Does the health care provider resuscitate if there is no written DNR order in the chart?*
   Yes. In most facility's policies and procedures, the requirement is that there must be a written order in the chart that should be renewed periodically.
4. *Is a do not resuscitate order the same as a do not treat order?*
   No. Explain to the patient the difference in the orders based on facility policies and procedures.
5. *What other medical treatments should be discussed with the patient when making a living will?*
   a. Radiation therapy
   b. Chemotherapy
   c. Antibiotics
   d. Intravenous lines (IVs)
   e. Diagnostic studies
   f. Surgical procedures
   g. Blood transfusions
6. *Can an advance directive be revoked?*
   Yes. It is not set in stone and can be revoked orally and in writing. The patient can tear it up or replace it with a new advance directive. (Check your state laws.)

Facts on DNRs (and Other Advance Directives) *(continued)*

7. *Is a living will in one state good in all states?*
   No, not necessarily. Depending on state law, the conditions and terms may be different. Also, some states require a notary to sign the living will, whereas others do not. (A national living will and health care agent form may be the solution, so that the advance directives can be upheld and honored in any state.)

8. *Are there some situations in facility settings in which DNRs are rescinded during surgical interventions?*[47]
   Yes, usually during surgical interventions. Check your policies and procedures.

9. *What does* euthanasia *mean? How many types of euthanasia exist?*
   a. *Euthanasia* means "good death." It allows for making a death essentially pain free for a patient.
   b. Four types exist: (1) *Voluntary* means the patient has consented; (2) *involuntary* means the person has not consented or cannot consent but there is a presumption he or she wishes to die; (3) *active* means steps or actions are actually taken to cause the person's death; and (4) *passive* means that nothing is done to hasten the person's death.[48]

10. *What is artificial nutrition and hydration? Is stopping this treatment legal and ethical?*
    a. Artificial nutrition and hydration are forms of life-sustaining treatments consisting of a chemically balanced mixture of nutrients and fluids given to the patient by placing a tube directly into the stomach, intestines, or veins.[49]
    b. Stopping this treatment is legally and ethically appropriate if (1) the competent patient refuses treatment or (2) there is no benefit (know your facility's policies and procedures).

11. *What was the first state to legalize physician-assisted suicide?*
    In 1997 Oregon legalized physician-assisted suicide. The patient requests a lethal prescription. A study done after the law passed indicated that concerns over loss of bodily functions and autonomy and pain control were the primary reasons for requesting the lethal prescription.[50]

    Dr. Jack Kevorkian (a retired pathologist) was convicted in March 1999 of second-degree murder for giving a fatal injection to a man with a terminal illness and amyotrophic lateral sclerosis (Lou Gehrig's disease). Kevorkian brought national attention to the issue of the right to assisted suicide and issues surrounding active, voluntary euthanasia. Claims exist that he assisted more than 130 people to commit suicide.[51]

KEEP IN MIND

▶ In most circumstances, a competent adult has the right to consent to or refuse medical treatment.

▶ A patient may become incompetent to make health care decisions, which would then be made by the health care agent. If and when the patient becomes competent again, he or she can resume making decisions about care and treatment.

▶ To be legally effective, a patient's consent to medical or surgical treatment must be what the law considers "informed consent."

▶ Assault and battery can occur when medical examination or treatment is provided without first obtaining the patient's consent.

▶ Today lawsuits alleging lack of informed consent are more likely to be based on professional negligence principles than on claims of assault and battery.

▶ Consent to treatment is informed consent when the patient has been provided with sufficient information to make an intelligent decision to accept or reject treatment that is based on a full disclosure of the relevant facts.

▶ It is the responsibility of the health care practitioner performing the procedure—the physician, nurse practitioner, or physician's assistant—to obtain the patient's informed consent.

▶ Signing as a witness does not subject the nurse to liability for failure to obtain informed consent.

▶ A court may require a very high standard of proof of an incompetent patient's desires before ordering the removal of life-sustaining treatment.

▶ An advance directive is made by the individual while he or she is competent but becomes effective only if and when the individual becomes incompetent to make health care decisions.

▶ By executing a living will, a competent individual can instruct his or her physician regarding the type of medical treatment the individual will accept or refuse if he or she becomes unable to make health care decisions in the future.

▶ A durable power of attorney for health care permits a competent adult to appoint a proxy health care agent to act on his or her behalf and to make health care decisions if the person becomes incompetent.

IN A NUTSHELL

Before the era of high-tech medicine, there was little if any need for courts and legislatures to be concerned about an individual's right to refuse treatment. This changed dramatically as it became possible to maintain such vital functions as respiration by artificial means and to provide nourishment via tubes and needles. Many people began to view the invasive procedures required to keep the body functioning as violations of their right to die with dignity. Initially these matters were handled by the patient or the immediate family and physician. If the patient (or the family of an incompetent patient) wished to forego artificial life-prolonging treatment, the physician complied by not ordering the treatment. Although this continues to be the practice in most situations today, the courts and legislatures are becoming increasingly involved in these matters.

As more laws are passed giving patients the right to refuse life-sustaining treatment and with the passage of the federal Patient Self-Determination Act, health care providers are at increased risk of liability for keeping patients alive against their expressed wishes. Some advocates of the right to die have proposed that health care providers who fail to honor patients' wishes be held liable for the patients' resulting "wrongful living." In drafting DPAHC and living will statutes, state legislators have recognized that some health care providers may not be able to honor the patient's desire to refuse treatment. Legislators have granted such providers immunity from liability as long as they do not prevent the transfer of the patient to a provider who will honor his or her wishes. This reasoning also applies to DNR orders; a physician should not oppose the transfer of a terminally ill patient who desires a DNR order to another physician if that physician cannot in good faith write the order.

The courts and legislatures are attempting to protect not only the patient's right to self-determination but also the rights of health care providers who now have the power to keep patients alive by technical and artificial means. Individuals, however, must exercise their rights to make decisions in advance regarding the health care they wish to receive in the future. In their role as educators in the community, nurses are in a unique position to inform individuals of their rights and to encourage the exercise of such rights.

AFTERTHOUGHTS

1. What information must be provided before the patient can give informed consent to treatment?
2. Define decision-making capacity as it relates to a patient's right to accept or refuse medical treatment.
3. Explain assault and battery in accordance with medical treatment and give an example of how it may apply to informed consent.
4. What basic elements must be proved before a physician may be found negligent for failure to obtain a patient's informed consent to medical or surgical treatment?
5. Describe two situations in which the consent to treat would be implied.
6. Describe five situations that are exceptions to the duty to disclose risks of a treatment.
7. Discuss the two basic standards relied on by courts for determining what information must be disclosed to the patient to obtain informed consent to treatment.
8. Explain what is meant by (a) an objective standard and (b) a subjective standard as each relates to what a patient must prove in a lawsuit involving informed consent.

9. What duty is imposed on health care facilities by the Patient Self-Determination Act?

10. Define advance directive and give examples of the two kinds of advance directives and how they relate to the concept of informed consent. Bring a copy of a form used in facilities for patients and discuss the language in the advance directives.

11. Does your state have statutory material risks that must be disclosed to the patient?

12. How can an advance directive be revoked according to your state laws?

13. Who should receive copies of your advance directives?

14. What are the types of euthanasia?

15. What is assisted suicide? What state or states have passed laws regarding assisted suicide? Is assisted suicide legal in other countries? Which ones?

ETHICS IN PRACTICE

Sarah Beam has told you that she wants to have all procedures and surgeries performed on her to keep her alive. Although she is 75 years old with lung cancer, she wants the chance to extend her life and does not believe in DNR orders.

As her nurse, you notice that after 2 weeks she has started having periods of lucidity and disorientation. The physician tells you that she should have another surgery to remove a large lesion on her liver to prevent further metastasis. The family has told the physician that he is not to discuss any surgeries with her and nothing is to be done.

1. What is the duty of the physician?
2. What is the duty of the nurse?
3. What are their potential legal and ethical dilemmas?

Other questions that should be clarified include the following:

4. Has a health care agent been appointed by Sarah?
5. Is this period of disorientation only temporary? What is the cause?

? What Would You Do?

Mr. S., 72 years old, was found at home by neighbors, unconscious, with multiple ecchymotic areas on his body and a fractured wrist. Because he lived alone, had no known relatives, and was unresponsive when he was admitted to the hospital, the history of the present illness was not obtained. Initially it was thought that he had been beaten by an intruder in his home.

What Would You Do? (continued)

He was admitted to the intensive care unit (ICU) and connected to a cardiac monitor. After several hours of monitoring, he began to have transient episodes of complete heart block with ventricular asystole. A diagnosis of Stokes-Adams syndrome was made. This diagnosis would account for his current injuries. Mr. S. also became more responsive, although he experienced episodes of disorientation.

The cardiologist was contacted by Mr. S.'s primary physician, and plans were made to insert a permanent pacemaker, a standard treatment for this condition. The cardiologist talked to Mr. S. briefly about the procedure and then told the nurse caring for the patient to have Mr. S. sign a surgical consent. The nurse brought the consent to the room and asked Mr. S. a few questions about what the physician had told him and his understanding of the pacemaker insertion procedure. Mr. S. seemed to have no understanding at all of the underlying disease process, the procedure, or the requirement for an informed consent.

The nurse proceeded to present some simple information to the patient about the procedure, its risks, and its benefits. After hearing this information, Mr. S. stated that he did "not want that thing inside of him" and refused to sign the consent form.

The nurse called the cardiologist later that evening and told him about what she had told Mr. S. and his refusal to sign the consent form. The cardiologist was furious, accused the nurse of undermining his authority, and demanded that she "get that consent signed" no matter what it took. He insisted that the patient was still somewhat disoriented and that the nurse's teaching had only confused him more.

What are the ethical issues involved in this case study? Was the nurse wrong in teaching this patient? What should the nurse do at this point?

References

1. Moskop, JC: Informed consent in the emergency department. Emerg Med Clin North Am 17(2):337–40, IX, X, 1999.
2. Salgo v. Leland, Stanford Jr. Univ. Bd. Of Trustees, 317 P2d 170 (Cal. Ap. 1957). Weintraub, "Documentation and Informed Consent." Neurol Clin 17(2):371–81, 1999.
3. Matter of McCauley, 409 Mass. 134, 565 N.E.2d 411 (1991).
4. Black's Law Dictionary, ed 6. West Publishing, St. Paul, Minn, 1991.
5. O'Keefe, ME: Nursing Practice and the Law: Avoiding Malpractice and Other Legal Risks. FA Davis, Philadelphia, 2001.
6. Ohio Revised Code Ann.;dw 2317.54 (Supp. 1988), for example, states: "A hospital shall not be held liable for a physician's failure to obtain an informed consent from his patient prior to a surgical or medical procedure or course of procedures, unless the physician is an employee of the hospital." In Robertson v. Menorah Memorial, 588 S.W.2d 134 (Mo. 1979), the Missouri Supreme Court rejected the plaintiff's argument that by having the patient sign the consent form, the hospital was responsible for informing the patient of the risks and benefits of treatment. The court held

that the physician alone was qualified to obtain the patient's informed consent. Clin Immunol 98:6–13, 1996. 5334-8 Anesthesiology 87:4, 1997.

7. O'Brien v. Cunord. S. S. Co., 154 Mass. 272, 28 N.E. 266.
8. Waisel, D, and Truog, R: Special articles. Anesthesiology 87:4, 1997.
9. Rice, B: The new rules on informed consent. Medical Economics, June 19, 2000.
10. Ibid., 152.
11. See, for example, Mroczkwski v. Straub Clinic and Hospital, 732 P.2d 1255 (Hawaii, App. 1987). See also Alaska Stat. §09.55.556, which provides for less than full disclosure if a health care provider reasonably believed that a full disclosure would have a substantially adverse effect on the patient's condition.
12. See, for example, Dessi v. United States, 489 F. Supp. 722, 727 (E.D.Va. 1980), applying Virginia law. The scope of a physician's duty to disclose typically is determined by the prevailing medical practice in the community—that is, what a reasonable physician in the community, of like training, would customarily disclose under the same circumstances.
13. Small v. Gifford Memorial Hospital, 133 Vt. 552, 349 A.2d 703 (1975). This rule and the medical community rule are discussed in greater detail in Section D, infra.
14. Clemons v. Tranovich, 589 A.2d 260.
15. Cobbs v. Grant, 104 Cal. Rptr. 505, 515, 516, 502 P.2d 1, 11–12 (1972).
16. Plutshack v. Univ. of Minn. Hospital, 316 N.W.2d 1, 3 (Minn. 1982).
17. Wright v. Hirsch, 572 So. 2d 783, 789–791 (La. App. 4th Cir. 1990).
18. Hondroulis v. Schumacher, 553 So2d 39 8 (La. 1988).
19. LaCaze v. Collier, 434 So2D 1030, 1048 (La. 1983).
20. Hezesau v. Pendleton Memorial, 71 S So2d 756 (La. Ap. Cir. 4-1/18/98).
21. Some states have enacted statutes prohibiting assault and battery lawsuits against health care providers. For example, Arizona Revised Statute §12–562 (1989) states, "No medical malpractice action brought against a health care provider shall be based upon assault and battery."
22. See Lacey v. Laird, 166 Ohio St. 12, 139 N.E.2d 25 (1956).
23. See, for example, Holten v. Pfingst, 534 S.W.2d 786 (Ky. 1975), in which the court held that a negligence cause of action would accrue where there is a failure of a physician to disclose a particular risk and the nondisclosure proximately injures the patient. See also Jones v. Howard University, Inc., 589 A.2d 419, 422 (D.C. App. 1991), in which the court pointed out that a breach of duty to disclose will not establish liability on the part of the physician; the unrevealed risk must actually materialize and injure the patient.
24. See, for example Hidding v. Williams, 578 So.2d 1192 (5th Cir. 1991).
25. In Truman v. Thomas, 27 Cal. 3d 285, 611 P.2d 902 (1980), the court held that where a patient indicates a refusal to undergo a risk-free test or treatment, a doctor must advise of all material risks of which reasonable persons would want to be informed before deciding.
26. Black's Law Dictionary.
27. Mroczkwski v. Straub Clinic & Hospital, 6 Haw. App. 563, 732 P.2d 1255, 1257 (1987).
28. Southland v. Temple University Hospital, 731 A2d 610 (Pa. Super 1999).
29. Hidding v. Williams, 578 So.2d 1192 (5th Cir. 1991).
30. Jefferson v. Griffith, Spalding County Hospital Authority, 247 Ga. 86, 274 S.E.2d 457 (Ga. 1981). See also Norwood Hospital v. Munoz, 564 N.E.2d 1017 (Mass. 1991). (The state's highest court reversed a lower court's order that a mother consent to a blood transfusion to save her own life to prevent her abandonment of a dependent child on the ground that the father had the financial resources to care for the child.)
31. Leach v. Akron General Medical Center, 13 Ohio App. 3d 393, 469 N.E.2d 1047 (Summit Co. 1984).
32. Ibid.
33. In re: Quinlan, 355 A.2d 647 (N.J. 1976).
34. Cruzan v. Director, Missouri Department of Health, 110 S. Ct. 2841 (1990). The Court did not distinguish between treatment with artificially administered food and water and other life-sustaining measures such as respirators. Some state laws make such distinctions. In the wake of the Cruzan decision, these laws may be challenged in the courts and found unconstitutional.
35. In re: Brown, 478 So. 2d 1033 (Miss. 1985).
36. Because every state statute is different and subject to be changed, it is important for the nurse to become familiar with the specific law of the state in which he or she practices.
37. Health Care Agents: Appointing One and Being One. Choice in Dying, Inc, 1998.
38. Omnibus Budget Reconciliation Act of 1990. This act has been called the Medical Miranda Act

because, like the Miranda rule, which requires police officers to read a list of rights to persons arrested, it requires health care providers to inform patients of their rights to accept or reject treatment.

39. 135 Cong. Record at 513567 (daily ed., Oct. 17, 1989).
40. Payne v. Marion General Hospital, 549 N.E.2d 1043 (Ind. App. 2 Dist. 1990).
41. Cruzan v. Director, Missouri Department of Health, 110 S. Ct. 2841 (1990).
42. In re: Milton, 29 Ohio St. 3rd 20, 505 N.E.2d 255 (1987).
43. "The essence of the Living Will is informed consent of the person to the status of irreversibility of dying or living maimed." Kutner: The living will—coping with the historical event of death. Baylor Law Rev 17:29, 1975.
44. Note, statutory recognition of the right to die: The California Natural Death Act. Boston Univ Law Rev Rev 57:148, 167, 1988.
45. See, for example, Cruzan v. Director, Missouri Department of Health, 110 S. Ct. 2841 (1990).
46. Poor, B, and Poirrier, G: End of life nursing care. Jones and Bartlett, Sudbury, Mass, 2001.
47. Ibid.
48. Ibid.
49. Ibid.
50. Ibid.
51. Ibid.

Recommended Reading

Ahronkeim, J, Moreno, J, and Zucherman, C: Ethics in clinical practice, ed 2. Aspen Publishers, Gaithersburg, Md, 2000.

Aiken, T: Advance directives. What health care professionals need to know. Long Term Care Network, 1999.

Badzek, L, Leslie, W, and Corbo-Richert, B: End of life decisions: Are they honored? J Nurs Law 5(2), 51–63, 1998.

Beauchamp, T, and Childress, J: Principles of biomedical ethics, ed 4. New York: Oxford University Press, 1994.

Choice in Dying, Inc.: Health Care Agents: Appointing One and Being One. Choice in Dying, Inc., New York, 1998.

Choice in Dying, Inc.: Advance Directives and End-of-Life Decisions. Choice in Dying, Inc., New York, 1996.

Choice in Dying, Inc.: Advance Directive Protocols and the Patient Self-Determination Act. Choice in Dying, Inc., New York.

Choice in Dying, Inc.: Artificial Nutrition and Hydration and End-Of-Life Decision-Making. Choice in Dying, Inc., New York, 1995.

Choice in Dying, Inc.: Cardiopulmonary Resuscitation, Do-Not-Resuscitate Orders and End-Of-Life Decisions. Choice in Dying, Inc., New York, 1995.

Choice in Dying, Inc.: Dying at Home. Choice in Dying, Inc., New York, 1996.

Choice in Dying, Inc.: Medical Treatments and Your Advance Directives, New York, 1996.

Choice in Dying, Inc.: The Physician Assisted Suicide Debate: Understanding the Issues. Choice in Dying, Inc., New York, 1997.

Durr, K: Ethics in Health Services Management. Health Professions Press, Baltimore, 1998.

Humphrey, D: Dying with Dignity: Understanding Euthanasia. Carol Publishing, New York, 1992.

Pozgar, GD: Legal Aspects of Health Care Administration, ed 7. Aspen Publishers, Gaithersburg, Md, 1999.

Resources

Partnership for Caring, Inc.
1035 39th Street, NW
Washington, DC 20007

Facility Liability: Employment Issues 12

Key Chapter Concepts

Nurse's bill of rights
Vicarious liability
Respondeat superior
Borrowed servant doctrine
Captain of the ship doctrine
Ostensible authority or agency
  doctrine
Inherent function
Control
Corporate negligence
Negligent hiring
Health Care Integrity and Protection
  Data Bank
Failure to fire
Employment at will
Just cause
Defamation

Conditional privilege
Loss of conditional privilege
Discrimination
Equal employment opportunity
  commission
Sexual harassment
Quid pro quo
Hostile work environment
Prima facie case
Age Discrimination and Employment
  Act
Civil Rights Act
Rehabilitation Act of 1973
Americans with Disabilities Act
Disability
Family and Medical Leave Act

Chapter Thoughts

When an employment arrangement is created, both the employee and the employer are bound by certain ethical rights and obligations. In the health care system, the majority of all nurses are employed in hospitals or nursing homes.

In an ideal world, the nurse's primary and only responsibility is to provide quality care to the assigned patients. The reality of the situation in the facility setting is that the nurse has multiple responsibilities: responsibility to the patient, responsibility to the facility, responsibility to the physician, and responsibility to self. Nurses experience continual conflict among these four responsibilities. This conflict takes many forms. Nurses are taught as students that they should develop high ideals and standards. One of the primary focuses of nursing as a profession is health maintenance and patient education. The facility setting, however, is not always the best place to express high ideals or to attempt to implement health maintenance and patient education. Nurses have little time to deal with patients individually because of short staffing ratios, shortened hospital stays, and restrictive facility policies that prevent the nurse from carrying out these important activities. Nursing as a profession has a strong tradition of humanizing health care through a holistic, personal approach to patient care that includes all the patient's problems and incorporates the patient's family. Yet the health care system tends to place a high value on and reward those nurses who master the new technology, develop more advanced medical skills, and spend less time with patients and their families. Nursing students are taught that they are colleagues with physicians in the provision of care for patients, yet to some persons the physician's role commands more power and prestige.

The employer-facility's obligations toward the nurses it employs appear to be rather limited. In general, these obligations fall into two categories: to provide a safe and secure environment for nurses to perform duties and to provide a fair wage. Although these categories can be expanded to include other factors, such as health care insurance, time off for maternity leave, hepatitis B vaccination, and so on, the extension of benefits appears more often to be an issue of recruitment and retention of nurses rather than an ethical issue of justice in employment.

All nurses are familiar with the patient's bill of rights. In many facilities, patients are provided with a copy of this document on admission. Although this document is not legally binding, it does provide some sense that patients are important individuals and recognizes their autonomy in the often impersonal health care system. In addition, the patient's bill of rights gives patients a feeling that they are "owed" certain elements of care and respect from the institution, as well as the institution's employees.

Are nurses ever given a nurse's bill of rights when they are hired by a facility, nursing home, or some other agency? Most nurses probably do not even know that such a document exists (Box 12–1). Like the patient's bill of rights, the **nurse's bill of rights** has no legal means of enforcement, but it does outline some fundamental ethical rights for nurses that should be recognized by the facility, nursing home, or other employing agency. Nurses work in extremely difficult circumstances because of their central role in patient care, close contact with families, dominance by the medical professions, and limitations from institutional policies. Yet without nurses to provide the hands-on, 24-hour-a-day care, facilities would have no way to deliver their often-advertised services. Nurses must be recognized as the valuable elements of the health care system that they truly are.

OBJECTIVES

Upon completing this chapter, the reader will be able to:

1. Describe how a facility can be held liable for the actions of its employees, independent contractors, and professionals.
2. Interpret events and issues in facilities, nursing homes, or other health care facilities that pose personal liability risks for nurses.
3. Identify the major protected groups in antidiscrimination statutes.
4. Discuss the rationale for developing and maintaining employee records, evaluations, and hiring applications.
5. Define the Americans with Disabilities Act.

6. Define the types of sexual harassment and understand the process for reporting them.
7. Specify and understand the other federal acts that attempt to combat various types of discrimination.

Introduction

In the majority of medical malpractice claims filed, the facility where the nurse or physician cared for the patient is named as a defendant. Facilities are named as defendants because of their deep pockets—meaning that they can pay larger settlements or judgments. **Vicarious liability** is the legal doctrine often cited when dealing with facility liability.

The first recognized legal duty of a facility is its responsibility for the acts of its employees under the doctrine of respondeat superior. The courts have also developed two other areas of liability for facilities, ostensible authority and corporate negligence (Box 12–2). Not only do facilities have to contend with lawsuits from the outside, they also get hit from within. Issues in hiring and firing, disability, and sexual harassment, to name a few, keep facility legal counsel busy as well.

Vicarious Liability

Respondeat Superior

Respondeat superior, mentioned in passing several times in previous chapters, is a Latin term handed down from English common law; it means "Let the master answer." When a nurse is hired by a facility, agency, nursing home, individual, or other

---

BOX 12–1

Nurse's Bill of Rights

1. The right to be treated with respect.
2. The right to a reasonable work load.
3. The right to an equitable wage.
4. The right to set your own priorities.
5. The right to ask for what you want.
6. The right to refuse without making excuses or feeling guilty.
7. The right to make mistakes and be responsible for them.
8. The right to give and receive information as a professional.
9. The right to act in the best interest of the patient.
10. The right to be human.

Source: Chenevert, M: Pro-nurse Handbook, ed 2. Mosby, St Louis, 1993, p 113, with permission.

BOX 12–2

Elements of Doctrines of Facility Liability

Respondeat Superior

1. Act or omission of the employee.
2. Occurs during employment relationship.
3. Negligent act occurred within the scope of employment.

Ostensible Authority

1. Patient looks to the facility for treatment.
2. Facility assigns the physician or nurse to treat.
3. Negligence of the physician or nurse causes injury.

Corporate Negligence

1. Facility knew or should have known.
2. Physician or nurse provides substandard care.

---

entity, the nurse owes a duty of care to the individuals under the care of the employer while the nurse is on duty and acting within the scope of employment.

If the nurse breaches a duty or standard of care owed to the patient and causes injury, the employer may be held legally liable under the doctrine of respondeat superior (Box 12–3).

Keep in mind that the nursing act in question must occur during the time of employment and while performing the duties required by the employer in order for the action to be even possibly considered within the scope of the nurse-employer relationship.

Examples of acts outside the nurse-employer relationship (which therefore do not fall under respondeat superior) include providing nursing care when not working for the employer, giving advice to neighbors, and responding to an emergency on the street. In addition, any procedure performed by a nurse that should only be done by a physician or nurse practitioner is also considered outside the nurse's scope of employment, and therefore the employer may argue it is not liable or responsible for the nurse's actions.

BOX 12–3

Acting Within the Scope of Employment— Further Inquiries

1. The time, place, and purpose of the act
2. Its similarity to what is authorized
3. The extent of departure from normal methods
4. Past dealings between the employer and employee
5. Whether the employer had reason to expect that such an act would be done

A CASE IN POINT

Improper Supervision

The Facts

In *Willinger v. Mercy Catholic Hospital,* a nurse-anesthetist failed to properly monitor anesthesia during a tonsillectomy, causing significant brain damage of a 5 year old. The nurse-anesthetist, an employee of the hospital, induced anesthesia under the supervision of the anesthesiologist. The anesthesiologist was then called to an emergency operating room to treat another patient. When the anesthesiologist returned, he found the patient without a heartbeat and the "color of a cadaver." The nurse-anesthetist was still administering a full dose of anesthesia and was not using a stethoscope to monitor the heartbeat.[1]

The Jury Decides

The hospital was held liable.

Liability

Under the principles of vicarious liability and the doctrine of respondeat superior, the nurse, as well as his or her employer, can be held liable. At the same time, the employer may be named in a suit with or without the employee and may be held liable because of the employer-employee relationship.

Borrowed Servant Doctrine

The **borrowed servant doctrine** is another theory of vicarious liability. In short, the doctrine says that if someone "borrows" an employee of someone else, the borrower is legally responsible for the "servant's" or employee's acts. For example, if a physician controls the acts of a nurse employed by a facility, the borrowed servant doctrine may be applied. This is no longer a widely used doctrine.[2]

Captain of the Ship Doctrine

Captain of the ship doctrine is also a form of vicarious liability. This doctrine holds that if a person supervises or controls another, he or she is legally responsible for that person. The common example is a surgeon in the operating room setting who "controls" the acts of the nurses in the suite. This doctrine is limited in many parts of the country. Nurses should be held accountable for their own acts or omissions, regardless of the orders given by a physician, according to the state boards of nursing and national nursing standards.[3]

Ostensible Authority or Agency

Under the **ostensible authority or agency doctrine** (also called doctrine of ostensible agency), a facility is liable for the negligence of an independent contractor if the patient has a rational basis to believe that the independent contractor is a facility employee.

Facilities may be held liable for the acts of independent contracting nurses, just as they are found liable for the wrongful acts of physicians who are independent contractors.

The courts have arrived at a test to establish ostensible authority, which includes the presence of these elements:

1. Subjective
2. Inherent function
3. Reliance
4. Control

Subjective

In *Grewe v. Mt. Clemens General Hospital*, a Michigan court held that the critical question in determining the existence of ostensible authority was whether the patient, at the time of the admission, looked to the hospital for treatment of his physical ailments or merely viewed the hospital as a place where his physician would treat him for his problem.[4] One factor was whether the hospital provided the physician to the patient or whether the patient and the physician had a patient-physician relationship apart from the hospital setting. The court ruled that when a patient looks to the facility for his or her treatment and is treated by medical personnel who are ostensible agents of the facility, the facility is held liable.

Inherent Function

An **inherent function** is one that exists in and is inseparable from the hospital. Ostensible authority is applied most commonly in situations involving emergency room physicians, even though the contract between the physician and facility usually identifies the physician as an independent contractor. Some courts have held that the physician is an agent of the facility because the emergency room physician performs an inherent function of the facility in providing emergency care.[5]

Reliance

A court may hold the facility liable if the patient relies on the facility's judgment (e.g., choosing to be admitted to that hospital for surgery rather than another) but is injured because of something the facility did or omitted doing.

Control

In certain circumstances, a facility may be liable for an independent contractor if a certain degree of **control** is exercised by the facility over the independent contractor. To identify whether or not control exists, a court examines and balances many factors, including the following:

1. The extent to which the employer determines the details of the work
2. The kind of occupation
3. The customs of the industry
4. Whether the work is generally supervised by the employer
5. Who supplies the place to work
6. Who supplies the instruments to work
7. The method of payment

Corporate Negligence

The courts have developed two separate and independent facility responsibilities that they consider under the doctrine of **corporate negligence:** the responsibility to hire qualified employees and the responsibility to monitor and supervise their performance and act upon substandard performances.

Under the theory of **negligent hiring,** the facility can be held liable for failure to:

1. Check references.
2. Perform criminal checks on applicants.
3. Confirm license status.
4. Determine skill and educational levels.

The facility will also be held liable for failing to investigate a physician's credentials before granting staff privileges.[6] In *Johnson v. Misericordia Community Hospital*, the Wisconsin Supreme Court found that there was sufficient evidence showing the facility's knowledge of a physician's incompetence for the jury to find the facility liable for granting the physician privileges and allowing him to practice orthopedic surgery.[7] This is likely to be applied to nurses in advance practice who may be required to apply for privileges to perform their duties, such as nurse-midwives and nurse-anesthetists.

Courts have held that the duty of the facility to reasonably investigate an applicant required that the facility check the health care provider's references, educational credentials, former practice, and prior claims. Facilities should also call the provider's former associates, as well as professional associations with which the provider is affiliated, and should ensure that the provider is licensed in the state. Failure to scrutinize a provider's credentials could foreseeably result in appointing an unqualified provider to the staff, creating an unreasonable risk of harm to the facility's patients.

As discussed earlier, the National Practitioner Data Bank (NPDB), which became operational in 1990, is a central repository for all actions taken by a state regarding a licensed health care practitioner. It was established to address problems caused by health care providers who, after losing their license or facility privileges, or being disciplined by their facility or by the state licensing board, move out of the state and practice in a new state. With the implementation of the data bank, each state and health care facility or provider is required to inform the data bank of actions taken regarding a licensee. This information is available to any facility requesting information about a practitioner. The bank provides information on medical malpractice payment reports, adverse licensure, clinical privileges, and professional society membership reports and Medicare/Medicaid exclusion reports.

Both the NPDB and the **Health Care Integrity and Protection Data Bank** (HIP-DB) are flagging systems used to facilitate comprehensive reviews of providers. The HIP-DB was created to combat fraud and abuse in the delivery of health care. It is a national data collection program for collecting information regarding health care–related criminal convictions, civil judgments, exclusion from participating in federal and state health care programs, licensure, and certification actions.

State medical boards also are required to report disciplinary actions, revocations of licenses, or other actions restricting a physician's right to practice. Self-insurers and insurance carriers also must report settlement payments or payments made as a result of a judgment. Failure to report can result in fines up to $10,000.[8]

It is the facility's duty is to protect the patient from health care providers who can cause harm. Facilities have been held liable for employees who have committed assault and battery on patients or visitors when the facilities failed to perform thorough and proper background checks.[9] Had they performed such checks in those cases, it would have been foreseeable to the facilities that the new employees might harm patients.

The facility must also monitor or supervise all medical and nursing personnel within the facility (whether the personnel are employees or independent contractors), including the quality of care. The facility is then liable for any injuries the patient suffers because of the facility's failure to monitor or supervise the physicians and nurses. The courts also expect the facilities to periodically review staff competency.

If a facility knows that an employee has harmed a patient but does not terminate that employee, it risks liability for **failure to fire** should that employee injure another patient.

Employment Law Liability

Employment Agreements

As an initial matter, the reasons for hiring personnel must be unbiased and fair and cannot be based on an individual's race, sex, national origin, religious preference, age, or handicap.

Except for in a few jurisdictions, most employment arrangements are employment at will, meaning there is no written contract specifying a term of employment.

A CASE IN POINT

Corporate Negligence

The Facts

In an Illinois case, *Darling v. Charleston Community Memorial Hospital*, plaintiff Darling, an 18-year-old man with a broken leg, was treated in an emergency room by an orthopedic surgeon. The patient charged that the resulting amputation was caused by the negligence of the physician and nurses.

The patient brought a suit against the hospital and the doctor under the theory of corporate negligence. At trial, the patient proved that the hospital did not require the following:

1. Orthopedic surgeons to review and update their surgical skills
2. Consultation in the event of surgical complications
3. The nursing staff to regularly examine patients recovering from surgery.

The patient also showed that the facility failed to enforce its policies requiring immediate reporting of patient complications by the nursing staff to the facility administrator.[10]

The Court Decides

In its opinion, the court clearly stated that, because of the hospital's failure to monitor the care provided by its attending physicians and nurses—through control of staff membership and clinical privileges—the facility was liable for the type of care provided.[11]

The Court Affirms the Decision

In *Bost v. Riley*, the court interpreted the Darling case as holding that a hospital could be held negligent for "failing to have a sufficient number of trained nurses attending the plaintiff, failing to require a consultation or examination by members of the facility staff, and failing to review the treatment rendered to the plaintiff."[12] The court held that a facility has a duty to make a reasonable effort to monitor and oversee the treatment that is prescribed and administered by physicians and nurses practicing in the facility.

Employment at will permits either the employer or the employee to terminate employment without cause or notice.

However, higher level nurses are more likely to deliver services under a written employment contract. For employees working under a contract, any reason used to terminate or discharge them before the term of the contract has expired may be considered unlawful. The only way to terminate a contractual employee is specified in the terms of the contract. If the contract does not provide terms for termination, then termination may occur only (1) at the expiration of the amount of time specified in the contract or (2) when the employee breaches the terms of the contract.

A few courts have found that contracts exist based on specific promises or words used in job announcements, application forms, and interviewing questions. Special care should be given to what is said in advertisements and applications. Consider interview questions in advance of the meeting. When closing an interview, the interviewer should indicate how or when the decision will be made and how the applicant will be notified. The interviewer should not indicate approval or disapproval with an applicant's responses.

Open questions are used to encourage the nurse applicant to talk and may call for a statement of position. Closed questions permit yes or no answers.

Open: What are your feelings about occasionally being asked to work on another floor?

Closed: Do you mind working on another floor on occasion?

Open: How is this position related to your goals and ambitions?

Closed: Would this position help you achieve any of your goals and ambitions?

"Why" questions used by the interviewer can make a question sound like a challenge and create unwanted defensive reactions. The question may be reworded in an open format to obtain the information.

Poor: Why do you think you can handle this job?

Better: What skills and management abilities do you have that would make you successful in this position?

Contract Arising After Employment

Handbooks and personnel and policy manuals can create an employment contract. Statements in employee manuals or company policies can be contractually binding and can alter an underlying employment-at-will status. An aggrieved nurse may successfully assert that the employment manual is a part of the contract, and the employer can be bound by it. For example, an employee who is terminated without notice or severance pay may allege that the employer did not abide by the employment manual, which provides for progressive disciplinary reviews and two weeks' notice of the termination.

Generally there are three theories used to determine whether an employee manual is contractually binding:

1. Employees' expectations;
2. A combination of employees' and employers' expectations; or
3. A unilateral contract theory.

The court can infer the employees' and employers' expectations from all the surrounding circumstances. A unilateral contract may be found as an offer of continued employment by the employer, and the employee's continued work converts the offer to a formal contract.

A CASE IN POINT

Wrongful Termination

The Facts

A plaintiff nurse moved from Michigan to North Carolina to accept a position at Duke Hospital. She was told, when accepting the Duke position, that she could only be discharged for incompetence. While she was employed at Duke, she refused to administer a drug that she believed would injure a patient. The patient was severely injured as a result of being given the medication by others. During a malpractice suit and prior to being deposed, the hospital and physicians who administered the drug warned the nurse "not to tell all." She testified truthfully and was fired immediately. She filed a suit for wrongful discharge.

At trial, she claimed wrongful discharge under two theories of law: contract and tort. In contract, she argued that assurances by Duke Hospital induced her to move from Michigan to North Carolina to take the position.

The Court Decides

The court held that the move constituted additional consideration, which removed her employment contract from one at will to one at contract.[13]

Manuals may state that they are subject to change. Words such as *fair, satisfactory,* and *reasonable* are subject to personal and legal interpretation because they are subjective and vague. If there is a correction to a current version of the manual, it should be referred to as a restatement, not a revision. All corrections or restatements should be distributed to facility employees. Employees should sign and date documentation to show that they have received notice of the changes.

Independent Consideration

When policies and procedures include disclaimers specifically stating that they do not represent an employment contract, most jurisdictions uphold the disclaimers. In *Thompson v. St. Regis Paper Co.*, the court stated that employers are not always bound by statements in employment manuals.[14] An employer can specifically state in a conspicuous manner that nothing contained in the manual is intended to be part of an employment relationship and that the manual merely contains statements of company policy. The employer may also specifically reserve the right to modify the policies.[15]

However, even when an employment contract or the policies and procedures appear to provide for termination at will, if an employer gives the employee extra or independent consideration (i.e., extra salary or benefits) beyond that which is stated in the contract or in the policies and procedures, that employment may not be terminable at will.

Evaluating Employee Performance

Failure to undertake appropriate performance evaluations and promote an individual based on those evaluations has been the basis of discrimination actions. To avoid claims of discrimination related to promotions, performance reviews must support the decision on promotion. Periodic employee evaluations are advisable. In conducting a written evaluation, facilities should use objective criteria to evaluate employees rather than subjective criteria. Be aware, however, that conducting periodic evaluations may lead to a **just cause** requirement for termination. With that in mind, if the evaluations do not reflect the reasons for termination, a facility may have a difficult time defending itself in a discrimination case—the evaluations did not reflect the just cause for terminating the employee.

Just cause requirements can be developed directly from the policy and procedure manual of the employer. In the manual, employers should spell out the types of offenses that will be disciplined, the types of warnings that are given, and the appropriate discipline to be administered. That way, the manual establishes the violations worthy of discipline (and that would lead to just cause), as well as the procedures by which to discipline. If the employer immediately terminates the employee, rather than following written procedure, there is no just cause for the termination. Similarly, if the employee commits an offense not stated in the manual, there is no just cause for termination.

Certain offenses may be established as cause for immediate termination. These offenses are generally lying, stealing, cheating, illicit drug use on the premises, and striking an employee or patient. If an employee is terminated for one of these offenses, the employer has just cause to do so.

Employee evaluations should describe significant performance problems and clearly state what kind of improvement is expected. Evaluations should be reviewed, signed, and dated by the appropriate superiors and employee. A copy of the evaluation should be maintained in the files of the nurse manager or supervisor, and the nurse should be given a copy. The evaluations should be based on observed and recorded employee performance during the period of the review. Supervisors should provide feedback on a continuing basis and not merely at the time of the review. Documentation should reflect feedback, record the achievement of set goals, and note discrepancies.

To ensure that performance evaluations are objective, facilities should establish (1) specific job-related standards, (2) guidance for use by evaluators, and (3) a review procedure by higher level management.

AUTHOR TIP: *Place disciplinary evaluations in a separate file from the nurse's personnel file. Personnel files can be requested by a plaintiff's attorney in a nursing malpractice case, and a disciplinary evaluation can be damaging and used against the nurse or facility in a malpractice suit.*

Terminating Problem Employees

How an employee is handled during the termination process, regarding reasons for the termination and conveying the news, can make a significant difference in his or her decision on whether or not to file a lawsuit.

If the employee belongs to a "protected group" (a member of one of the groups protected under the antidiscrimination acts), the likelihood of successful legal action increases. Detailed documentation should reflect the facts, reasons, and actions supporting the termination decision. In addition, facilitators should review how other similarly situated employees have been handled. If another individual's situation has been handled differently, the facility must distinguish between the two situations and justify the discrepancy. Their termination interview presents a forum for forthright discussion about the reasons for termination; outline those reasons for the employee. Any hint of cover-up or unfair treatment could result in the employee's taking legal action. A facility policy may also be developed requiring the employer to give written notice with the reasons for termination, so that there is no room for misunderstandings.

Standards for Dismissal

Courts across the nation have arrived at a variety of rules on appropriate standards for dismissal.

In *Toussaint v. Blue Cross and Blue Shield of Michigan,* the court indicated that an employer should be permitted to establish its own standards for job performance—as well as standards for dismissal based on nonadherence to those standards—even though another employer or a jury might have established lower standards.[16]

And in *Pugh v. See's Candies, Inc.,* a corporate vice president with 32 years of service was terminated without explanation. The court found an implied agreement that the company had to prove good cause for the termination. The court based its decision on the extreme length of service, chain raises, bonuses and promotions, the president's repeated assurances that employment would continue if the employee did a good job, the company's acknowledged practice of not terminating executive personnel except for cause, and the company's failure ever formally to criticize or warn the plaintiff that his job was in jeopardy.[17]

Other examples of situations where courts have found just cause include the following:

1. Depressed market conditions
2. Financial need for the business to reorganize and relocate operations[18]
3. Open defiance and insubordination

4. Fighting[19]
5. Excessive absenteeism[20]

NOTE: Clear violation of a company policy is a question for the court and not for the jury.[21]

Executives, managers, supervisors, and creative employees are generally evaluated by more subjective considerations that can often be difficult to quantify, measure, or objectively compare, particularly in a small company. Although cases do not tend to require broader company discretion for terminating higher-level or special employees, there appears to be some recognition that a different standard applies.[22]

Exceptions to At-Will Employment

The employee also has the right to leave the employer without notice or cause. When an employee cannot show that a contract was formed, there are still several exceptions to the strict at-will rule. The two major categories of exceptions are as follows:

1. Implied covenant of good faith and fair dealing
2. Public policy

Implied Covenant of Good Faith and Fair Dealing

Termination itself does not constitute a breach of the covenant of good faith and fair dealing, unless it is done specifically to deprive the employee of earned compensation. Several jurisdictions hold that employment relationships, like commercial relationships, require an obligation between the parties. This obligation prevents an employer from terminating an employee for the sole reason of depriving the employee of earned but not received compensation (commissions, salary, company benefits) for services already performed.[23]

Public Policy

An employee at will may not be terminated for reasons inconsistent with established public policy. Termination is prohibited by public policy if it is done "in retaliation for performing an important and socially desirable act, exercising a statutory right, or refusing to commit an unlawful act."[24] Employees have a claim under public policy if they are terminated (1) for asserting a statutory right, such as filing a workers' compensation claim; (2) for doing what the law requires, such as serving on a jury; or (3) for refusing to do what the law forbids, such as committing perjury.

Under the nomer of public policy, many states have laws that protect "whistleblowers." These laws protect employees who disclose alleged illegality about or within their employment and then are terminated by the employer.

A CASE IN POINT

Public Policy

The Facts

A psychiatric nurse provided information to a state agency about a patient confined in a state hospital. She also testified on behalf of the patient at his commitment hearing. The nurse was terminated. Her employer said she was terminated for failure to support hospital programs, insubordination, insults to superiors, mistreatment of patients, and failing to limit her damages by refusing to take a demotion.

The Court Decides

The court found that the nurse had been terminated—in contravention of public policy—because she had provided information to the state agency.[25]

Post-termination

Once an employee has been terminated, the issue of references arises. An employer must have a definite policy on giving out or serving as a reference to a terminated employee to prevent potential liability for defamation or negligence. Today many facilities develop policies to avoid these potential problems or litigation when discussing former employees or other sensitive information. During the termination interview, the reference policy should be discussed. The policy should allow the employer to reveal only that the employee worked for the employer for a specific period of time and performed a particular type of work.

Defamation

Defamation, as discussed earlier, occurs when the plaintiff is exposed to public hatred, ridicule, or contempt, through oral or written publication of false statements. The "public" is generally considered to be the more limited, professional community in which the plaintiff works. Publication occurs when there is any kind of communication to any individual other than the plaintiff. The person to whom the defamatory statements are made must have heard and understood the remarks to be about the plaintiff. If an employer giving a reference, for instance, knows that a published statement is false, or recklessly disregards a statement's veracity in disseminating it, the employer may be liable for defamation. Half-truths may be as misleading and are as actionable as whole lies.[26] This rule is subject to the qualified privilege discussed later.

Conditional Privilege

An employer may have a conditional privilege to disclose defamatory information concerning an employee. A **conditional privilege** renders nondefamatory an employer's statements concerning the character and abilities of former employees if directed to a prospective employer.[27] This defense usually applies when information is sought from an employer regarding the qualifications or character of a former employee.[28] Similarly, entries on internal personnel documents are generally considered conditionally privileged.

Loss of Conditional Privilege

Loss of conditional privilege occurs if the employee can prove recklessness. This may occur if the employer recklessly disseminates statements, disregards truth or falsifies information, fails to verify information, or, where it is practical, fails to safeguard against error. Actual bad faith, ill will, or improper purpose or motive inconsistent with social policy or interests may constitute actual malice and cause an employer to lose conditional privilege. Willful false statements destroy the conditional privilege and constitute malice unless the employer has a reasonable belief in the truth of a statement.

Negligence

An employee about whom a reference was given may not only have an action under defamation but may also have a separate negligence claim. The employer may not be legally obligated to provide references but is bound to exercise due care in providing references it gives voluntarily. If due care is not used and causes damages to the former employee, the elements of negligence are met.

◢ Discrimination and Harassment

As more nurses become responsible for employment decisions within a facility, they have increased liability for these employment decisions. Nurses' actions on behalf of their employers, or on their own behalves, expose them to potential liability for wrongful termination, wrongful failure to hire, or wrongful failure to advance employees.

Antidiscrimination statutes protect employees and should be integrated fully into employee management procedures, including hiring, planning and conducting performance reviews of employees, managing problem employees, and terminating unacceptable employees (Box 12–4).

An example of a bona fide occupational qualification is demonstrated in an Illinois case. In *Garcia v. Rush-Presbyterian Medical Center*, the court found that employment at a complex medical center required the ability to speak English.[29]

BOX 12–4

Overview of Antidiscrimination Statutes

Statutes exist to protect people on the basis of the following:

1. Race
2. Color
3. Religious preference
4. National origin
5. Pregnancy status
6. Age
7. Disability
8. Gender

Exceptions

1. A religious entity may consider religious background.
2. These factors can be considered if they constitute a bona fide occupational qualification.
3. These factors can be considered if they constitute a business necessity.

Discrimination

Title VII 42 U.S.C. 2000 e-1 et seq., the Civil Rights Act of 1964, protects employees from **discrimination** based on race, color, religion, sex, or national origin and provides that pregnant women receive the same protection as other employees and applicants. See Box 12–5 for a brief history of Title VII.

The **Equal Employment Opportunity Commission** (EEOC), which enforces Title VII, also has guidelines that provide protection from sexual harassment, including conduct in which:

1. Submission to sexual advances is implicitly or explicitly considered a condition of employment.
2. Submission to sexual advances is used as a basis for employment decisions.
3. Sexual harassment interferes with job performances, even if it only creates an intimidating, offensive, or hostile atmosphere.

Sexual Harassment

The issues of **sexual harassment** concern the misuse of power and control over others in "lower" positions of the power structure in both academic and clinical settings. Sexual harassment can be heterosexual or homosexual. Sexual harassment is unlawful if submission to it meets any of the following conditions:

BOX 12-5

A Sexual Harassment Timeline

1972: Title IX of the Education Amendments extended the prohibition regarding sex discrimination to educational institutions receiving federal funds.
1980: The EEOC issued sexual harassment guidelines for the workplace, applying to supervisors, employees, and nonemployees.
1987: Title IX was clarified, making the entire institution subject to the requirements, not just the section of the institution receiving federal funding.

---

1. Is a condition of employment
2. Interferes with performance
3. Is the basis for employment decision
4. Creates a hostile and intimidating work environment

There are two types of sexual harassment: quid pro quo and hostile environment.

Quid Pro Quo

Quid pro quo claims stem from implicit requests for sexual favors and from requests for sexual favors that are used as a condition for employment decisions such as promotions.

To prove a quid pro quo case, the following elements must be present:

1. Sexual advances are unwelcome.
2. Harassment is sexually motivated.
3. Plaintiff is a member of a protected group (i.e., employees of a hospital that are in a lower position in the power structure).
4. Plaintiff's reactions to the superior's advances affect an aspect of his or her employment or advancement, such as promotion, salary increase, or productivity.

An example of quid pro quo harassment is as follows: An institution's administrator tells a nursing faculty member that he loves good looks and brains in a woman. The educator ignores the administrator's remarks and walks away from him in disgust after the comment. The administrator then suddenly finds fault with her work with no basis and fires her. See *Chamberlain v. 101 Realty, Inc.*, which illustrates the elements of quid pro quo sexual harassment.[30]

Hostile Work Environment

In a **hostile work environment,** offensive behavior creates a hostile or intimidating work environment, which interferes with the work performance of the plaintiff. To

A Case in Point

Sexual Harassment and Discrimination

The Facts

A female registered nurse (RN) worked full-time in an intensive care unit (ICU). Shortly after being hired, a male RN was hired to work the same shift. Not long after he was hired, he began sexually harassing the female RN with offensive sexual comments and jokes, suggesting a threesome with another nurse, requesting oral sex, and physically touching her breasts and buttocks. She rejected his advances and requested that the harassment cease.

She complained to her supervisor, the director of nurses, and the human resources director. She asked hospital administration to speak with him, and they stated it could not be done without filing a formal complaint. She hesitated, wanting the incident to be handled confidentially because she needed to continue to work with him. When she did decide to file the formal complaint, she notified her supervisor several times and was told that the supervisor was too busy. She contacted human resources and was told to make an appointment, but she never followed through.

The hospital administration met with the male nurse and informed him of the accusations, that if a formal complaint was filed an investigation would need to be done, and that, if the allegations were true, he must cease his actions. The female nurse was subsequently fired based on allegations that she had committed five serious errors and that she missed 2 weeks of work due to illness.

The nurse filed a suit against the hospital for sexual harassment and retaliation.

The Jury Decides

The jury found for the plaintiff nurse based on the fact that the defendant hospital knew or should have known about the sexual harassment and failed to take swift remedial action. Although the nurse died before the case was settled, her estate was awarded compensation for emotional pain and suffering, lost wages and benefits, punitive damages, and attorney fees.[31]

establish that a hostile work environment exists, it is not necessary to show that the offensive conduct was directed specifically at the plaintiff; it is enough that the behavior was observed or known by the plaintiff and affected his or her psychological and emotional status and well-being.

Outside of these two defined categories, sexual harassment can take many forms. Subtle action, such as requesting a person to have drinks or dinner after work, may

A CASE IN POINT

Hostile Work Environment

The Facts

In *Meritor Savings Bank v. Vinson*,[32] the victim alleged that the supervisor made repeated demands for sexual favors, fondled her in front of other employees, forcibly raped her on numerous occasions, and exposed himself to her.

The Court Decides

The court found that the allegations were sufficient for a case of sexual harassment.

The Facts

A cardiologist was accused of verbally and physically abusing female employees, creating a hostile work environment. He also verbally insulted male employees. Numerous instances of abuse reported included shouting, cursing, throwing objects, using vulgarity, shoving female employees, and striking a female employee with a defibrillator paddle to give her an electric shock to get her to move more quickly. The evidence contained allegations of abuse over an extended period made by 4 male and 10 female employees.

The Court Decides

The court found that there was sufficient evidence to support the allegations[33]

qualify. The EEOC looks at the totality of the circumstances and focuses on several factors to determine if the conduct was unwelcome. It considers the following:

1. Type of conduct (physical, verbal, or both)
2. Hostile or offensive conduct
3. Frequency of conduct
4. Consistency of the victim's conduct
5. Category of offender (supervisor, coworker, or other)
6. Others who were part of the harassment or who assisted[34]

In a recent case, the court found that the alleged acts of a physician did not support a sexual harassment claim by a nurse who was both an employee and patient. The physician allegedly bit a cake shaped like a breast at an office party, made unwanted sexual advances to a staff worker, commented to a staff worker she looked "really hot today," and said an employee looked sexier after breast surgery. None of the alleged acts of sexual harassment was directed at the nurse.[35]

Victims' Redress

The first line of redress for victims is to consult their employer's sexual harassment policy. These policies are a requirement for receiving federal funding. The policy must include the EEOC language on sexual harassment. The following items must be described in the policy:

1. A grievance procedure
2. The type of forms that need to be completed
3. To whom the incident is reported
4. The hearing procedure and an alternative in case the person in charge of the hearing is the offender
5. The resolution process

The policy must protect the legal rights of all parties involved by ensuring confidentiality and due process. The policy is applicable to on- and off-campus placements, including clinical areas.

A sexual harassment complaint by a faculty member or nursing student against an employee or professional at the clinical site implicates the clinical facility and the educational institution. For example, if the complaint is against a physician, he or she is held accountable to the clinical facility's policy manual even when the physician is not an employee of the hospital. The facility itself may be liable for the actions of those who work for it. The facility is also responsible for complying with the grievance procedure stated in its sexual harassment policy. Because the educational institution has a contract with the facility, the school has an obligation to make the clinical facility aware of a sexual harassment complaint by a nursing student. If the school fails to monitor the clinical facility for any further signs or incidents of sexual harassment, it may be liable to the student if further problems occur.

If the internal policies and procedures of the academic institution or the clinical facility fail to address the sexual harassment complaint, victims have the right to sue in federal court to resolve their problems.

Filing a Claim

The plaintiff must first exhaust all state and federal administrative remedies prior to filing a civil court action. Sixty days after filing with the state authority, the plaintiff may file a complaint with the EEOC, although some states permit filing in both the state agency and the EEOC at the same time. An EEOC complaint must be filed within 180 days of the alleged violation. The EEOC then investigates and resolves the violation through conciliation or court action. If the employee is not satisfied with the EEOC resolution, the employee may file a claim with the trial court.[36]

In a Title VII claim, the plaintiff has the burden to prove, by a preponderance of evidence, a **prima facie case** of discrimination (Box 12–6). A prima facie case means that on its face, if the employer offered no evidence at all, the employee's claim would prevail in proving discrimination.[37]

BOX 12–6

How to Make a Prima Facie Case of Discrimination

1. There is direct evidence that there is discrimination such as a "smoking gun" or a letter stating a discriminatory reason for failing to hire or to terminate the employee.
2. Discriminatory treatment can be inferred by the plaintiff employee if the plaintiff shows that:
   a. He or she is a member of a protected group.
   b. He or she is qualified for the job for which the plaintiff applies or from which the plaintiff is discharged.
   c. He or she is rejected or terminated.
   d. The position remains open or someone outside the protected group has replaced him or her.
3. In age discrimination, statistical patterns from which an inference of discrimination may be drawn.

Age Discrimination and Employment Act

The **Age Discrimination and Employment Act** (ADEA), 29 U.S.C. 621 (1967), also enforced by the EEOC, prohibits discrimination by an employer against anyone 40 years old or older in decisions involving hiring and promotions. It exempts public safety employees, top managers, and, until 1994, tenured college professors over 70 years old because age is a factor in those positions. The proof and allocation of proof in an ADEA matter are similar to a Title VII case. Besides the "smoking gun" and "inferred" proof of discrimination, statistical patterns can establish proof from which a reasonable inference of discrimination can be drawn.[38]

Civil Rights Acts

The **Civil Rights Act** of 1866, 42 U.S.C. 1981, prohibits discrimination on the basis of race, lineage, and national origin in the formation and enforcement of employment contracts. On-the-job racial harassment is not included because the act does not apply to discrimination that does not impair the formation of the contract. There must be proof of "purposeful discrimination" in forming the employment relationship, and the burden of proof is the same as in Title VII.

The Civil Rights Act of 1871, 42 U.S.C. 1983, provides the right to sue a person who deprives another of a right under the Civil Rights Act of 1866. The deprivation must occur "under the color of statute, ordinance, regulation, custom, or usage." "Under the color of statute" essentially means that there must be some action by the state or a publicly supported entity that deprives another of the right to form and enforce an employment contract. A facility receiving federal or state financial assistance, such as a college receiving federal funding, may be considered to be acting under the color of statute by virtue of the public assistance.

Rehabilitation Act of 1973

The **Rehabilitation Act of 1973** outlaws discrimination based on disability. According to the Rehabilitation Act, a handicap is a physical or mental impairment that substantially limits one or more major life activities. The handicap does not necessarily have to be a long-term disability; it can be a short-term handicap. The Rehabilitation Act applies to employers who receive federal financial assistance or who have contracts with the federal government.

Americans with Disabilities Act

Congress passed the **Americans with Disabilities Act** in 1990 to eliminate discrimination against United States residents with physical or mental disabilities. This act applies to all employers, not just those receiving federal funding.

Historically, disabled individuals have been discriminated against and isolated. They face disadvantages and unequal opportunities in such vital areas as employment, health services, telecommunications, public accommodations, entertainment, and housing. Unlike other groups, the disabled have not had legal recourse to address these issues. Congress passed the Americans with Disabilities Act in 1990 to improve equality of opportunity, full participation in the activities of daily living, and economic self-sufficiency.

The goal of the Americans with Disabilities Act is to eliminate discrimination against people in the United States who have physical or mental disabilities so that they can participate more fully in the workplace and social life. This act not only prohibits discrimination but also delineates clear, enforceable standards through its accompanying regulations.

What Is a Disability?

The term **disability** is defined in the ADA as any physical or mental impairment that limits any major life activity. This broad-based definition covers all individuals with obvious physical disabilities but also includes individuals with such disabilities as diabetes, cancer, human immunodeficiency virus (HIV), or acquired immunodeficiency syndrome (AIDS), as well as recovering alcoholics and drug addicts. The act does not cover any individual who is, at present, using illegal drugs. The "illegal use of drugs" means possession, distribution, or use of drugs that violates the Controlled Substance Act. Also covered by the ADA are individuals who have a work, social, or family relationship with disabled individuals. Because of the broad definition of

---

BOX 12–7

Who Is Covered by the ADA?

1. All individuals with one or more physical or mental disabilities that limit any major life activity.
2. Those who have a record of such a disability.
3. Those who are regarded as having a disability.
4. Individuals who have a work, social, or family relationship with a disabled person.

---

impairments, there is an ongoing process of identifying additional covered disabilities. Specifically excluded from coverage are homosexuals, bisexuals, transvestites, transsexuals, pedophiliacs, exhibitionists, voyeurs, those with gender identity disorders, gamblers, pyromaniacs, and kleptomaniacs, unless they have identified disabilities that are covered (Box 12–7).

Title I, Employment, and the ADA

All employers, employment agencies, labor organizations, and joint labor management committees fall under the rubric of the ADA. No discrimination is allowed against any qualified applicant with a disability or against disabled individuals regarding any terms and conditions of work. This includes promotions, salary, discharge, transfer, and all other conditions of work. See Box 12–8 for criteria for discriminatory practice.

The ADA has affected the workplace in numerous ways. Employers have eliminated most pre-employment medical inquiries. Medical questionnaires have also changed because employers can no longer ask about prior injuries, employee compensation claims, and diseases.

The ADA prohibits any question seeking to identify the nature or severity of any individual's disabilities. Employers are restricted to asking only about a candidate's ability to do the job safely. If a physical examination is required, it must be job specific. Employers also have the responsibility of educating all employees about the ADA's requirements.

BOX 12–8

Discriminatory Practice

1. Denial of participation to a disabled person
2. Unequal benefit
3. Failure to provide settings suitable for use by the disabled
4. Denial to someone affiliated with a disabled person
5. Exclusion because of lack of insurance coverage

The essential functions of the job have to be clearly identified by the employer, who must determine whether an applicant is qualified. Many disputes have arisen in this area.

A qualified individual with a disability is someone who can safely perform all aspects of a job with or without reasonable accommodations. The employer has the right to require that the individual does not pose any threat to the health and safety of him- or herself or others. Keep in mind that an employer does not have to hire a disabled applicant if there are other equally qualified applicants.

Reasonable accommodation refers to the employer's responsibility to provide the necessary restructuring, reassignment, equipment modification or devices, training materials, interpreters, and other accommodations for any disabled individual. Employers are required to make all reasonable accommodations necessary for a disabled employee to function in the workplace. This is applicable to all job applicants and employees. Disabled individuals should be prepared to seek appropriate modifications by asking the employer specifically to meet their needs. For example, a disabled person who requires an interpreter should make this need known to the employer. If the person is hearing impaired, appropriate telephone devices may be requested. And the need for reasonable accommodation cannot impact a decision to hire someone. Much litigation surrounds the definition and implementation of reasonable accommodation.

Defenses to ADA Claims

There are several defenses to ADA claims and to the enforcement of ADA requirements.

UNDUE HARDSHIP DEFENSE

The undue hardship defense is an exception to the mandate that employers deliver reasonable accommodations to disabled employees. If an accommodation is too expensive or difficult to implement, it may be considered an undue hardship; however, the employer must thoroughly investigate and offer data to prove this defense. A determination of undue hardship is made based on cost, the resources of the employer, the size of the employer, the number of employees, and the type of operation or function of the employer.

QUALIFICATION STANDARD AND HEALTH AND SAFETY DEFENSE

Another defense to an employment claim based on ADA violation is that the health and safety of the individual or others is compromised. All qualification standards require that applicants safely perform their jobs. Employers can ask questions about any applicant's ability to do the job and perform safely all necessary job-related functions. If an employer can prove that an applicant or employee who is disabled could not safely perform the job, the employer may prevail.

RELIGIOUS ENTITIES DEFENSE

Employers that are religious entities are not prohibited from giving preference to individuals of a particular religion.

PUBLIC SAFETY DEFENSE

Public safety is a priority, and it can be a defense to an employment claim if a reasonable accommodation cannot eliminate the risk of transmittal of infectious or communicable diseases to others. For example, if a nurse's aide is hired for a job and through a physical exam it is discovered that he or she has active tuberculosis, the job offer can be rescinded based on the public safety defense.

The Hiring Process and the ADA

An individual who cannot, with a reasonable accommodation, perform an essential job function is not considered a qualified individual with a disability under the ADA (Box 12–9). An unqualified individual is not protected by the ADA. It is important for employers to determine whether job applicants are in fact qualified. This requires an affirmative answer to two questions:

1. *Does the individual satisfy the prerequisites for the position?* You will need to review whether the applicant has the appropriate educational background, employment experience, skills, licenses, or other job-related requirements for the position. The facility does not have to provide an accommodation to an individual with an impairment who has not met the initial selection criteria. An individual is not entitled to a reasonable accommodation until the applicant satisfies the first prerequisite.
2. *Can the individual perform the job's essential functions with or without a reasonable accommodation?* This prong of the test requires consideration of candidates who passed the first selection criteria but who may need a reasonable accommodation to pass the second. *Essential functions* refers to fundamental job duties intrinsic to the position she holds or desires. For example, if an applicant cannot hear but has graduated from an accredited nursing school and passed the board examination, the facility might be required to provide an accommodation in order for her to perform the job's essential functions.

An accommodation is not required if it imposes an undue hardship on the facility. An undue hardship often means a significant increase in operating expenses or disruption to the business.

BOX 12–9

Mental and Physical Disabilities Potentially Covered by the ADA

Mental Impairments

1. Personality disorders
2. Major depression
3. Bipolar disorder
4. Anxiety disorders
5. Schizophrenia

Physical Conditions

1. Cancer
2. Drug addiction
3. Alcoholism
4. Heart disease
5. Blindness
6. Diabetes
7. Deafness or hearing impairment

Essential and nonessential job functions should be identified and descriptions prepared. Preparing a written job description before advertising for a position or interviewing candidates assists in identifying a qualified individual. Inaccurate, vague, or overly general job descriptions can do more harm than good and should be discarded.

Employment applications should be reviewed to make sure they comply with federal and state laws. Questions about the facility's prerequisites should be included. Questions regarding an individual's disability status, health, past medical problems, and workers' compensation claims should be deleted. Specific job-related questions to help determine whether applicants can perform the essential functions of the job should be provided where practicable.

An employment test that would screen out individuals with disabilities should not be used unless the test is shown to be job related for the position in question and consistent with business necessity. An employment test must be selected and administered in a manner that ensures that the test results accurately reflect the skills, aptitudes, or other factors the test is designed to measure. A test designed to measure sensory, manual, or speaking skills when those skills are job related may be used. A facility should administer written tests orally to applicants who are blind or visually impaired or who have a learning disability.

The only preoffer drug test that should be required is one that solely detects the use of illegal drugs. No drug tests may be given that attempt to detect a disability prior to extending a conditional offer of employment.

If a medical examination is a required part of the hiring process, the examination should be administered to all entering employees receiving conditional job offers in the same category. The exam results must be kept confidential. Only those people with a need to have that type of information should be informed.

The major requirement of the ADA is that during the pre-employment interview, applicants may not be asked if they have a disability, nor may they be asked about the nature or severity of a disability. It is permissible to ask about an applicant's ability to perform job-related functions. The personnel policy manuals must be updated to reflect the ADA policy. At a minimum, facilities should review the following policies:

Attendance and Lateness

Neutral policies concerning attendance and lateness distributed to all employees should be drafted and enforced consistently. If an employee violates a neutral policy, he or she may be terminated even if the reason for the violation is excessive absenteeism to care for his or her disabled spouse. An employee with a disability may be disciplined if the violation exceeds the facility's attempts at reasonable accommodation.

Leave of Absence

A facility should review its leave-of-absence policy, particularly with respect to leaves with pay. The ADA does not entitle individuals with disabilities to have more paid leave time than nondisabled employees.

Work Schedules

Facilities should consider part-time or modified work schedules to help accommodate all employees, not only those with disabilities.

Interview, Discipline, and Performance Forms

Interview, discipline, and performance forms should be prepared objectively. They must indicate why an individual was hired, disciplined, demoted, and so on. They should provide a nondiscriminatory record should an individual bring a claim alleging discrimination based on disability or on some other protected basis, such as age, race, sex, national origin, marital status, or veteran status.

The facility should develop a disability policy in compliance with procedure. A written policy that explains the facility's commitment to adhere to and enforce its obligations under the ADA and other relevant nondiscrimination laws should be distributed. It should contain a procedure for job applicants and employees to file complaints if they feel they have been discriminated against on the basis of the disability. This may prevent an employee from filing complaints with a government agency or in court and will provide a sound employee relations practice.

A facility is not liable for failing to provide an accommodation that was not requested. If no request is received, it is inappropriate to provide an accommodation. A facility must have knowledge of the limitations of an applicant or employee before a duty to accommodate arises. However, if an employee or applicant with a known disability is having problems performing his or her job, it would be reasonable of the facility to discuss the possibility of an accommodation with the employee. The employee with the disability is not required to accept the accommodation.

Once you are aware that an individual has a disability:

1. Consider discussing possible accommodations with the individual.
2. Identify the barriers to job performance resulting from the particular disability.
3. Assess the reasonableness of each accommodation in regard to its effectiveness, equal opportunity, and hardship.
4. Implement the accommodation that is most appropriate to the individual and imposes the least hardship on the facility.

An effective accommodation does not have to be the most expensive or the most difficult to implement. As long as it provides a reasonable solution to an employment obstacle, it may be the least expensive or easiest to implement. Reallocation of essential functions is not required in order to provide a reasonable accommodation.

Family and Medical Leave Act

The **Family and Medical Leave Act** (FMLA) is enforced by the United States Department of Labor. It guarantees, under specific circumstances, up to 12 weeks of unpaid leave per year for an employee to care for the health of a family member or his or her own health or after the adoption of a child. The act maintains job protection for these individuals.

For the FMLA to kick in, the following conditions must be met:

1. The employee must have been employed at the business for at least 1 year.
2. The employee must have worked at least 1250 hours.
3. The business must have at least 50 employees who live no more than 75 miles from the business and have worked at least 20 weeks during the current or proceeding year.

KEEP IN MIND

▶ Four bases for facility liability are respondeat superior, ostensible authority, corporate negligence, and employment liability.
▶ *Respondeat superior* means "Let the master answer."

▶ *Scope of employment* refers to acts that describe what an employee is hired to do to accomplish the employer's goals.

▶ Ostensible authority is when the facility is held liable for the negligence of an independent contractor if the patient has a rational basis to believe that the independent contractor is a facility employee.

▶ Antidiscrimination statutes protect people from discrimination based on race, color, religious preference, or national origin, as well as protecting pregnant women, people ages 40 and older, and persons with disabilities.

▶ The Age Discrimination and Employment Act does not protect public safety employees and top managers.

▶ The general rule in the United States is that if there is no employment contract, an employer is free to terminate an employee at any time for any reason or for no reason (i.e., fire at will).

▶ Whistleblowers are defended in many states by laws that protect employees who disclose illegality and then are wrongfully terminated by the employer.

▶ The Americans with Disabilities Act's goal is to eliminate discrimination against persons in the United States who have physical or mental disabilities, so that they can participate more fully in the workplace and social life.

IN A NUTSHELL

There are a number of legal risks to health care facilities outside the traditional malpractice realm. Both from a rights and a liabilities perspective, nurses should keep all these issues in mind while practicing, particularly those interested in taking on administrative roles that involve hiring and terminating other employees. Not only do facilities stand to lose on the basis of vicarious liability and corporate negligence, but as large employers, all the other employment law and discrimination interests come into play as well. Over the course of a career, and from varying standpoints, most nurses will be privy to some type of employment-related or discrimination-based lawsuit. Understanding the basics of some of these claims will prove worthwhile in the future.

AFTERTHOUGHTS

1. When can the facility be liable for the acts of a nurse even if the nurse is not sued?

2. How can a facility be held liable for the acts of a nurse who is an independent contractor?

3. Identify and describe the legal theories that a court may use to extend liability to a facility for a nurse's actions.

4. Define the roles and positions that nurses have or may develop that lead to their increasing liability in employment decisions.

5. What type of questions should never be on an interviewer's list?

6. Describe three situations that illustrate a policy that appears neutral but has a discriminatory impact.

7. When, if ever, can an employee with a drug or alcohol problem be terminated?

8. What are the advantages and disadvantages of being an employee at will?

9. What steps can a facility take to prevent a terminated employee from filing a wrongful termination suit?

10. Contact the EEOC and learn what is needed to file a claim; discuss this with the class.

11. Develop a sexual harassment scenario and present it to the class. Have the class discuss how it should be handled.

12. Discuss a recently reported medical malpractice case in your state. Outline the elements of negligence and breaches by the facility, nurse, and others.

13. Is the facility liable when a nurse who is going home from work injures someone in a traffic accident? Give reasons for your answer.

14. Role play an interview with a new applicant or a nurse who has been terminated.

15. Consider the following scenarios:

(A) A 65-year-old female patient is admitted to the local hospital because of dizziness, blackout spells, and vomiting of blood. The provisional diagnosis is "R/O seizures v. gastrointestinal bleeding." The patient is admitted at 1900 hours (7 PM) to the medical-surgical floor for observation.

At 2200 hours (10 PM), the patient vomits 100 ml of bright red emesis. Her vital signs are deteriorating. However, the nurses fail to call the attending physician. The patient complains of abdominal tenderness and has abdominal guarding.

At 0300 hours (3 AM), the patient's vital signs have worsened and the physician is called, who orders a stat type and match for blood. (There is a 3-hour delay before the blood is given.) No further communication takes place between the staff and physician.

When the physician makes rounds, he rushes the patient to the intensive care unit (ICU) to stabilize her internal bleeding. She codes in the ICU and expires. Who has breached a standard of care? Who can be held liable? What doctrines of law may be used?

(B) Does the residential health care facility owe to the spouses of the facility's nursing assistants any duty of care to control infections or warn of the danger of infection?

Two married nursing assistants were employed by a convalescent and long-term residential care facility. Both contracted skin rashes and were treated for a staphylococcal infection. Both workers filed workers' compensation claims, and it was determined that their infections were work related.

Spouses of the nursing assistants both contracted *Staphylococcus* bacterial infections, and one physician opined that they contracted their skin infections from their wives.

Both spouses filed a personal injury complaint alleging that the facility owed them and their families a duty of care to maintain the facility free of staphylococcal or other infectious diseases. The cases were consolidated.

The facility moved for summary judgment arguing that no duty was owed to protect nonpatients from infectious diseases routinely found in the general community.

The court granted the facility's motion and ruled that no duty of care was owed.

Plaintiffs appealed. The Supreme Court of Alaska looked at the issue of foreseeability and concluded that it was foreseeable that spouses of the nursing assistants could be infected by diseases if the facility did not take reasonable measures to minimize the spread of diseases or warn the nursing assistants to take precautions to avoid infecting their spouses. The facility allegedly disregarded sanitary, health, and infection control practices. The court reversed the summary judgment and remanded the case for further proceedings.[39]

ETHICS IN PRACTICE

Julie C., registered nurse (RN), had worked the 11 AM to 7 PM shift in the neonatal intensive care unit (NICU) for 2 years. Today, as she finished her last entry in the progress notes for Baby L., a 1-pound, 4-ounce premature infant, she could hear the sounds of her nurse colleagues outside the window as they prepared to picket the hospital in a strike for better pay, better working conditions, and better staffing.

Over the past several months, the nursing staff had organized as a group and attempted negotiations with the hospital administration. The very traditional hospital administration had always viewed any attempt to organize any of the staff, but particularly the nurses, as unprofessional and insubordinate. The history of the hospital was replete with stories of nurses who had been fired because they had attempted to unite the nurses in an organized manner to seek better working conditions. Consequently the administration viewed this strike as a major violation of their unwritten policy and threatened all the nurses who participated in the strike with employment termination.

Although Julie C. recognized that the working conditions were poor and that the pay scale was the lowest in the relatively small city, she still felt a strong obligation to the hospital and the patients. Many of the patients who could be discharged or moved to other facilities were already gone from the hospital, but a small number of the patients, such as Baby L., could not be moved without extreme risk to their health and lives.

The leader and organizer of the strike was one of Julie L.'s classmates and best friends. She had stressed to Julie that without the support of 100% of the nursing staff, the strike would be a failure and the hospital would win again. The hospital had already begun hiring some aides to provide care while the nurses were on strike. Julie felt that the care provided by these untrained aides was substandard and probably dangerous to the patients' lives. Julie's friend made the point that it was really the hospital's responsibility to provide adequate care for the patients and that the administration could have the whole nursing staff back as soon as they began negotiating in good faith.

Julie was tempted to sign out her charts and join the strike at the end of her shift. Yet she felt an obligation to stay for another shift and care for Baby L. and the several other infants who could not be moved. What should she do? What ethical issues are involved in her decision?

References*

1. Willinger v. Mercy Catholic Hospital, 362 A.2d 280 (Penn. Supp. 1976).
2. O'Keefe, ME: Practice and the Law: Avoiding Malpractice and Other Legal Risks. FA Davis, Philadelphia, 2000.
3. Ibid., 124.
4. Grewe v. Mt. Clemens General Hospital, 273 N.W.2d 429 (Mich. 1978); 51 A.L.R. 4th 235 (1990).
5. Adamski v. Tacoma General Hospital, 20 Wash. App. 98, 579 P.2d 970 (1978); 51 A.L.R. 4th 235 (1990); Mduba v. Benedictine Hospital, 52 A.D. 450, 384 N.Y.S.2d 527 (1978).
6. O'Keefe, ME: Practice and the Law: Avoiding Malpractice and Other Legal Risks. FA Davis, Philadelphia, 2001.
7. Johnson v. Misericordia Community Hospital, 99 Wis.2d 708, 301 N.W.2d 156 (1981).
8. American Medical Association and National Health Lawyers Association: Physician's Survival Guide—Legal Pitfalls and Solutions. AMA, NHLA, Washington, DC, 1991, pp 41–60.
9. O'Keefe, ME: Practice and the Law: Avoiding Malpractice and Other Legal Risks. FA Davis, Philadelphia, 2001.
10. Darling v. Charleston Community Memorial Hospital, 33 Ill.2d 326, 211 N.E.2d 253, 14 Atl.3d 860 (1965).
11. Idem.
12. Bost v. Riley, 262 S.E.2d 391 (N.C. App. 1980); 51 A.L.R. 4th 235 (1990).
13. Sides v. Duke, 74 N.C. App. 331, 328 S.E.2d 818 (1985); 75 A.L.R. 4th 13 (1990).
14. Thompson v. St. Regis Paper Co., 102 Wash. 2d 219; 685 P.2d 1081 (1984).
15. 79 Mich. App. 93; 261 N.W.2d 222 (1977), rev'd, 402 Mich. See also Karie v. General Motors Corp., 282 N.W.2d 925 (1978).
16. Toussaint v. Blue Cross and Blue Shield of Michigan, 408 Mich. 579, 292 N.W.2d 880 (1980); 33 A.L.R. 4th 129 (1990).
17. Pugh v. See's Candies, Inc., 116 Cal. App. 3d 311, 171 Cal. Rep. 917 (1981), modified on other ground, 117 Cal. App. 3d 502a (1981).
18. Cutterham v. Coachman Industries, Inc., 169 Cal. App. 3d 1223, 215 Cal. Rep. 795 (1985); 677 F. Supp. 1021 (N.D. Cal. 1988).
19. Grozek v. Ragu Foods, Inc., 63 A.2d 858, 406 N.Y.S. 2d 213 (4th Dept. 1978).
20. Shah v. S.S. Kresge Co., 166 Ind. App. 1, 328 N.E.2d 775 (1975); 33 A.L.R. 4th 120 (1990).
21. Helsby v. St. Paul Hospital and Casualty Co., 195 F. Supp. 385 (D. Minn. 1961), aff'd, 304 F.2d 758 (8th Cir. 1962); 80 A.L.R. 4th 421, 433 (1990).
22. Supra, 19.
23. Maddaloni v. Western Massachusetts Bus Lines, Inc., 386 Mass. 877, 438 N.E.2d 351 (1982); 44 A.L.R. 4th 1145 (1990).
24. King v. Mannesmann Tally Corp., 847 F.2d 907 (1st Cir. 1988).
25. Witt v. Forest Hospital, 450 N.E.2d 811 907 (1st Cir. 1988).

*NOTE: Cites to American Law Review, fourth edition (A.L.R. 4th), have been provided as a potential source for identifying the law in individual jurisdictions.

26. Glaz v. Ralston Purina Co., 24 Mass. App. Ct. 386, 509 N.E.2d 297 (1987) 12 A.L.R. 4th 544 (1990); Tameny v. Atlantic Richfield Co., 27 Cal. 3d 167; 164 Cal. Rptr. 839 (1980).
27. Doane v. Grew, 220 Mass. 171, 107 N.E. 620 (1915).
28. Sheehan v. Toban, 326 Mass. 185, 93 N.E.2d 524 (1950).
29. Garcia v. Rush Presbyterian Medical Center, 660 F.2d 1217 (7th Cir. 1981).
30. Chamberlain v. 101 Realty, Inc., 915 F. 2nd 777 (1st Cir. 1990).
31. Hanley v. Doctors Hospital of Shreveport, 821 So 2d 508 (L.A. App Cir. 2 6/06/2002).
32. Meritor Savings Bank v. Vinson, 477 U.S. 57 (1986).
33. Fiesta, J: When sexual harassment hits home. Nursing Management 30(5):16–18, 1999 (Kopp v. Samaritan Health System, Inc.).
34. Aiken, TD: Sexual harassment. In Dochterman, J, and Grace, H (eds): Current Issues in Nursing, ed 6. Mosby, St. Louis, 2001.
35. Ibid, 581.
36. Equal Employment Opportunity Commission, 2401 E Street, NW, Washington, DC, 20210.
37. McDonnell Douglas Corp. v. Green, 411 U.S. 792 (1973).
38. Marshall v. Sun Oil, 605 F.2d 1331 (5th Cir. 1979); Schultz v. Hickok, 358 F.Supp. 1208 (N.D. Ga. 1973).
39. Boileu and Oliver, Appellants v. Sisters of Providence in Washington and/or DBA Our Lady of Compassion Care Center, Appelles. Supreme Court No. 507575 (Alaska 2/23/98).

Resources

National Practitioner Data Bank and Health Care Integrity and Protection Data Bank
P.O. Box 10832
Chantilly, VA 20153-0832
http://www.npdb-hipdb.com

American Nurses Association
600 Maryland Avenue, SW
Suite 100 West
Washington, DC 20024

Guide to Nurses Rights, 1998
http://www.nursingworld.org
1-800-274-4ANA

Liability of the Nurse Manager 13

JEAN M. FARQUHARSON, RN, JD

Key Chapter Concepts

Accountability
Personal accountability
Public accountability
Direct liability
Short staffing
Independent contractor
Abandonment
Wrongful discharge
Wrongful transfer
Consolidated Omnibus
    Reconciliation Act (COBRA)

Emergency Medical Treatment and
    Active Labor Act (EMTALA)
ORYX initiative
Adverse sentinel event
Root cause analysis
Immediate jeopardy
Outcome and Assessment
    Information Set (OASIS)

Chapter Thoughts

New graduate nurses, as well as nurses who are in their first few years of practice, seldom consider the possibility of becoming a nursing manager. Most would answer that they do not have the knowledge or the skill level to be a manager or head nurse and are not ready to assume the increased responsibility of such a position. Most, likely, would be right. However, the reality of the workplace is that many good bedside nurses do go on to become nursing managers in a variety of different roles, ranging from head nurse to vice president of nursing.

In the patient care setting, nurse managers are primarily problem solvers. When difficult or unusual situations arise that the floor nurses are unable to deal with, the nurse manager is called on to resolve the difficulty. Nurse managers also function as administrators and are instrumental in resolving conflict on and off the unit. They are often responsible for staffing and arranging work schedules to ensure adequate patient care. When a problem arises with a nurse or staff member who is not performing at an acceptable level, it is the responsibility of the nurse manager to facilitate and create other options that can enable both the staff member and the unit to achieve its goals. The nurse manager also promotes staff development and department efficiency to ensure high-quality, cost-effective patient care.

The ethical concept of accountability means that the nurse is answerable or responsible for his or her actions. **Accountability** in nursing takes two forms. **Personal accountability** is the responsibility that the nurses have to themselves and to the patient or patients entrusted to their care. **Public accountability** is the responsibility the nurse has to the employer and to society in general. The primary goals of professional accountability in nursing are to maintain high standards of care and to protect the patient from harm.

All nurses are accountable for the proper use of their knowledge and skills in the provision of care. Nurse managers have an additional accountability to those whom they supervise. A key element in accountability is the nurse's willingness to accept the consequences for decisions made and actions taken. As professional autonomy increases, so does the level of accountability.

Both ethically and legally, nursing managers are held to higher standards than the nurse who is not in a nursing management role. What would be acceptable as a reasonable and prudent course of action for a non–nurse manager may not be acceptable for a nurse manager.

OBJECTIVES

Upon completing this chapter, the reader will be able to:

1. Describe in detail the nurse manager's role in establishing and maintaining facility standards of care.
2. Identify situations in which a nurse manager is liable for the actions of another.
3. Describe the difference between vicarious and direct liability as they affect the nurse manager.
4. Describe the common areas of direct or personal liability of the nurse manager, including the duty to train, orient, supervise, and delegate.
5. Describe how potential liability from the effects of short staffing can be minimized by determining the reasonableness of actions under the circumstances.
6. Describe the nurse manager's role in minimizing potential liability situations.
7. Define abandonment and wrongful discharge or transfer and discuss how they can arise in the facility setting.

Introduction

Whenever there is a problem on a hospital unit, such as an unexpected change in a patient's condition, medication not received from the pharmacy, or a difficult physician, one cry is heard: "Call the nurse manager in charge." Nursing managers have unique positions in facilities. They have supervisory responsibility, and inherent in that responsibility is potential legal liability.

In this chapter, the term *nurse manager* is used generically to include all levels of nurse managers from head nurses to supervisors and directors of nursing to vice presidents of patient services. This chapter addresses several areas of potential liability for the nurse in a management position.

Supervisors Establish Facility Standard of Care

In previous chapters, the four basic elements of nursing malpractice were discussed in detail. A plaintiff must prove all these elements—duty, breach, proximate cause, and damages—to establish malpractice. Nurse managers have the primary responsibility for establishing and maintaining standards of care that the staff must follow. Although nurses must meet basic national, state, and perhaps specialty group standards, each individual facility establishes standards for its nursing service personnel that it spells out in its nursing service policy and procedure manuals.

In a malpractice lawsuit, the plaintiff's counsel tries to show that the nurse failed to meet a standard adopted by his or her institution. If asked under oath, nurses must admit that the staff is bound to follow the policies and procedures adopted by their institution and that they are required to be familiar with institutional policies and procedures.

The nursing manager must make sure that the nursing standards described in the policy and procedure manuals are reasonable and that the staff knows and understands the standards (Box 13–1).

Crafting and Drafting Standards of Care

Managers must avoid language that creates unrealistic expectations or "ensures" patient safety when drafting policies and procedures. The law requires that nurses be reasonable under the circumstances, not that they be perfect. Although nurses try to provide optimal care and follow the highest standards, it can be argued that when less than optimal care occurs, a breach of the standard has taken place. Even if lower standards apply universally to a specific situation, if the facility policy establishes a higher standard, the facility policy applies for that individual case.

The language used and the responsibilities outlined in policy and procedure manuals must be reasonable and generally accepted within the nursing or medical profession.

Legal counsel should review policies and procedures to determine whether they are reasonable from a legal standpoint.

BOX 13–1

Defining Policy and Procedures

Policy: Overall plan or series of steps to accomplish or coordinate the general goals and acceptable procedures in a facility.
Procedures: The tools used to implement the policies.

Nursing managers have an obligation to have the following:

1. Manuals available on each nursing unit
2. Staff members periodically review the manuals
3. Staff members perform procedures in accordance with the manuals
4. Manuals periodically updated to the current national standards

The words and expectations expressed in your facility's policy and procedure manual establish your institution's standard of care. Make certain that the standard is reasonable and does not promise a higher standard than the law requires.

Liability for Nurse Managers

When accepting the role of a nurse manager, one issue that often surfaces is how the new role increases personal liability and exposure to lawsuits (Box 13–2).

Liability for the Acts of Others

The most often asked question from nursing supervisors is: "Can I be held liable if a nurse I am supervising commits malpractice?" The short answer is: "It depends."

Although everyone is held responsible for their own acts of negligence, there are certain limited instances when the law imposes liability for the acts of another. This is known as vicarious liability. Under a theory called respondeat superior, the employer is held responsible for injuries or damages that occur when the employee is negligent in carrying out duties in the "course and scope of employment."

Based on this theory, if a nurse commits malpractice while on duty, the facility, not the nursing manager, is liable for the damage.

If, however, a nurse owns a service that supplies sitters and employs individuals to sit with patients in the facility or in the home, vicarious liability may attach. For example, if one of the sitters falls asleep on duty and the patient falls out of bed and fractures a hip, the nurse employer can be held liable. Even if the owner–employer–nurse supervisor is not present, the nurse employer is liable under respondeat superior.

UNLICENSED PERSONNEL AND THE MANAGER'S LICENSE

A commonly asked question is: "Am I at risk of losing my license if the unlicensed personnel I supervise are negligent?" The answer is: "No." Only the person awarded the license can lose the license. Student nurses, aides, orderlies, technicians, assistants, or any other unlicensed personnel do not work under the protection of the nurse manager's license. They are working within the confines of a health care facility and under the license of the facility, not of a specific nurse.

The nurse manager has an obligation to ensure that unlicensed personnel do not perform functions that require a license. They must also supervise and be sure that

A Case in Point

Well Baby Assessment Policy

The Facts

In *Parker v. Southwest Louisiana Hospital Association,*[1] the hospital's policy exceeded national standards; however, the policy was not followed by the staff. An apparently well baby had a cardiac and respiratory arrest approximately 24 hours after birth. Even though resuscitative procedures were instituted immediately, the infant sustained severe brain damage and died 9 months later.

Hospital policy required that well babies be visually observed every 10 to 15 minutes, even though the American Academy of Pediatrics standards required visual observation only every 20 to 30 minutes.

The Jury Decides

Because the hospital required a more rigorous standard in its written policies, the staff's failure to adhere to those policies resulted in hospital liability for this tragic death.

BOX 13–2

Areas of Potential Liability for the Nurse Manager

1. Failure to properly delegate
2. Failure to properly assign tasks or duties to a nurse or other nurse extenders
3. Failure to check off staff on skill levels
4. Failure to properly train or educate staff
5. Failure to require or obtain additional education and retraining for staff
6. Failure to provide proper patient care
7. Failure to perform duties as a nurse manager (e.g., failure to call treating physician when notified by staff of patient's deteriorating condition)
8. Failure to ensure that the staff knows procedures on how to operate equipment safely
9. Failure to orient staff to the unit
10. Failure to provide assistance for nursing staff
11. Possibility of abandonment claims against the nurse manager and staff
12. Lack of documentation showing attempts to rectify short staffing problem on a unit

A CASE IN POINT

Respondeat Superior

The Facts

The case of *Bowers v. Olch*[2] illustrates the theory of respondent superior. A surgical nursing supervisor assigned two nurses to assist in the patient's operation, one as a circulating nurse and the other as a scrub nurse. Several days after the surgery, a needle was discovered in the patient's abdomen. The patient sued the supervisor, the hospital, the operating room nurses, and the physicians.

The Court Decides

The court dismissed the nursing supervisor from the lawsuit because the theory of respondeat superior was not applicable to her. The supervisor did not employ the nurses she supervised and was not legally responsible for their actions.

tasks assigned to subordinates are appropriately carried out. For example, a manager allows a nurse's aide to administer medication, but the aide administers it to the wrong patient. Most likely, the nurse manager will be found negligent in his or her own right and the hospital, as the employer of both, will be held responsible. The nurse manager breached a duty and would be liable for failure to provide adequate supervision. The manager might also face disciplinary actions from the state Board of Nursing for improper delegation of nursing tasks.

Even if the tasks assigned are appropriate to the training of the personnel, it is the manager's obligation to ensure that the tasks are performed correctly.

Nurse managers must be sure that unlicensed personnel:

1. Do not perform functions that require a license, and
2. Perform assigned functions in an appropriate manner.

Personal Liability

RENDERING NEGLIGENT PATIENT CARE

Although nursing managers are not usually held responsible for the acts or omissions of the staff that they supervise, they are always held responsible for their own acts or omissions. This is known as **direct liability.** Because the job description of a manager includes many more "acts" to be performed than the job description of a staff nurse, there is more opportunity for the manager to "fail" to do something. The clearest example of personal liability occurs when a manager renders direct patient care and causes an injury.

A CASE IN POINT

Unlicensed Personnel and the Manager's License

The Facts

In *Hicks v. New York State Department of Health*,[3] a nurse was found guilty of patient neglect because of her failure to properly train and supervise the aides working under her. A security guard found an elderly nursing home patient lying in the dark, partially in his bed and partially restrained in an overturned wheelchair. He was undressed and covered in dried urine and feces.

The Court Decides

The court found that the nurse failed to assess whether the nursing aides had delivered proper care to the patient, which led to inadequate care of the patient.

FAILURE TO PERFORM SUPERVISORY DUTIES

Nurse managers can also be held liable for a failure to carry out their supervisory responsibilities. For example, certain institutions require staff nurses to notify the supervisor of unfavorable patient responses to treatment. It is then the supervisor's responsibility to notify the attending physician. This procedure is followed especially during the night shift. If the supervisor's failure to notify the physician of an important change results in injury to the patient from delayed treatment, then the supervisor may be liable. If the physician fails to call or respond and the supervisor is aware of the patient's declining condition, the supervisor must go through the chain of command to get the treatment needed by the patient, even if it means going over the treating physician's head to the director or administrator.

DELEGATION AND THE NURSING MANAGER

When delegating and working with unlicensed assistive personnel (UAP), the nurse must look at the following areas:

1. What is the training and experience of the UAP?
2. Has the UAP been "checked off," or approved for the tasks delegated?
3. Is there documentation that the UAP has the skills and training required?
4. Are the lines of communication clear between the UAP and nurse? Does the UAP know when the nurse should be called, paged, or reported to with concerns relating to the patient?
5. Is there a clear line of communication between the nurse and UAP?

A CASE IN POINT

Rendering Negligent Patient Care

The Facts

In *Norton v. Argonaut Insurance Co.*,[4] an assistant director of nursing made the rounds on a busy pediatric unit and offered to transcribe physicians' orders and carry them out. The physician's order for a 3-month-old infant was "Lanoxin 3 c.c.," but the order did not indicate per os, by mouth (PO), or intramuscular (IM) administration. This supervisor was unaware that a pediatric elixir of Lanoxin existed and knew only of the injectable liquid.

She questioned the order with two physicians but never called the physician who ordered the medication. She also failed to check the *Physicians' Desk Reference* or call a pharmacist to determine the correct dosage. She administered 3 cc (ml) of IM Lanoxin to the 3 month old, who died from an overdose. The supervisor was found negligent, and the hospital's insurer was held liable.

The Court Decides

The nurse was found negligent not in her supervisory duties, but in her regular nursing duties. She failed to know the appropriate pediatric dosage and did not take appropriate actions to determine the correct dose.

6. If the UAP needs additional training, is it available in the facility?
7. What are the policies and procedures of the facility concerning the UAP's job description, skill requirements, and educational requirements?

Nurse managers are required to delegate or assign tasks to nursing staff and other staff. The state Board of Nursing should be consulted if there is a question of what can be actually delegated by the nurse manager (Box 13–3).

Some state boards of nursing offer assistance in determining when it is safe to delegate by providing a delegation decision-making flowchart (Figure 13–1).

FAILURE TO TRAIN, ORIENT, AND EVALUATE

Another area of expanding nurse manager liability arises from the manager's obligation to train, orient, and evaluate the ability of staff nurses to perform specific functions and procedures. Most major facilities have in-service education departments to orient new nurses and assist in the continuing education of nurses. The manager's responsibility is to determine on a day-to-day basis whether nurses are capable of performing necessary procedures.

BOX 13–3

Delegation and the Manager

The National Council of State Boards of Nursing (NCSBN) published five rights of delegation for nursing managers:
1. Right task
2. Right circumstances
3. Right person
4. Right direction and communication
5. Right supervision and evaluation

The key to the manager's functioning is reasonableness. It is considered reasonable to check periodically to make certain that procedures are being followed and that the nurses working in an area know the procedures used routinely.

Issues Handled/Encountered by Nurse Supervisors

Short Staffing

Aside from handling direct patient care and supervisory and training responsibilities, nurse managers must also handle numerous administrative tasks. A major problem is **short staffing,** a situation on a unit or in a facility in which there is not sufficient staff for the number of patients to be cared for at various acuity levels. Problems such as the nursing shortage (Box 13–4), the increased demand of the aging population, continuing budget constraints, and the focus of reducing the cost of providing care mean that this will continue to be an issue that nurse managers must resolve. Units are constantly functioning with less than the optimal number of nurses. Attempting to resolve short staffing by assigning nurses to areas where they have little or no expertise may temporarily solve the staffing problem but can open the facility and affected personnel to potential liability. To avoid liability situations caused by short staffing, the supervisor must be reasonable and staff nurses must be flexible.

Reasonableness under the circumstances requires close attention to any situation involving patient safety. Although there may not be sufficient staff to monitor patients constantly, there are reasonable alternatives that would lessen the risk of injury to the patient. For example, a medicated patient has special safety concerns. Side rails must be up so that the patient can avoid serious injuries. The patient must be instructed not to get out of bed and fall, and warning devices should be in place if needed. The call light must be placed within the patient's reach. These are all simple measures that can prevent serious injuries. Above all, these measures should be documented.

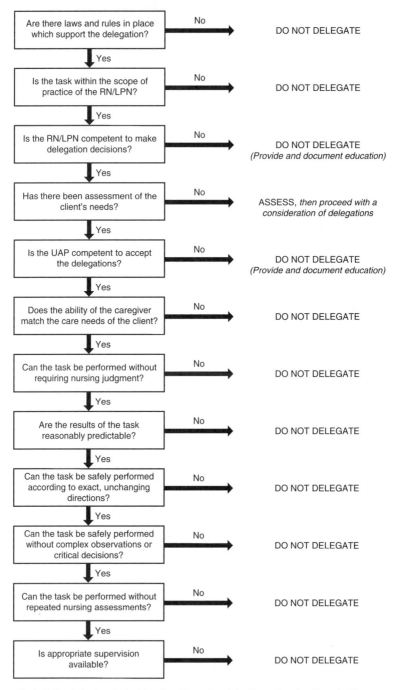

Figure 13–1. Delegation decision-making tree.

A CASE IN POINT

A Breakdown in Orientation

The Facts

One case involved a 1-day-old infant who became a paraplegic when air was pumped into a scalp vein, crossed the infant's patent foramen ovale, and lodged in vessels in his lower spine. At least five nurses who rotated through the neonatal intensive care unit (NICU) checked the pump and intravenous (IV) line and failed to place an end-line filter on the IV tubing as it entered the child. The pump had neither an alarm nor an automatic shutoff device in case the fluid ran out. The only mechanism to prevent air from being pumped into the patient if the fluid ran out was the end-line filter. When wet, the filter became an air barrier.

The nursing procedure manual for the operation of the pump clearly stated that this end-line filter must be used during the setup of the pump and at all times when the pump was in operation. Five nurses who took care of the infant did not know that, when using the pump, the end-line filter was required. None of the five nurses who worked in the NICU knew that the procedure existed or how to operate the pump.

The Court Decides

The head nurse of the unit and the supervisor were found negligent for failing to make sure that the staff nurses knew the procedures for their unit and could implement them safely. The jury concluded that it was not reasonable for so many nurses to be ignorant of the safe operation of the pump. Following the incident, a procedure was developed to determine each nurse's knowledge of the use of the pump.

One measure of reasonableness in short staffing situations is how closely accepted guidelines and standards have been followed. The nursing manager must be aware of the guidelines concerning staffing requirements. The Joint Commission on Accreditation of Healthcare Organizations (JCAHO) provides certain standards for staffing that generally require "a sufficient number of qualified registered nurses" and "sufficient nurses to assure prompt recognition of any untoward change."[5] As yet, no specific numbers have been assigned by the JCAHO as to what constitutes a sufficient number of qualified staff; however, this may change. California recently passed a law that requires a specific number of nurses, depending on the acuity of the patient.

In California, Assembly Bill 394, Health Facilities: Nursing Staff, was passed and signed by the governor. The bill requires the state Department of Health Services (DHS) to adopt regulations establishing minimum nurse-to-patient ratios by licensed nurse classification and by hospital unit for all licensed hospitals. This bill was in

---

BOX 13–4
Recruiting Nurses in a Nursing Shortage

According to the Bureau of Labor Statistics, there will be approximately 1 million nursing positions open between 2002 and 2010. A decrease in nursing school enrollments and an increase in the number of retiring nurses is creating a nursing shortage just at the time that the population is aging. As the nursing shortage continues, facilities must find new ways to attract and keep their staff. Recruiting nurses has changed with the help of the Internet. There are approximately 100,000 Web sites with job listings and 600,000 jobs posted on-line.[6]

The following information should be available on an institution's Web site to encourage recruitment:

- A description of the staff and nursing practice environment
- Professional responsibilities
- Organization union or nonunion
- Mission statement of the facility
- Philosophy of nursing: Are nurses involved in clinical, research, and ethics committees?
- Demographic and location information: what patient population is served
- Types of services offered by the facility
- Salary range and differentials, along with benefits such as 401K plans, disability benefits, sick leave, child or elder care, and educational benefits
- On-line resume submission
- Credentialing requirements
- Organization information—corporate structure, growth potential or downsizing possibilities
- Nursing personnel—key players and their biographical sketches and positions
- Other links that may be helpful
- Contact person to speak to regarding questions[7]

The federal government has made a move to assist with the nursing shortage. On August 1, 2001, President George W. Bush signed the Nurse Reinvestment Act into law. The law authorizes the following:

- Nursing student scholarships and loan repayment programs
- Career ladder programs
- Grants for long-term care training to develop and to add a gerontology curriculum to nursing programs
- Nursing administration best-practice grants
- Public service announcements to inform and encourage persons to enter the profession
- Loan repayment programs for nurses who prepare and agree to teach in nursing schools

response to the health care crisis, managed care issues, facility downsizing, and reduction of the licensed nursing staffs, resulting in a decline in the quality of patient care.

Courts have not provided numbers because what is reasonable under one set of facts may not be reasonable under another. Similarly, most health care organizations have been reluctant to say precisely what number constitutes an adequate staff. Certain specialty areas such as obstetrics have established standards requiring specific staff-patient ratios. These standards must be consulted in determining staffing requirements in these specialty areas.

Factors that affect the reasonableness of staffing include the following:

1. Acuity of the patients
2. Intensity of care
3. Qualifications and experience of the staff available
4. Attempts to secure adequate staffing (which should be clearly documented)
5. Utilization of alternatives (such as family members, friends, and outside nurses)
6. Use of ancillary staff
7. Utilization of safety measures (side rails, restraint jackets, or, in certain limited circumstances, restraints and documentation)
8. Increased frequency of rounds
9. Ability to close units and float staff to other needed areas

Floating

Because of the need to provide competent nursing care, not just care, floating (sending a nurse from one unit to work on another) as a means of relieving short staffing of units raises questions for nurse managers. Is the nurse competent to perform the duties required on the unit? For example, it may not be appropriate to send a registered nurse (RN) with no intensive care experience to a pediatric intensive care unit (ICU). In fact, some nurses and state nurses' associations are using an assignment despite objection (ADO) form (Figure 13–2) in an attempt to protect the nurse and make administration aware of the short staffing problem so that it can be dealt with before a patient is injured.

Nurses are aware of the need to document their work related to patient care, but they also must be aware of the need to document workplace occurrences that affect themselves or general patient care. The ADO form is a tool that can be used by the RN to document an unsafe or potentially unsafe environment, relating either directly to the patient or to the nurse, and provide a written report of the issue to institutional administration. The form documents that the RN is not refusing the assignment but that he or she has cause for concern. This form does not become part of any patient record, and the RN has no control over what the institution administration does with the form. Although the form does provide a record of an occurrence that causes the nurse concern and confirms her role as a patient advocate, it does not prevent the institution from terminating him or her as an employee. The RN completing the form should give one to the supervisor, keep one for personal records, and send one to the

A Case in Point

Short Staffing

The Facts

In *Bossier v. DeSoto General Hospital*,[8] a patient who had been given a narcotic sustained injury when she fell on her way to the bathroom. Only half side rails were in use, and no one told the patient not to get out of bed. No one suggested to the family that the patient needed constant supervision while receiving the medication. The hospital was short staffed and did not have the staff to provide the patient with constant supervision.

The Court Decides

Reasonable measures under the circumstances were not employed, and the hospital was held liable.

state Board of Nursing. More information on which state boards of nursing offer the form can be found on American Nurses Association's (ANA's) Web site at *http://nursingworld.org/wpa/infolnks.htm.*

Still, an experienced RN working in an unfamiliar area is better qualified than no nurse at all. Perhaps the best solution to floating is to cross-train nurses in specific, related areas, such as labor, delivery, and postpartum care; surgery and postanesthesia care; pediatrics, nursery, and neonatal intensive care unit (NICU). Cross-training increases the number of nurses who can perform in a patient care area while increasing the confidence of the nurses providing care in these areas.

Agency or Pool Nurses

Another reasonable quasi-solution to short staffing issues is the use of agency or outside pool nurses and in-house pool nurses. Outside pool nurses are not employees of the facility; they are employed by an agency whose function it is to provide temporary nurses to facilities with short staffing problems. In-house pool nurses are employed by the facility, are not assigned a permanent unit, and agree to float. They may also be part-time employees or nurses seeking overtime work who are willing to work on any hospital unit. Pool nurses must be oriented to units and must be evaluated by managers to determine whether they meet facility requirements for the position. Pool nurses should not be made charge nurses, except in rare circumstances, and only after there has been adequate orientation to facility policies and procedures. Because charge nurse responsibilities include supervising other personnel, qualifications and training must be well documented before a pool nurse is allowed to assume those responsibilities.

ASSIGNMENT DESPITE OBJECTION

PURPOSE
The purpose of this form is to notify hospital supervision that you have been given an assignment that you believe potentially unsafe for the patient or staff. This form will document the situation. LSNA may use it to identify statewide frauds.

INSTRUCTIONS - PLEASE PRINT. FORMS MAY BE PHOTOCOPIED.
One or more RNs may complete this form. Give one copy to your supervisor, one copy to your facility and keep one copy for yourself. You may also send one copy to LSNA at 5700 Florida Blvd. Suite 720, Baton Rouge, LA 70806.

Section 1: *Before accepting the assignment and completing this form, you must give your supervisor (not the Charge nurse) notice of your objection to the assignment. Please put the complete name and title of the person making the assignment and receiving the objection. Please complete the response section with the supervisor's response, as well as the date and time of the response. If you do not receive a response from your supervisor, submit a copy of this completed form to the next level(s) of administration. Complete the sections "Other persons notified" below if you notified any other persons (head nurse/clinical manager of the unit).*

I/We

Registered nurse(s) employed at _____ Facility _____ on _____ Unit _____ Shift _____

Hereby protest my assignment as: ☐ Primary Nurse   ☐ Charge Nurse   ☐ RN pulled to unit   ☐ Other _____ despite my objection.

Made to me by _____ at _____ Date/Time _____

Supervisor's Name/Title _____

Supervisor's Response _____ Supervisor's Signature: _____

Other persons notified:

_____ Name _____ Date/Time _____ Response _____

_____ Name _____ Date/Time _____ Response _____

Section 2: *Please check all appropriate statements.*

Although I agree to accept this assignment, I am objecting to this assignment on the grounds that:

☐ Staff is not trained (or inexperienced) in area assigned.
☐ Staff not given adequate orientation to the unit.
☐ Inadequate staff for acuity (short-staffed).
☐ New patients transferred/admitted without adequate staff.
☐ Unit staffed with excessive registry personnel.

☐ Assignment poses a serious threat to health and safety of staff.
☐ Assignment poses a potential threat to health and safety of patients.
☐ Staff involuntarily forced to work beyond scheduled hours.
☐ Unit staffed with unqualified/inappropriate personnel.
☐ Other (please explain)

Section 3: *Complete, to the best of your knowledge, the patient census at the time of your objection. From your assessment indicate for each acuity level, the number of patients on the unit that fit into the category. If there are acuity factors not listed, please specify.*

Patient census: Start _____   End _____   Unit capacity _____   Admits _____   Discharges _____

Figure 13–2. The Assignment Despite Objection Form. Used with permission from the Louisiana State Nurses Association. Tawna Pounders, Executive Director.

Faculty levels: High _____   Average _____   Low _____

Factors influencing acuity. Check those that apply.

☐ on respirators   ☐ complete care   ☐ isolation precautions   ☐ restrained

☐ frequent VS   ☐ frequent assessments   ☐ receiving blood products   ☐ receiving IV drips/TPN/Chemo

☐ Other _____   ☐ <4 hrs post-op

Section 4: *Complete, to the best of your knowledge.*

PATIENT CARE STAFFING COUNT	RN	LPN	AIDE	ANCILLARY	PREVIOUS # STAFF FOR EQUIVALENT CENSUS
Start of shift					
End of shift					

Section 5: *Complete this section if the situation cannot be explained adequately in Sections 2 or 3, or if additional information is relevant.*

Brief statement of the problem _____

Section 6: *Complete this section at the conclusion of your assigned shift.*

Did you receive any additional considerations (admits redirected, etc.) during your shift?   ☐ No   ☐ Yes, describe _____

Were there any negative patient outcomes on your shift?   ☐ No   ☐ Yes, describe _____

What was your greatest patient care challenge during your shift and how did you handle it? _____

What planned follow-up can assist in reducing or avoiding the occurrence of similar assignments? _____

Section 7: *Demographic data. If you plan to submit a copy of the form to LSNA, please complete the following information.*

yrs as RN _____ # yrs in current position _____ Age _____ Gender _____

_____ # yrs in current specialty area _____

Are you a member of a professional nursing organization?   ☐ No   ☐ Yes, (please identify organization) _____

As a patient advocate, in accordance with the Nurse Practice Act, I/we have utilized this agency's chain of command to notify the appropriate individuals that, in my/our professional judgment(s), this assignment is potentially unsafe and may place patients or staff at risk. I/We indicate acceptance of the assignment despite described objection(s). It is not my/our intention to refuse to accept the assignment or raise questions of either insubordination or of failure to meet obligations to the patient(s). However, I/we give notice to the employer of the above facts and indicate that for the reasons listed, responsibility for the consequences of the assignment rests with the employer.

_____   _____

RN signature(s)   Print name(s)

LSNA WORKPLACE ADVOCACY 1-800-457-6378   Revised 12/99

Figure 13–2. The Assignment Despite Objection Form. Used with permission from the Louisiana State Nurses Association. Tawna Pounders, Executive Director. *(continued)*

Floating

You are the nurse manager for the ICU and are short staffed for the 3-to-11 shift. You know a new postoperative patient is coming from the operating room and that the only available registered nurse (RN) to staff your unit is from the labor and delivery unit. She has had only 3 months' experience on an ICU.

What are possible solutions or options?

1. Who can be held liable if a patient is injured under the care of the labor and delivery nurse?
2. What can be done now so that in the future dilemmas such as this can be avoided?

In-house pool arrangements can provide nurses familiar with the institution; however, the number of shifts a registered pool nurse works should be monitored. Guidelines should be put in place limiting the number of additional shifts an in-house person can work as a pool nurse. Tired nurses make mistakes that can harm or endanger patients. The same concerns apply when supervisors ask nurses to work overtime.

Independent Contractors

Outside pool nurses who work in facilities are not employees of the hospital, but **independent contractors.** According to the Internal Revenue Service, generally an independent contractor is one who the payer has the right to control or direct only the result of the work but not the methods or means of accomplishing the results.[9] In some instances, the nurse is hired by the patient or the patient's family.

Vicarious liability, as discussed earlier, is imposed because of the relationship between the persons. In a true independent contractor situation, there is no vicarious liability.

If a nurse is employed by an outside agency or pool and injures a patient in the health care facility, then, more often than not, the employer (the pool agency, not the health care facility) is liable. There are exceptions, however, where facilities may be held accountable for the actions of a pool nurse. For example:

1. If the nurse manager fails to orient the pool nurse to the unit and this leads to injury, the facility is liable for breaching its duty to provide the necessary training.
2. If the facility or agency fails to ensure that the nurse is licensed and is competent to perform procedures, the facility and agency both may be held liable if the pool nurse injures a patient.
3. If the nurse manager fails to make the necessary rounds and provide assistance to the pool nurse and this failure results in patient injury, the facility will most likely be held responsible.

The nurse's employer will likely be held liable, under a theory of respondeat superior, for the actions of the nurse, its employee. Note that even if a pool nurse is an independent contractor, a patient may sue the health care facility on the grounds that the facility "vouched" for the pool nurse or that the pool nurse was an "apparent agent or employee" of the facility. Although the pool agency may ultimately pay the monetary damages in the case, the existence of an independent contract does not necessarily shield the health care facility from being named in a lawsuit and having to more expensively defend it. (See the discussion on ostensible authority in the next chapter.)

To insulate health care facilities from vicarious liability for independent contractors, contracts between the pool agency and the facility should provide that the agency will indemnify or reimburse money to the facility if the facility is found liable for the actions of the pool nurse.

Abandonment

Traditionally, **abandonment** is a premature termination of the professional treatment relationship without adequate notice to the patient. The failure to adequately monitor patients on in-patient units may lead to allegations of abandonment. Claims for abandonment are generally made against physicians. It is much harder for a plaintiff to sustain an abandonment cause of action against a facility providing in-patient services. However, situations can and do exist where abandonment claims brought against facilities are successful, such as abandonment of a patient in the postoperative area or by the home health agency.

The emergency room, especially at large inner-city hospitals, can be a source of abandonment claims, because patients can "fall through the cracks" in the system. or instance, a patient could be triaged, placed on a gurney, put in the hall, and not seen again until some staff or visitor notices that he is not breathing. Therefore, it is vital that nurse managers in emergency rooms know that once a patient is in the facility's system, it is their responsibility to be sure the system provides adequate follow-up. Even when triage determines that a patient can wait to be seen, the patient must not be left without someone responsible for reasonable, periodic follow-up.

To be sure, if a nurse leaves a unit without adequate coverage or before relief arrives and something happens to a patient, an abandonment argument can be made.

Transporting Patients

Transporting patients for in-house testing, x-rays, or surgery can also lead to situations where the patient is left alone. Managers must be sure that facility transportation departments are not leaving patients without adequate supervision. It is not reasonable to leave an unattended patient waiting anywhere in the facility. If that patient falls, the facility will probably be held responsible for the injuries.

A CASE IN POINT

Independent Contractor

The Facts

In *Briggins v. Shelly Medical Center*,[10] the Supreme Court of Alabama ruled that whether a hospital was vicariously liable for the acts of a certified registered nurse anesthetist (CRNA) employed as an independent contractor was a question to be decided by the jury.

A CRNA was employed by Alabama Anesthesia Associates and was serving as an independent contractor in a hospital where she administered anesthesia to Ms. Briggins, who aspirated during the course of surgery and died a few days later. The decedent's husband sued both the hospital and the anesthesia group as the employers of the CRNA. The hospital filed a motion for summary judgment alleging that because it was not the employer of the CRNA, it could not be held vicariously liable for his actions.

The Court Decides

The Alabama Supreme Court ruled that the inquiry regarding whether the hospital could be liable went beyond the mere fact of employment and sent the question to the jury to decide the decision. The jury held that the existence of the independent contract was not enough to insulate the facility from potential liability for the acts of an independent contractor

COBRA/EMTALA and Wrongful Discharge

Related to the theory of abandonment is the theory of **wrongful discharge** or **wrongful transfer.** This situation can arise when a person with no health insurance goes to the emergency room of a private hospital. Even though it is likely that the hospital will not recoup payment for services, those emergency services must be provided if the patient arrives in an unstable condition.

The **Consolidated Omnibus Reconciliation Act (COBRA)** and an act called the **Emergency Medical Treatment and Active Labor Act (EMTALA),** found at 42 U.S.C. 1395 §(dd), implicate hospitals that receive federal monies (Medicare) and that provide emergency services. Under these acts, such facilities are required to provide a screening examination and all services necessary to stabilize serious medical conditions, including active labor, before the hospitals may discharge or transfer patients, regardless of a given patient's insurance coverage.

Known as the "antidumping acts," these acts are intended to relieve the tremendous burden on charitable institutions by requiring private institutions to provide necessary emergency services without regard to an individual's ability to pay. For

A CASE IN POINT

Nurse Abandonment

The Facts

In *Eyoma v. Falco*,[11] a postanesthesia nurse on duty left the unit, asking another nurse to "keep an eye" on her postoperative patient. There was no indication that this second nurse heard the nurse or observed the patient. When the anesthesiologist made rounds, he saw that the patient was not breathing and began resuscitative efforts. The patient remained in a coma for 1 year and then died.

The Jury Decides

A jury exonerated the anesthesiologist and held a postanesthesia nurse 100% at fault for the death of a patient.

---

noncompliance, EMTALA specifically authorizes civil suits for damages, loss of Medicare monies, access to federal court, and a 2-year statute of limitations in which to bring any action.

At a minimum, hospitals must adopt a written policy that reflects the language of the statute. Each transfer from the emergency room should be reviewed to determine compliance. If the institution does not provide maternity services, this fact should be clearly posted in the emergency room. Even without maternity services, if a pregnant woman in the late stages of active labor enters the emergency room, a physician must certify that the patient is stable before a transfer can take place.

Minimizing Potential Problems Before They Arise—The Nurse Manager's Role

JCAHO

Each hospital accredited by the JCAHO has to implement an overall quality assurance program. The standards require evaluations of the quality and appropriateness of patient care, suggestions on how patient care can be improved, and resolutions of identified problems.

Generally, nursing supervisors are asked to implement this program. In this unique capacity, a nurse supervisor can act as a liaison among nurses, other departments within the facility, and the medical staff.

JCAHO's ORYX Initiative

Each hospital accredited by JCAHO has to implement an overall quality management program. Lately facilities have been executing quality management plans that include outcome-based systems that focus not only on established criteria but also on specific problems. All JCAHO facilities must participate in what it calls the ORYX program.

In 1997 JCAHO introduced the **ORYX initiative.** This program was designed to integrate outcomes and other performance measurement data into the accreditation process. Organizations with a census of 120 patients or more are required to select measures from a changing list of performance measurements.

During the accreditation process, the organization is asked to explain how well these performance-based measures have been integrated in the organization's performance improvement activities. Each organization must explain why the particular measure was chosen, how the ORYX data has been integrated into the performance improvement program, and its results.

As of 2001, more than 15,000 performance measures from nearly 300 performance measurement systems have been cataloged in JCAHO's database. In the future, JCAHO intends to move into the next phase of its ORYX initiative by identifying certain core performance measures that can be monitored. Such measures may include clinical performance, patient perception of care, health status, and administrative or financial measures. JCAHO is continuing to work on modifiying applicable core measures, and updates are likely.[12]

In addition to the collection of ORYX data, all JCAHO organizations must monitor adverse sentinel events. As defined by JCAHO, an **adverse sentinel event** is "an unexpected occurrence—involving death or serious physical or psychological injury, or the risk thereof. Serious injury specifically includes the loss of limb or function."[13] JCAHO refers to these as "sentinel" because they send a signal or warning to the organization that it must take immediate action. When an adverse sentinel event occurs, the organization must conduct a **root cause analysis.** A process for identifying the "most basic or causal factor or factors that underlie variation in performance, including the occurrence of an adverse sentinel event." In conducting a root cause analysis, a team is appointed to ask difficult and critical questions regarding how the event occurred, what was actually done, what should have been done, and what can be done in the future to prevent such events from occurring again. Understandably, root cause analyses can increase staff anxiety due to the fear of blame and potential disciplinary actions.

Centers for Medicare and Medicaid Services

If your facility is not JCAHO accredited but is a qualified Medicare/Medicaid provider, the Centers for Medicare and Medicaid Services (CMS, formerly Health

Care Financing Administration [HCFA]) conditions of participation will apply. These conditions require facilities to analyze whether any "immediate jeopardy triggers" exist. As defined by CMS, **immediate jeopardy** "is a situation in which the provider's noncompliance with one or more requirements of participation has caused, or is likely to cause, serious injury, harm, impairment, or death to a resident." (See 42 CFR Part 489.3; Guidelines for Determining Immediate Jeopardy may be found in Appendix Q to the *State Operations Manual* and may be accessed through the Centers for Medicare and Medicaid Services Web site [*http//:www.cms.hhs.gov*]).

Surveyors will determine whether an immediate jeopardy situation exists, identify what the organization did to determine its existence, and explain the steps taken to correct the situation. Failure to adequately prevent or correct immediate jeopardy issues may result in the loss of provider status.

For those nurse managers in the specialty of home health, CMS requires an **Outcome and Assessment Information Set (OASIS).** OASIS performs many functions for the government. Answers to certain OASIS questions determine what Medicare will pay for and whether or not admission to home care is appropriate.

These monitoring programs supplement the quality improvement programs that should already be in place in your facilities. They should not be used as a substitute for programs already established. Implementation of the numerous new initiatives required by JCAHO and CMS will require more effort on the part of the nurse managers to convey the information to those nurses they supervise.

Hospital Quality Improvement Programs

Quality improvement programs developed by facilities that the nurse manager must be aware of include, but are not limited to, the following:

1. Nursing orientation programs, continuing education requirements for nurses, and periodic monitoring of continuing education hours by supervisors.
2. Identification of high-risk areas for patient injuries or the potential for injuries utilizing immediate jeopardy and adverse sentinel event guidelines.
3. Identification of high-risk areas for patient injuries.
4. Identification of high-risk areas for potential liability.
5. In-service education programs on adequate and appropriate documentation in the medical record.
6. Periodic chart audits to determine whether staff nurses, as well as physicians, are charting appropriately and actually communicating the medical information necessary for good patient care.
7. Effective communication mechanisms to handle complaints made by patients, their families, physicians, and other departments with the facility.
8. Findings from the programs should not be used to punish health care workers.

9. Conducting immediate investigations when an adverse event occurs and implementing the necessary changes to prevent these events from occurring in the future.

The effectiveness of any quality improvement program is a three-step process: development, implementation, and follow-up.

KEEP IN MIND

▶ Nurse managers have the primary responsibility for establishing and maintaining standards of care that the staff must follow.

▶ The language used and the responsibilities outlined in policy and procedure manuals must be reasonable and generally accepted within the nursing profession.

▶ If a nurse is an employer, owner, or supervisor, the nurse employer can be held liable for negligent acts of employees under the theory of respondeat superior.

▶ Unlicensed assistive personnel do not work under the nurse's license.

▶ Nurse managers must be sure that unlicensed personnel do not perform functions that require a license.

▶ Nurse managers can be held personally and professionally liable if they fail to properly render direct patient care.

▶ Nurse managers can also be held liable for failure to properly delegate, train, orient, and evaluate staff or failure to properly supervise.

▶ Floating or "pulling" a nurse to another unit can be dangerous if the nurse does not have the experience and knowledge required to extend care to patients in that type of unit.

▶ Abandonment is a premature termination of the professional relationship without adequate notice to the patient.

▶ COBRA affects hospitals receiving federal monies that provide emergency services and requires under EMTALA that hospitals provide emergency services to stabilize patients with our without insurance.

▶ The effectiveness of a quality improvement program is a three-step process: development, implementation, and follow-up.

IN A NUTSHELL

Nurse managers have a monolithic task. Because of their roles as teacher and manager, nurses are often the first to recognize how patient care can be improved and what steps are necessary to accomplish those changes. Very often, nurse managers are faced with conflicting concerns about the delivery of good patient care and the reality of financial constraints imposed either by their institution or by third-party payers. It is the skillful nurse manager who can recognize how to effect reasonable change without increasing cost. No one can prevent all adverse outcomes. The goal is to recognize the ones that can be prevented. Striving for the optimal patient care should be the goal of the health care system in this country.

AFTERTHOUGHTS

1. Discuss how the facility's policy and procedure manual can be used by plaintiff's counsel to establish negligence.

2. Define the concept of respondeat superior, and describe under what circumstances it is applicable.

3. What are the nurse manager's responsibilities in supervising unlicensed personnel?

4. Discuss the nurse manager's duty to train, orient, and evaluate staff and how the breach of these duties can result in liability.

5. Name five factors that affect the reasonableness of the nurse manager's actions in a short staffing situation.

6. Before determining whether a nurse should be floated to another floor, what factors must the nurse supervisor consider?

7. Define abandonment, and give examples of situations where a claim for abandonment may be made in a hospital setting.

8. What criteria must be met under COBRA and EMTALA before an emergency room patient may be transferred to another institution or facility?

9. What is ORYX? What is OASIS?

10. Create your own policy and procedures on a new treatment. Discuss the resources used to develop your own written policy and procedures.

11. Create your own checklist for "checking off" staff on a treatment or procedure required on the unit. Will it stand up in a court of law to protect you as a nurse manager?

12. Discuss the delegation decision-making process.

13. Discuss three ways to deal with the short staffing problem.

14. List the five rights of delegation.

15. Discuss what quality improvement programs for facilities may include.

ETHICS IN PRACTICE

Maggie C., registered nurse (RN) and head nurse of a busy neurologic intensive care unit, was reviewing the weekend staffing for the unit on a Friday afternoon. As usual, the unit's nine beds were full with patients in various levels of recovery from brain surgery or head injuries. The staffing on the weekend was short, with only enough staff to safely care for eight patients. After spending a great deal of time reworking the schedule, calling nurses on the phone, and trading days off, Maggie finally managed to arrange sufficient coverage for the unit.

As Maggie was closing her office for the weekend, Dr. West, a neurosurgeon, approached her and related the following situation. Mrs. P., a 63-year-old patient with a brain tumor, had been scheduled for surgery 3 days earlier. Because she had a very rare blood type that was difficult to match, the surgery had been delayed. Although a few days' wait was not expected to worsen her condition drastically, Mrs. P. had become anxious when informed about the delay. Although the blood bank had just obtained the necessary units for the surgery and had informed Dr. West that he could now operate, Dr. West was wondering if the neurologic unit would be able to safely care for Mrs. P. over the weekend.

This unit was the only unit in the hospital equipped to monitor brain surgery and provide appropriate nursing care for this type of patient. Because the neurologic stepdown unit was also full, it would be difficult to transfer one of the patients on the neurologic unit to make a bed available for Mrs. P. Mrs. P. would most likely require one-to-one care for 18 to 24 hours after surgery.

Should Maggie tell Dr. West that he can go ahead with the surgery and that she will make the adjustments to provide care for this patient? What ethical obligations does Maggie have to the patient? How about her obligations to Dr. West and the facility?

References

1. Parker v. Southwest Hospital Association, 540 So.2d 1270 (La. App. 3d Cir. 1989).
2. Bowers v. Olch, 120 Cal. App. 2d 108, 260 P.2d 992 (1953).
3. Hicks v. New York State Department of Health, 570 N.Y.S.2d 395 (A.D. 3 Dept. 1991).
4. Norton v. Argonaut Insurance Co., 144 So.2d 249 (La. App. 1st Cir. 1962).
5. JCAHO Nursing Services N.R. 4.1 and N.R. 4.2.
6. Curtain, L, and Simpson, R: 10 tips for recruiting nurses on the web. Health Management Technology, December 2000.
7. Ibid., 40.
8. Bossier v. DeSoto General Hospital, 442 So.2d 485 (La. App. 2d Cir. 1983).
9. http://www.irs.gov/businesses/small/article/0,,id=99921,00.html, accessed November 8, 2002.
10. Briggins v. Shelly Medical Center 585 So.2d 912 (Ala. 1991).
11. Eyoma v. Falco, 589 A2d 653 (N.J. Super. A.D. 1991).
12. http://www.jcaho.org/accredited+organizations/long+term+care/oryx/index.htm, accessed November 8, 2002.
13. Conducting a Root Cause Analysis in Response to a Sentinel Event. Joint Commission on Accreditation of Healthcare Organizations, Oakbrook Terrace, IL, 1996.

Resources

Joint Commission on Accreditation of Healthcare Organizations
One Renaissance Boulevard
Oakbrook Terrace, IL 60181
(630) 792-5000
http://www.jcaho.org/

Core Measure Information for Healthcare Organizations
(630) 792-5085
http://www.jcaho.org/pms/core+measures/index.htm

ORYX Information for Healthcare Organizations
(630) 792-5085
http://www.jcaho.org/accredited+organizations/long+term+care/ltc+update/2002issue1/
    programnotes.htm

Sentinel Event Hotline
601 13th Street, NW
Suite 1150 North
Washington, DC 20005
(630) 792-3700 (JCAHO—Sentinel Event Hotline, Illinois Office)
(202) 783-6655 (JCAHO—Washington Office)
(202) 783-6888 (Fax)

Centers for Medicare and Medicaid Services
http://cms.hhs.gov/

The Nurse and the Medical Malpractice Lawsuit 14

Key Chapter Concepts

Plaintiff

Defendant

Special damages

Punitive damages

Prelitigation panel

Complaint

Answer

Contributory negligence

Comparative negligence

Assumption of the risk

Good Samaritan laws

Unavoidable accident

Defense of the fact

Sovereign immunity

Request for production
   of documents and things

Interrogatories

Depositions

Parties

Fact or material witness

Expert witness deposition

Independent medical examination

Admissions of fact

Legal research

Mediation

Arbitration

Voir dire

Peremptory challenge

Challenge for cause

Chapter Thoughts

For many years those involved in nursing have strived to be recognized by medicine as belonging to a separate and distinct profession. Over the course of these years, nursing has gained a great deal of power, independence, and influence in the health care industry. However, these gains have been accompanied by an increase in, and stricter interpretation of, the legal accountability associated with nursing practice. Nurses have a professional obligation to use this long sought after power, independence, and influence to increase the quality of patient care, as well as to promote legal and ethical nursing practice.

As the fear about legal liability and legal actions against nurses increases, concern for the law has become a major preoccupation. Indeed, all practicing nurses must recognize what types of actions increase their risk of malpractice suits.

Yet the law and the legal system have a narrow view of nursing practice. Legally speaking, those aspects of patient care called nursing can be limited to activities that are specifically covered in the nurse practice act and scope of practice. In reality, the practice of nursing involves all the activities, both tangible and intangible, that nurses do whenever they enter into a relationship with a patient. This broader view of the nurse-patient relationship is the concern of ethics.

In most situations, ethics includes or exceeds the law where questions of nursing practice are involved. Ethical nursing practice is almost always legal nursing practice. If nurses are aware of the ethics involved in nursing practice and follow the ethical code, they should have little to be concerned with from the legal system.

OBJECTIVES

Upon completing this chapter, the reader will be able to:
1. Describe defenses to medical malpractice claims.
2. Discuss how to prepare for a deposition.
3. Outline the various types of discovery techniques.
4. Identify the stages of the trial process.
5. Discuss alternatives to lawsuits, such as mediation, arbitration, and facilitation.
6. Define common documents and items used in litigation.

Introduction

This chapter discusses how the legal system operates, how nurses can best protect themselves if they are sued, and the role of the nurse as an expert, fact, or material witness in malpractice litigation.

In a lawsuit, a **plaintiff** is the person or entity initiating the lawsuit who is claiming harm or damage by the defendant. In cases where a patient has died, the next of kin or legal guardian of the decedent may take the role of plaintiff on behalf of the estate of the deceased. The **defendant** is the person or entity that is sued. Defendants in a medical malpractice action can include but are not limited to the following: nurse, physician, health maintenance organization (HMO), insurance company, hospital or care-providing institution, equipment or pharmaceutical company, and other health care providers such as physical therapists and nursing assistants.

The Litigation Process: Initial Stages

Negligence Defined

To maintain a medical malpractice claim, the elements of negligence must be present. To be successful in a lawsuit, the plaintiff has the burden of proving the following:

1. The defendant owed a duty to the plaintiff

2. The defendant breached this duty through an act of omission or commission
3. The defendant caused damages to the plaintiff
4. There is a proximate cause between the breach of duty and the damages or injuries suffered by plaintiff

Specifically, damages can include, but are not limited to, pain and suffering; emotional distress; mental anguish; severe disfigurement; loss of chance of survival; decreased life expectancy; loss of nurturance; loss of consortium; past, present, and future lost wages and medical expenses; and premature death.

If all elements of negligence are not established, the plaintiff will not be successful in pursuing the claim. If the judge or jury decides that the plaintiff has proven the elements necessary to establish liability, the specific amount of the award for the damages is decided.

Types of Damages

A plaintiff can sue for various types of damages.

Special damages are based on actual monetary losses, such as past, present, and future lost wages and medical expenses, that are caused by the defendant's acts or omissions.

General damages are awarded for the plaintiff's pain and suffering caused by the defendant's acts.

Punitive damages are intended to punish the defendant for the egregious nature of the tort. The defendant's actions must be willful and wanton, and the numerical amounts are not based on the plaintiff's actual monetary loss. Usually the award is doubled or tripled to punish the defendant economically, so that this type of behavior will never occur again. State laws vary regarding what types of actions are compensable with punitive damages. Not every state permits awards of punitive damages for malpractice actions.

Preparing the Case

Once a plaintiff decides to seek legal redress for a perceived harm and seeks an attorney, the malpractice claim goes through a long and intensive process (Box 14–1).

Prelitigation Panels

The majority of malpractice cases are tried in state courts. Prior to litigating the case in state court, the plaintiff may have to present the case to a **prelitigation panel,** medical tribunal, medical review panel, or arbitration panel to determine if negligence has occurred. The panel renders an opinion based on its review and evaluation of the materials submitted by plaintiff and defendant.

BOX 14–1

The Legal Process: Initial Stages of a Malpractice Claim

1. Pretrial preparation is begun (review of medical records by the plaintiff's attorney and expert witness: retrieval of all medical and office records, patient bills, and other pertinent documents).
2. A procedural process may be required by state law (e.g., prelitigation panels such as medical review panels, medical tribunals, or arbitration panels).
3. Petition for damages or complaint is filed in court by the plaintiff's attorney.
4. Complaint or summons is sent to the defendant health care provider by certified mail or served by a sheriff or process service company.
5. Defendant health care provider contacts insurance company to notify it of the claim.
6. The insurance company assigns an attorney or law firm to the defendant health care provider.
7. Answer to the complaint or counterclaim is filed by defendant; defenses are alleged.

The filing process and prelitigation panels differ from state to state. If a prelitigation panel is required, the plaintiff usually submits evidence to a panel of health care providers, attorneys, and/or judges (depending on the state law) that demonstrates how the injury was caused by the defendant and the extent of the injury.

Evidence submitted to the members of the medical review panel, for example, can include medical records, affidavits, expert reports, treatises, authoritative texts, journal articles, photographs, medical illustrations, depositions, medical or legal memoranda, or position papers. This varies from state to state.

Arguments are made for and against the existence of such panels or tribunals. Defendants contend that they reduce frivolous suits, whereas plaintiffs argue that they merely prolong the legal process and increase expense by requiring a "trial" submission to the tribunal prior to actually litigating in court. Most malpractice cases take approximately 3 to 5 years to be tried, mediated, or settled. In those states with prelitigation panels, the process is delayed by approximately 6 to 18 months, depending on the state and the panel process.

Filing a Lawsuit

Complaint

After the panel or tribunal reviews the case, the plaintiff files a lawsuit with the court. If there is no requirement for a prelitigation panel, the complaint is filed directly with the appropriate court. A sheriff or process service company serves defendants named in the petition or complaint. The **complaint** outlines the following:

- Names of the plaintiffs and defendants
- Allegations of breaches of duty
- Damages or injuries
- Demand for an award

Some states do not allow specific amounts for damages demands to be specified in the complaint. This practice avoids publicity for malpractice suits that demand huge awards. See Appendix A, Sample Complaint, at the end of this chapter.

As soon as nurse defendant receives notification of a suit, that nurse should notify the facility administrator and contact the insurance company. The insurance company will retain the attorney or law firm that will represent the nurse. Typically, attorneys or law firms are retained by insurance carriers and handle all the lawsuits filed against the insured. In some instances, nurses are able to choose their own attorneys. See Box 14–2 for tips on selecting the right attorney. See Appendix B for a Sample Fee Agreement and Authority to Represent.

Although some nurses believe that if they have insurance, they are more likely to get sued, in reality, most attorneys do not have access to a central national data bank that supplies information on nurses' insurance policies. The lawsuit filed against a nurse should be based on nursing negligence found in the medical records. Unfortunately, some attorneys use the "shotgun" approach and sue everyone who was treating or caring for the patient, rather than limiting the number of defendants to those who treated the patient negligently, as indicated by medical records.

The nurse must refrain from consulting with anyone except his or her attorney, facility attorney, risk manager, or supervisor. The nurse should not speak to staff members, the plaintiff's attorney, or the plaintiffs about the circumstances surrounding the lawsuit.

Answer

After a defendant receives the complaint, the defense attorney files an answer on behalf of a defendant. The **answer** admits, denies, or declines to answer the allegations in the complaint, and then offers defenses to the allegations.

Defenses to a Malpractice Claim

There are numerous avenues that an attorney can take to prepare a defense, depending on the evidence reviewed. Common defenses may be based on any of the following:

1. Contributory or comparative negligence
2. Statute of limitations
3. Assumption of the risk
4. Good Samaritan laws
5. Unavoidable accident

6. Defense of fact
7. Sovereign immunity

Contributory Negligence Versus Comparative Negligence

The states vary regarding whether they accept the defense of contributory negligence or that of comparative negligence. This distinction may be the decisive factor for a malpractice claim. In a **contributory negligence** state, plaintiffs are not allowed to

---

BOX 14–2

Selecting the Attorney Who Is Right for You

To find the right attorney for you and your case takes some time and research. Locate potential candidates using the following methods:

1. The national and state nurse attorney associations (e.g., The American Association of Nurse Attorneys)
2. The local bar association
3. The national and state trial lawyers associations
4. The state bar associations
5. The state boards of nursing
6. Referrals from families and friends
7. Referrals from other attorneys
8. Attorneys who present seminars
9. Directories, yellow pages, special listings
10. Legal clinics
11. Pro bono legal clinics
12. Prepaid legal services

Ask the following questions:

1. How long have you been practicing in this field?
2. Have you had any cases similar to mine and what was the outcome?
3. What are your other areas of practice?
4. If you cannot take my case, can you refer me?
5. What is the fee arrangement?
6. What is the time line and overall process of the case?
7. Do you represent plaintiffs, defendants, or both?
8. Who will be working on the case? What is their fee arrangement?
9. What is the actual process and cost for each stage (e.g., medical review panel, trial, appeal)?
10. What areas of law cannot be handled by you or your firm?
11. Will you keep me updated by phone, mail, fax, and so on?

> **BOX 14–2**
>
> ## Selecting the Attorney Who Is Right for You *(continued)*
>
> Make sure you feel comfortable with the attorney.
>
>   When you meet with the attorney for the first time, bring the following with you:
>
> 1. A chronological list of events
> 2. All bills pertaining to the issue
> 3. All medical records or pertinent documents
> 4. All correspondence pertaining to the issues
> 5. A detailed narrative
> 6. Photographs if applicable
> 7. Policies, procedures, and evaluations
> 8. Letters of termination, letters of recommendation (if pertaining to a nursing board action)
> 9. A check if a retainer is required
> 10. Death certificate
> 11. Autopsy

recover damages if they contributed to their injuries in any manner. Suppose, for example, a physician failed to perform a surgical procedure properly. However, the plaintiff increased his injuries by not taking the medication ordered by the physician and thus contributed to his own damages. That plaintiff cannot recover because the defendant physician can successfully argue contributory negligence.

In a **comparative negligence** state, the award is based on the percentage of fault on the respective parts of the plaintiff and the defendant. For example, if the award is $100,000 and plaintiff is found to be 40% at fault for her injuries, she receives only $60,000 for damages. Usually, in comparative negligence states, if a plaintiff is deemed to be 50% or more at fault, no award will is given.

Statute of Limitations

The statute of limitations defines the period allowed by law for filing a lawsuit. If the malpractice suit is not filed within the time limits mandated by law, the plaintiff loses the right to sue the defendants. In most states, a suit must be filed within a specified period from the date of the breach of duty or from the date on which the patient knew or discovered that malpractice caused the injury. Every state has different time limits and different guidelines for determining the time frame within which a lawsuit must be filed. Some states base the period from the date of the last treatment, whereas others allow a minor or a child's parents or guardian to file a malpractice claim until a child reaches the age of 18 or 18 plus 2 years. State laws vary; be sure to check your individual state laws.

Assumption of the Risk

The **assumption of the risk** defense states that the plaintiff, by agreeing to have a procedure or treatment performed by a health care provider, has assumed either expressed, voluntary, or implied risks. Under this theory, the plaintiff, as a result of assuming the risk, has virtually waived the right to sue for damages that result from the risk. This theory is based on the informed consent of the patient.

Good Samaritan Laws

Good Samaritan laws are enacted to protect those who render health care at the scene of an accident, emergency, or disaster. Good Samaritan laws usually cover health care providers who practice using the appropriate standards of care as guidelines. They will not cover negligent acts that occur during the course and scope of employment. If a fee is received for services rendered, the Good Samaritan Statute cannot be invoked. Also, if a patient is intentionally harmed, or there is gross negligence (based on accepted standards of care), the Good Samaritan Statute cannot be used as a defense. Depending on the state, laws may apply differently to nurses and physicians.

Unavoidable Accident

The **unavoidable accident** defense is used when nothing other than an accident could have caused the plaintiff's injury. For example, a patient walks down a hall, slips, and breaks an ankle. Nothing on the floor caused the accident. The patient was capable of ambulating without assistance, and a health care provider did not breach any standards. Documentation in an incident report or chart that the floor is clean may save the facility from exposure and a damage award.

Defense of the Fact

Defense of the fact contends that the health care provider's treatment was not the cause of the damage to the plaintiff. The facts belie attributing fault to the defendant. For example, the plaintiff has a minor eye procedure performed and claims that she is paralyzed and has a debilitating muscle disease from the surgery, a result that is highly unlikely.

Sovereign Immunity

Historically, federal and state governments used the legal doctrine of **sovereign immunity** to prevent negligence suits from being filed against them. Note, however, that the federal government can be sued under the Federal Tort Claims Act. Likewise, many states are also no longer immune from tort liability actions.

Captain of the Ship Doctrine

The key case on the Captain of the Ship Doctrine dates back to 1949. The surgeon was held vicariously liable for the negligence of a nurse and anesthesiologist. Historically, under the captain of the ship doctrine, case law decisions held that physicians could be held liable for negligence of other members of the surgical or health care team. However, this doctrine has eroded and many states no longer recognize it.

Borrowed Servant Doctrine

In a 1956 Pennsylvania case, the court found that the incorrect placement of a hot water bottle during surgery while the patient was on the operating room table was a medical duty. The nurse was considered a "borrowed servant" of the surgeon. This doctrine also has eroded and is rarely recognized.

■ The Litigation Process: Discovery

Discovery is the stage in a lawsuit during which all information, facts, and circumstances surrounding the alleged malpractice incident are "discovered" by plaintiff and defendant. Discovery tools include requests for production of documents and things, interrogatories, depositions, physical and mental examinations, and admissions of facts (Box 14–3).

Discovery is the most time-consuming stage of litigation and can take years to complete. There are several "tools" used by trial attorneys to "discover" all the information surrounding the claims alleged in the complaint or petition for damages.

BOX 14–3

The Legal Process: Discovery

1. Discovery stage (subpoenas and subpoenas duces tecum may be used)
   - ■ Requests for production of documents and things
   - ■ Interrogatories
   - ■ Depositions
   - ■ Physical or mental examination
   - ■ Admissions of fact
2. Pretrial hearing
3. Mediation (possibly)
4. Settlement negotiations (possibly)
5. Pretrial conference

Discovery "tools" include:

1. Requests for production of documents and things
2. Interrogatories
3. Depositions
4. Independent medical examination
5. Admissions of fact

Requests for Production of Documents and Things

Requests for production of documents and things are requests by the plaintiff or defendant for items from the other party that pertain to the issues of the lawsuit and may lead to discoverable information. See Appendix C, Sample Request for Production of Documents.

Interrogatories

Interrogatories are written questions sent by one party to the other requesting information about issues and witnesses surrounding the incident of alleged malpractice. The information requested can be very general, such as "List all employers and reasons for leaving employment." Interrogatories can also seek very detailed and medically oriented information, such as "What are the common signs and symptoms of sepsis?" Such information can later be used at the trial during cross-examination of the witnesses. See Appendix D, Sample Interrogatories and Answers, at the end of this chapter.

Interrogatories may request information that is privileged and confidential. The client's attorney should argue that such information is confidential and therefore protected from disclosure. Depending on the state laws, privileged information can include correspondence, notes, documents, incident reports, and conversations between the attorney and the client. This is considered attorney work product. Clients have a right to speak freely without fear that information given to their attorney is available to the opposition.

Attorneys can make objections to interrogatories, such as "Objection to Interrogatory No. 1 because it would cause undue hardship and burden to obtain the information." If the attorney refuses to answer interrogatories within the allowed time, opposing counsel can file a motion to compel answers to interrogatories. A hearing may be set so that a judge can decide whether to grant or deny the motion to compel. The judge will decide whether the interrogatories must be answered and whether the party would be severely hindered in presenting the case without the requested information or if the information can be obtained through another discovery avenue.

Depositions

Although many malpractice suits are settled prior to trial, nurses often have to endure the anxiety and tension of having their depositions taken. A **deposition** is a structured interview by opposing counsel during which the person being interviewed (the deponent) is placed under oath and asked questions about issues of the lawsuit. See Appendix E, Excerpts from a Deposition, at the end of this chapter.

Why Are Depositions Taken?

Depositions are done to:

1. Gather all available discoverable information about the case.
2. Assist attorneys in assessing strengths and weaknesses in their cases.
3. Assist attorneys in formulating settlement and trial strategies.
4. Evaluate the credibility, knowledge, demeanor, and appearance of the witnesses.
5. Determine the existence and substance of pertinent documents.
6. Determine the availability and limits of insurance coverage.
7. Discover the facts and circumstances of the alleged malpractice and breaches of the standard.
8. Preserve the testimony of a witness who may be unavailable at the time of trial because of relocation or death (called a deposition for perpetuation of testimony).
9. Determine the cause of the plaintiff's injuries.
10. Determine the extent of the injuries and types of injuries sustained by the plaintiff and his family.
11. Be used prior to or during trial to refresh the witness's memory.
12. Be used during trial to impeach a witness's credibility. Did the witness commit perjury?

See Box 14–4 for examples of the types of questions that may be asked in a deposition.

Who Can Be Deposed?

Parties (plaintiffs or defendants) to a lawsuit are routinely deposed. **Fact or material witnesses,** who are persons having knowledge about the circumstances surrounding the events of the alleged malpractice, may also be deposed. For example, a circulating nurse who is not a defendant may be deposed to determine if he or she knows anything about the events involving the birth of a brain-injured infant. Persons who the attorney wishes to depose who are not a party to the suit are generally issued a subpoena indicating the time and place the deposition will be held. The subpoena compels the person to attend. See Appendix G, Sample Subpoena, at the end of this chapter.

BOX 14–4

Types of Questions Asked in a Deposition

Through depositions, attorneys attempt to elicit information from the plaintiff, defendant, or fact witnesses on the following:

1. General background and marital status of the deponent
2. Educational background
3. Certifications and advanced degrees
4. Professional and social organizations
5. Employment history
6. Basic medical and nursing knowledge information, such as common signs and symptoms of fetal distress or common nursing care and treatment given to alleviate pressure sores
7. Continuing educational courses attended
8. In-service courses attended
9. Specific information related to the case at issue, such as "What specific symptoms of lithium toxicity did Mr. Beam exhibit on October 26, 2003?"
10. Teaching positions
11. What would be done differently, if anything
12. If you have ever been disciplined; if your license has ever been probated, suspended, or revoked; or if you received an informal or formal letter of reprimand (if you are a health care provider)

If you are an expert, questions can be asked concerning the following:

1. General background
2. Marital status
3. Educational background
4. Employment history
5. Professional and social organizations
6. Teaching positions
7. Seminars, lectures, and presentations
8. Textbooks, journal articles, treatises, or research papers written or authored
9. Clinical experience in the areas of alleged malpractice
10. Certifications or advanced degrees
11. Number of times you have testified in a deposition and at trial as an expert for plaintiff or defendant
12. The fee for evaluating the case, testifying at a deposition, and testifying at trial
13. How you were contacted by the attorney to review the case
14. What texts you view as authoritative in the field
15. Whether you personally examined the patient
16. Your relationship with the attorney or law firm

Types of Questions Asked in a Deposition (continued)

17. Your opinion on hypothetical situations
18. Breaches of the standard by each defendant
19. Causal connection between the breach and the plaintiff's injuries
20. The elements of malpractice
21. Whether any court has ruled that you are qualified to testify as an expert in a case and in what specialty area
22. The standard of care in effect at the time the patient received care
23. The standard of care for other health care providers
24. Questions attempting to discredit you: "When is the last time you actually worked as an OB nurse?" "Why have you changed jobs so often?" "When were you hired by the plaintiff to testify on his behalf?"
25. Repetitive questions to see if you change your answer
26. If you have ever been disciplined; if your license ever been probated, suspended, or revoked; or if you have received an informal or formal letter of reprimand (if you are a health care provider)

Expert Depositions

In medical malpractice and personal injury cases, the plaintiff uses medical and nursing expert witnesses to assist the judge and jury in understanding the standards of care and causal connections between breaches of the standard and damages sustained. **Expert witness depositions** are some of the most common because expert testimony is crucial to sustaining a claim. Also, each side must understand the strengths and weaknesses of their cases according to expert opinions. Attorneys routinely retain expert witnesses to evaluate medical records to determine if a standard of care has been breached and, if so, what damages have been caused by the breach. Expert witnesses in a malpractice suit may be nurses, physicians, economists, physical therapists, or hospital administrators, depending on the allegations of negligence. For someone to qualify as an expert, attorneys consider the following points:

1. Is the expert currently practicing? If not, is the expert teaching students in the specialty area that is at issue in the lawsuit?
2. Has the expert published journal articles or textbook chapters?
3. Is the nurse an officer in professional organizations or associations?
4. Has the expert testified previously in a deposition or trial? Has this testimony been primarily for plaintiffs or defendants?

AUTHOR TIP: *Lawyers should be cautious in hiring expert witnesses. For instance, experts who have testified numerous times, in numerous different lawsuits, sometimes lose their credibility and garner the reputation of "selling their opinions" and are considered "hired guns." In other words, they will give their clients whatever opinion the client wants if the money is high enough. For the most part, however, experts who testify often provide a valuable service to both plaintiffs and defendants in malpractice cases.*

As another matter, if your expert has testified in other malpractice cases, it is crucial to check his or her testimony in those cases to ensure that it does not contradict the testimony he or she will be providing in your case.

Counsel can request that the expert witness list and produce all documents—that is, treatises, textbooks, journal articles, depositions, and any other material used to develop the expert opinion of the case.

Another type of deposition commonly taken is that of the custodian of documents, for example, an operating room director who is in charge of maintaining the operating room log.

Remember, it is important to reserve the right to read and sign the deposition after it is taken. This gives the nurse an opportunity to review the deposition for accuracy.

PREPARING FOR THE DEPOSITION

- Review all medical records and pertinent information.
- If you are a defendant and have kept a diary of the events surrounding the incident, notify your attorney. If you review this diary to prepare for your deposition, opposing counsel can request that a copy be attached to the deposition.
- Be careful about materials you bring to your deposition that may be discoverable.
- Review incident reports with caution prior to a deposition. Some health care providers avoid the potential of having the incident report produced at the deposition by discussing—rather than actually reviewing—the report with the attorney. The attorney-client privilege may then be invoked to prevent the production of the incident report. Some states allow opposing counsel to obtain the incident report.
- Insist that your attorney clue you in on what to expect. Ask for guidance on what to cover. Your attorney cannot tell you what to say but can direct you on the best way to say it.
- Dress comfortable and professional.
- Arrive early to become comfortable with your surroundings.

DURING THE DEPOSITION

- Speak slowly and clearly.
- Do not be intimidated.
- Maintain eye contact only with the questioning attorney.
- Be honest. Tell only the truth.
- Be straightforward and concise.
- Answer verbally because a court reporter is recording your answer verbatim. Keep in mind that what you say will be recorded exactly as you say it. Using slang will not appear professional when others are reading the deposition.

- Do not answer a question you don't understand. Ask for clarification if needed.
- Think before answering the question. Take as much time as necessary. Remember, it is your deposition.
- Do not volunteer information. Remember, the purpose of the deposition is to allow the opposing attorney to discover information.
- If the question can be answered by "yes" or "no," then do so unless you are an expert (in which case you are expected to explain in detail your findings).
- Be cautious of the yes-or-no trap. Attorneys who cross-examine witnesses do not want them to explain away problems in the evidence, so they will ask questions that look bad for the witness or party. In these cases, answer "yes" or "no" but always explain. For example: Q: "Isn't it a fact that you failed to take vital signs every 15 minutes as ordered?" A: "Yes, but only one time because the nurse's aid took vital signs instead of me at 11:15 PM."
- Keep a mental note of the questions being asked. If the same question is asked twice, have the court reporter read back your previous answer.
- Do not rush to answer. Before answering, take 5 seconds to allow your attorney to make any objections that are needed to preserve the record for trial.
- Do not volunteer additional information if the attorney remains silent for a time after you answered. This is a common attorney deposition tactic called "the pregnant pause."
- Listen to your attorney when he or she makes objections to questions. Follow his or her lead if you are instructed to answer the question or not to answer the question.
- Do not make assumptions or exaggerations.
- Do not speculate. Base your answers on the facts of the case.
- If you do not know or cannot remember, simply state, "I don't know" or "I don't remember."
- If you are an expert witness, be cautious if a hypothetical question is asked. Many times the hypothetical question does not state exactly the facts in the case at hand.
- Provide a resume or curriculum vitae if requested.
- Maintain your composure.
- If you are tired or confused, take a break.
- Do not argue, get angry, or be sarcastic with the opposing attorney.
- Avoid using absolutes, such as "I always take vital signs on a post-op patient every 30 minutes."
- Do not make excuses for other people's actions.
- You have the right to read and correct the transcripts of your deposition. Never waive the right to do so.
- Caution: Be sure you have read your deposition prior to testifying at trial.

If you change your testimony at trial, the following type of scenario could occur:

ATTORNEY: "On March 31, 2003, your deposition was taken by me?"
NURSE: "Yes."

ATTORNEY: "And you were sworn under oath to tell the truth. Isn't that correct?"

NURSE: "Yes."

ATTORNEY: "On March 31, you stated that you contacted Dr. Alexes about the patient's decreased pedal pulses, cyanotic skin coloring, and coldness to the extremity seven times during the 7-to-3 shift of July 31, 2001. Is that correct?"

NURSE: "Yes."

ATTORNEY: "Today you are again under oath to tell the truth. Is that correct?"

NURSE: "Yes."

ATTORNEY: "Today you are telling the jury that you only contacted the physician one time as documented in the record? When were you lying, March 31 or today?"

Videotape Deposition

If your deposition is being videotaped, your attorney should do a trial run prior to your actual deposition. Be very conscious of body language, looking at the camera, and your appearance (color and style of clothes, makeup, type of jewelry). If a glare bounces off your glasses, take your glasses off so that the judge or jury can see your eyes. It is very disturbing when you cannot see a person's eyes and facial expressions.

Practice so that your videotape is an asset to the case. This may be the only way that the judge or jury will see or hear you if you cannot be at trial for whatever reason.

Independent Medical Examination

An **independent medical examination** (IME) is another tool used to discover information about the plaintiff's mental and physical condition. For example, if a person is claiming severe pain or loss of use of an arm from a surgical procedure, an examination by physicians chosen by the plaintiff and the defendant may be obtained to get a second opinion regarding the type and extent of injuries or to see if the patient is just a malingerer.

Admissions of Fact

Admissions of fact are written requests to admit or deny facts regarding issues of the lawsuit. This technique attempts to limit the number of facts that must be disputed and argued at trial. See Appendix F at the end of this chapter for an example of admissions of fact.

Legal Research: Foundation of a Lawsuit

In facing or bringing a lawsuit, **legal research** almost always plays an integral role. Nurses who are familiar with the basic methods of performing legal research will find themselves one step ahead should litigation pose a threat. Legal nurse consultants, nurse paralegals, paralegals, nurse attorneys, or attorneys may perform research for numerous reasons. One main purpose of research is to find case law on specific issues and understand the development of the line of cases on a given issue. Legal research is also conducted to assess liability and the value of a case, by comparing it with cases with factual and legal similarities. Research also serves to determine how courts have ruled on various issues, to evaluate opposing counsel's experience in trials or in certain legal practice areas, to see if the plaintiff is litigious, and to discover how often the defendant has been sued in the past.

Computer-Assisted Legal Research

The use of the Internet, Web sites, and software in legal research has allowed easier access to case law, statutes, citations, and legal decisions.

Many state and federal statutes and case law can be obtained on CD-ROMs. If you are interested in obtaining either CD-ROMs or on-line services, contact your local law library or bar association to see what they recommend.

Case Law Research

Many times the most important research done is on case law and previous decisions rendered that have given rise to the body of law on which your case is based. When you pull a case from a book or on-line, it has the following citation structure and contains the following elements:

Citation: *John Smith v. Brown Medical Center,* 376 So. 2d 992 (La. 2003).

1. Case name
2. Case citation (includes decision date, docket number, and name of court).
3. Brief case summary that describes lower court decisions and why and how the case was brought to the higher court.
4. Headnotes or subject notes, written by the publisher of the case, that refer to specific areas of interest and law that are discussed in the case opinion (e.g., tort, negligence, statute of limitation).
5. Names of attorneys representing plaintiff and defendant.
6. Names of judges who decided the case.
7. Names of judges who did not take part in rendering the decision.
8. Text of the case opinion.

The text of the opinion includes the facts of the case, both substantively and procedurally, the issues of the case, a discussion of each issue and the law as it applies to each issue, the decision in the case, and the court's reasoning for the decision.

A case must be checked to determine if it is still good law and has not been overturned by more recent case law. The term commonly used is *shepardizing*. The researcher uses *Shepard's Case Citations* to determine if the case in question has since been overturned, remanded, or cited in other case opinions.

Statutory Research

Statutes are also commonly researched to determine current laws. An example of a statutory citation is 42 U.S.C. 1322(a).

The Litigation Process: Trial

The discovery process can take 1 to 3 years or longer, depending on the number of plaintiffs, defendants, fact or material witnesses, and expert witnesses.

After the discovery is complete, cases are set for trial. Some claims may be settled through mediation or arbitration rather than going through the trial process. **Mediation** or **arbitration** can be quicker and less expensive than a full-blown trial (Box 14–5).

BOX 14–5

Alternative Methods of Resolving Conflicts

Mediation and arbitration can be more efficient method or resolving disputes than using litigation.

Mediation

Mediation is a process in which a neutral third-party facilitates and assists parties who have a conflict or dispute in finding a mutually beneficial and acceptable resolution. Mediation allows the parties to:
- Discuss the issues in a nonthreatening environment.
- Make informed and voluntary decisions.
- Discuss the causes of the conflict and needs of the parties in a confidential manner.
- Address past conflicts and future relationships.
- Resolve conflicts in less costly and time-consuming manner.
- Have access to legal counsel.
- Have power over the process.

Mediators may be nurse attorneys, attorneys, legal nurse consultants, paralegals, social workers, judges, health care providers, or others who have been trained in mediation techniques.[1]

Arbitration

Arbitration is a process of resolving conflicts in a more structured setting similar to the litigation process. With this method, discovery is allowed and witness lists are provided. There can be one arbitrator or a panel of arbitrators who can award damages, interest, attorney fees, and punitive damages if allowed by law.[2]

If a case does go to trial, preparation is intense. The trial itself may last days to months, depending on the complexity of the issues of the case. After the trial at the lower court level, the losing party may choose to appeal the case to the appellate court or Supreme Court, a process that can take months to years to complete. The trial process is both long and expensive (Box 14–6).

To shorten the trial, judges hold pretrial hearings so that they can decide such issues as the qualifications of witnesses, admissibility of evidence, and expert qualification.

Preparing for the Trial

When meeting with your attorney:

1. Develop a chronology of events and circumstances, with times, dates, and important events.
2. Provide a list of nurse experts who can be used in your defense.
3. Ask how you fit into the entire picture.
4. Ask about types of questions you can expect to be asked.
5. Ask about possible defenses to the lawsuit allegations.
6. Review statements or depositions previously taken from you or others involved in the lawsuit.
7. Review statements made by others in depositions or affidavits about actions taken by you.
8. Discuss allegations of negligence by each defendant in the lawsuit.
9. Review documents such as medical and office records, radiographs, videotapes, policies and procedures, national standards for your specialty, or authoritative texts and journal articles.
10. Know the weak spots in your testimony and how to handle them.

BOX 14–6

The Legal Process: Trial

1. Jury selection
2. Opening statements by plaintiff and defendant
3. Case presentation by plaintiff
4. Case presentation by defendant
5. Motion by defendant for directed verdict against plaintiff
6. Closing statements by plaintiff and defendant
7. Jury instructions by the judge
8. Jury deliberations
9. Verdict
10. Appeal (optional)

11. Be open and honest with your attorney about facts and circumstances surrounding the alleged malpractice. Don't leave your attorney open to surprises and ambush.

12. Educate your attorney about nursing and medical terms or conditions, national standards, facility and unit policies and procedures, job descriptions, and other information that can help your case.

13. In preparation for your trial, your attorney may videotape you in a mock direct examination or cross-examination. Review and study your demeanor, appearance, and presentation.

14. During the trial, write notes to your attorney if there is an important point that is missed or information that should be brought out before the jury or judge.

15. Do not express emotion verbally or in the form of fidgeting, rolling your eyes, nodding, pencil tapping, knuckle cracking. Remember, the jurors are watching you on and off the stand.

16. Dress conservatively. Do not wear heavy makeup or excessive jewelry.

17. Wear a suit, dress, or business attire.

18. When testifying, look at the jury or judge and not at your attorney so that you can build a rapport with the trier(s) of fact.

19. When sitting at the trial table, sit up, look interested, and look at the witness who is testifying.

20. Do not talk about the case in hallways or elevators. Do not talk to the jurors or a mistrial may be declared.

21. If you are an expert witness, use demonstrative evidence to "teach" the judge or jury. Examples of demonstrative evidence include the following:
    a. Medical charts
    b. Medical illustrations
    c. Skeletons and anatomic body parts
    d. Videotapes with medical graphics
    e. Medical models
    f. Blowup charts of policies, procedures, standards, and the medical records.

22. In most states, you have to convince the jury that more probably than not a breach of the duty owed caused damages to the plaintiff.

Jury Selection

On the day of a jury trial, the first step is to select a jury. Jurors are selected from a jury pool of citizens from the area. The attorneys or judge ask questions of the potential jurors to determine whether there are any biases, prejudices, or relationships between jurors and plaintiffs, defendants, attorneys, or significant others. This judicial process is called **voir dire.**

Each side has peremptory challenges or can challenge a potential juror for cause. A **peremptory challenge** is a way to eliminate a jury candidate without the attorney having to show cause for his or her removal.

Challenge for cause means that an attorney can ask that a juror be dismissed from the jury because of bias or prejudice. For example, if one juror states that her daughter is a nurse and that she would never find another nurse liable for medical malpractice, then this potential juror would be excused by reason of bias. In most malpractice claims, 12 jurors and 1 or 2 alternates are selected.

Presentation of Evidence

After the jury is selected, plaintiff and defense counsel present their opening statements. The opening statements summarize what the parties will try to present and prove through evidence and witnesses during the trial. Because the plaintiff has the burden of proof, the plaintiff presents his or her case first. Evidence must be sufficient and relevant to prove the elements of negligence. Demonstrative evidence (e.g., photography, anatomic models, charts, medical illustrations) and expert witnesses may be used.

The plaintiff presents evidence in the form of such things as standards, policies, procedures, medical records, and expert and fact testimony. Defense counsel then has the opportunity to conduct a cross-examination of witnesses used by plaintiff to discredit the witnesses and punch holes in their testimony. The plaintiff's counsel can then do a redirect examination to clarify new points brought out during the cross-examination or to rebuild the witness's credibility.

After the plaintiff has presented all the evidence and witnesses in an attempt to prove the elements of negligence, the plaintiff rests. Defense counsel then proceeds by presenting evidence and witnesses to refute the plaintiff's allegations and to refute the evidence presented. Direct examination, cross-examination, and redirect of a witness are also allowed during the defendant's presentation. After all the evidence, witnesses, and examinations are completed, the defendant rests. Both sides then present closing arguments.

Each attorney summarizes the evidence presented, points out important testimony presented by fact and expert witnesses, and tries to persuade the jury that the burden of proof has or has not been met. Closing arguments are prepared by counsel and may be rehearsed to provide the most effective argument for the attorneys to persuade the judge or jury. The judge then instructs the jury on the laws pertinent to the case.

Deliberation and Finding

The jury retires to deliberate the evidence presented during trial. A foreperson is selected to maintain control of the deliberations. Jurors are not allowed to speak to anyone during deliberations. Material admitted into evidence during the trial can be taken into the deliberations to be reviewed by jurors. If the jury has questions, the foreperson sends a message to the judge for an answer. After jury deliberation is complete, the jurors return to the courtroom and the judge reads the verdict regarding liability and the award for damages.

If the trial is a judge trial, the judge renders a judgment immediately or takes the matter under advisement and renders a judgment after reviewing trial materials or trial briefs submitted by counsel.

In many courts, after the verdict judges allow the attorneys to speak to the jurors about how they decided the verdict, concentrating on the strong and weak points of the case, the credibility of the witnesses, and other issues related to the trial presentation.

The plaintiff or defendant may then appeal the verdict. This process can take several years if it goes to the court of appeals and Supreme Court levels.

Keep in Mind

▶ Elements of negligence are duty, breach of duty, proximate cause or causal connection, and damages.
▶ In some states, prelitigation panels must be completed prior to pursuing a claim in court.
▶ Some defenses to malpractice claims are contributory or comparative negligence, statute of limitations, assumption of the risk, Good Samaritan laws, unavoidable accident, defense of the fact, and sovereign immunity.
▶ Discovery is the stage in a lawsuit where facts and information are gathered through various techniques, such as depositions, interrogatories, requests for production of documents and things, and independent medical examinations.
▶ The deposition is a structured interview under oath that is used to discover facts and circumstances surrounding the allegations.
▶ The following persons may be deposed in a lawsuit: plaintiff, defendant, expert witness, material or fact witness, and custodian of important records.
▶ Before your deposition, prepare, review important documents, and meet with your attorney.
▶ Medical malpractice claims may be tried in state or federal court by a judge or jury. The majority of cases are filed in state courts.
▶ Attorneys retain expert witnesses to discuss the breaches of the standards of care, causation, and extent and types of damages.

In a Nutshell

Nurses benefit from familiarity with the litigation process, not only from a defense perspective, but also from the point of view of a fact or expert witness. For the most part, this process impacts nurses under the guise of negligence. To be sure, attorneys will guide you through litigation, from a prelitigation panel to trial, and through motions of discovery, depositions, and the appeal process. But a nurse who is knowledgeable about the process, as well as about the clinical aspects of a case, will prove to be a valuable collaborator with the attorney on the case and may ultimately help the case to be resolved in a more positive manner.

AFTERTHOUGHTS

1. List the elements of negligence that a plaintiff's attorney must prove to successfully litigate a malpractice suit.
2. Discuss the types of damages that may be awarded to plaintiff.
3. Discuss (a) the purpose of the prelitigation panel and (b) the pros and cons of the prelitigation panel.
4. Outline the steps in a medical malpractice lawsuit.
5. Outline and give an example of the various types of discovery methods used in malpractice litigation.
6. List and discuss defenses to a malpractice claim.
7. Define the purposes of depositions.
8. Outline recommendations on how to prepare a nurse for a deposition.
9. Discuss tips on what to do if you are testifying at trial.
10. Can opposing counsel discover correspondence between a nurse and his or her attorney involving the case? Why or why not?

ETHICS IN PRACTICE

Mr. Steven S. is a 76-year-old retired scientist who lives by himself in a small apartment. He is admitted to the medical-surgical unit of the community hospital with a diagnosis of weakness, dehydration, electrolyte imbalance, and malnutrition. He has no close family, but a neighbor who accompanied Mr. S. to the hospital informed the nurse that she felt he had a preoccupation with his bowel movements and took large quantities of over-the-counter laxatives.

During the admission interview, Mr. S. was mildly disoriented to place and time but denied taking any over-the-counter medications. He was started on intravenous (IV) electrolyte and fluid replacement and placed on a high-calorie diet and bedrest. He was very compliant with the treatments, except that he frequently visited the bathroom for bowel movements.

On entering the room, one of the nurses on the evening shift noticed that Mr. S. was hurriedly returning what appeared to be a small bottle of laxative pills to his shaving kit. The nurse asked him about it, but was told "It's none of your business—just stay out of my stuff!" by a very irate Mr. S. The nurse later informed Mr. S.'s physician of the episode. The physician ordered the nurse to obtain the shaving kit and see if there were any laxatives in it. He reasoned that if the patient was taking large doses of laxatives and having diarrhea, all the treatments being given him would do no good.

Initially the nurse agreed with the physician, but after thinking about the situation further and remembering some basic principles of law she had been taught in school, she questioned the legality of searching a patient's belongings without permission. What should she do? What laws or ethical principles is she violating by searching this patient's belongings without permission? Does the principle of beneficence ever excuse breaking the law?

References _____

1. Aiken, J, Aiken, T, Grant, P, and Warlick, D: The basics of alternative dispute resolution. In Legal and Ethical Issues in Health Occupations. WB Saunders, Philadelphia, 2002.
2. Ibid.

Resources _____

Aiken, T: The plaintiff's perspective. In Iyer, P: Nursing Malpractice, ed 2. Lawyers & Judges, Tucson, 2000.
Fish, R, Ehrhardt, M, and Beckett, JS: Preparing for Your Deposition. A Comprehensive Guide to the Deposition Process for Physicians and Other Professionals. PMIC, Los Angeles, 1994.
O'Keefe, M: Nursing Practice and the Law: Avoiding Malpractice and Other Legal Risks. FA Davis, Philadephia, 2001.

Associations:

American Arbitration Association
335 Madison Avenue
Floor 10
New York, NY 10017-4605
(212) 716-5800
(800) 778-7879
(212) 716-5905 (Fax)
http://www.adr.org

American Bar Association
Section of Dispute Resolution
740 15th Street
Washington, DC 20005
(202) 662-1680
(202) 662-1683
http://www.abanet.org/

Association for Conflict Resolution
1527 New Hampshire Avenue, NW
Washington, DC 20036
(202) 667-9700
(202) 265-1968
http://www.acresolution.org/

American Association of Legal Nurse Consultants
4700 West Lake Avenue
Glenview, IL 60025-1485
(877) 734-2562
(877) 734-8668
http://www.aalnc.org

The American Association of Nurse Attorneys
7794 Grow Drive
Pensacola, FL 32514
(877) 538-2262
(850) 484-8762 (Fax)
http://www.taana.org/

Appendix A
Sample Complaint

9TH JUDICIAL DISTRICT COURT FOR THE PARISH OF JUMONVILLE
STATE OF LOUISIANA
No. 2003-200   DIVISION "F"
ALEXES ANTHONY AND BRETT ANTHONY, Individually and on behalf of their
deceased mother, Shirley Anthony
VERSUS
SAFE MEDICAL CENTER, TINA D'ANDREA, RN, AND
JAMES WRONG, M.D.
Filed: Dy.
Clk. _____

PETITION FOR DAMAGES

The complaint of Alexes Anthony and Brett Anthony, individually and on behalf of their deceased mother, Shirley Anthony, persons of the full age of majority and residents of the parish of Jumonville, State of Louisiana, represent that:

I.

Made defendant herein is Safe Medical Center, which, upon information and belief, is duly licensed and authorized to do business as a health care facility in the Parish of Jumonville, State of Louisiana, and, at all times material herein, rendered care to decedent, Shirley Anthony.

II.

Made defendant herein is James Wrong, MD, who, upon information and belief, is a physician duly licensed and authorized to and practicing in the State of Louisiana and was the attending physician at Safe Medical Center at the time of Mrs. Anthony's admission to the facility.

III.

Made defendant herein is Tina D'Andrea, RN, who, upon information and belief, is a registered nurse duly licensed and practicing in the State of Louisiana and was the nurse rendering care to the deceased, from 0700 hours until her death twelve (12) hours later on September 30, 2003.

IV.

On September 30, 2003, Shirley Anthony was admitted to Safe Medical Center surgical unit through the emergency department with complaints of bleeding from mouth and fainting. The provisional diagnosis was "R/O Seizure Disorder or GI bleeding."

V.

Twelve (12) hours later, Mrs. Anthony expired. The cause of death listed on the death certificate was "gastrointestinal bleeding and shock." The autopsy confirmed the cause of death.

VI.

Safe Medical Center is liable unto petitioners for the acts and/or omissions and/or breach of contract of their agents and/or employees and/or independent contractors under the Doctrine of Respondeat Superior including but not limited to:

1. Failure of the emergency room staff physician to timely recommend and obtain a gastrointestinal consult upon presentation to the facility;
2. Failure of the nursing staff to recognize obvious signs and symptoms of gastrointestinal bleeding;
3. Failure on the part of the nursing staff to properly document;
4. Failure to timely and properly monitor, observe, and assess a critically ill patient;
5. Failure to obtain a thorough medical history;
6. Failure to properly establish a nursing diagnosis and identify health care needs;
7. Failure to timely and properly evaluate Mrs. Anthony's responses to interventions;
8. Failure of the nursing staff to obtain the care and treatment needed by Mrs. Anthony by going through the chain of command;
9. Failure to report to the treating physician the deteriorating condition and signs and symptoms associated with same;
10. Failure of the staff to timely and properly intervene;
11. Failure of the staff to timely recommend and perform the appropriate diagnostic tests and consultations;
12. Failure to properly document;
13. Any and all other breaches of the standards of care determined prior to trial.

James Wrong, MD, is liable unto your petitioners for acts and/or omissions and/or breached contract, including but not limited to:

1. Failure to timely and properly treat;
2. Failure to recognize, diagnose, and treat obvious signs and symptoms of gastrointestinal bleeding;
3. Failure to timely perform the appropriate diagnostic studies and consultations; and
4. Any and all other acts of negligence which may be proven at the trial of this matter.

Tina D'Andrea, RN, is liable unto your petitioners for her acts and/or omissions and/or breach of contract including, but not limited to:

1. Failure to recognize obvious signs and symptoms of gastrointestinal bleeding;
2. Failure to properly monitor;
3. Failure to timely notify the treating physician of deteriorating condition;
4. Failure to notify the treating physicians of obvious signs of GI bleeding documented in nurses' notes.
5. Failure to timely and properly intervene;
6. Failure to properly assess seriousness of the patient's condition;
7. Failure to properly establish a nursing diagnosis and identify health care needs;
8. Failure on the part of the nursing staff to properly document;
9. Failure to timely and properly evaluate Mrs. Anthony's responses to interventions;
10. Failure of the nursing staff to obtain the care and treatment needed by Mrs. Anthony by going through the chain of command;
11. Failure to report to the treating physician the deteriorating condition and signs and symptoms associated with same;
12. Failure of the staff to timely recommend and perform the appropriate diagnostic tests and consultations;
13. Any and all other acts of negligence which may be proven at the trial of this matter.

VII.

As a result of the actions of James Wrong, MD, Tina D'Andrea, RN, and Safe Medical Center's employees and/or agents and/or independent contractors, Alexes Anthony and Brett Anthony, sustained emotional distress, mental anguish, loss of consortium, funeral expenses, and all other damages that may be determined prior to the trial of this matter.

VIII.

The decedent, Shirley Anthony, suffered severe pain and suffering, emotional distress, mental anguish, past medical expenses, diminution of the enjoyment of life, loss of life expectancy, loss of chance of survival, and premature death.

IX.

Petitioners demand damages as are reasonable in the premises in accordance with Louisiana law; however, they reserve their right to demand a specific dollar amount at the trial of this matter.

X.

The medical review panel rendered an opinion on June 6, 2003. The members of the panel found that the evidence supported the conclusion that James Wrong, MD, Tina D'Andrea, RN, and Safe Medical Center failed to meet the applicable standard of care.

WHEREFORE, Petitioners pray that defendants, Safe Medical Center, Tina D'Andrea. RN, and James Wrong, MD, be served with a copy of this Petition for Damages; that they be required to answer same, and that after due proceedings had, there be judgment herein in favor of petitioners and against defendants, for damages as are reasonable in the premises, interest from date of judicial demand, and for all general and equitable relief.

Respectfully submitted:

Jean Borders (12345)
222 Main Street
New Orleans, LA 93458
(981) 364-2380

Please Serve:

1. Safe Medical Center
   Through their Agent for Service of Process
   Thomas G. Zeringue
   450 Treadway Street
   New Orleans, LA 93528

2. James Wrong, MD
   91111 8th Street
   New Orleans, LA 93821

3. Tina D'Andrea, RN
   4524 Poplar Street
   New Orleans, LA 93821

Appendix B
Sample Fee Agreement and Authority to Represent

I, the undersigned client (hereinafter referred to as "I", "me," or the "Client"), do hereby retain and employ (Attorney's name) and her law firm (hereinafter referred to as "Attorney"), as my Attorney to represent me in connection with the following matter:

_____

_____

1. **ATTORNEY'S FEES.** As compensation for legal services, I agree to pay my Attorney as follows:

Contingency   ____YES   ____NO

(Attorney shall receive the following percentage of the amount recovered before the deduction of costs and expenses as set forth in Section 2 herein)

_____% if settled without suit
_____% in the event suit is filed
_____% in the event a trial actually starts
_____% in the event an appeal is filed by any party

It is understood and agreed that this employment is upon a contingency fee basis, and if no recovery is made, I will not be indebted to my Attorney for any sum whatsoever as Attorney's Fees. (However, I agree to pay all costs and expenses as set forth in Section 2 herein, regardless of whether there is any recovery in this matter. In the event of recovery, costs and expenses shall be paid out of my share of the recovery.)

Hourly Fee—No Advance Deposit   ____YES   ____NO

I agree to pay Attorney's Fees at the rate of $____per hour and paralegal or legal nurse consultant fees at the rate of $____per hour. I agree that time is billed in increments of 10 minutes. Attorney shall provide me with itemized Statements for Professional Services Rendered (including costs and expenses), and I agree to promptly pay each statement. If I fail to pay each statement within ten (10) days of Attorney's request, Attorney shall have, in addition to other rights, the right to withdraw as my Attorney based on my failure substantially to fulfill an obligation to Attorney.

Hourly Fee—With Advance Deposit   ____YES   ____NO

I agree to pay Attorney's Fees at the rate of $____per hour and paralegal or legal nurse consultant fees at the rate of $____per hour. I agree that time is billed in increments of 10 minutes.

It is understood and agreed that I shall pay my Attorney an initial advance deposit of $____due upon Attorney's acceptance of this agreement, which deposit shall be applied toward the payment of attorney's fees and costs and expenses. This deposit shall be deposited into Attorney's trust account and Attorney is authorized to pay Attorney's fees and costs and expenses out of the existing deposit, at least on a monthly basis. Periodically Attorney shall provide me with itemized statements for professional services rendered (including costs and expenses). Should the work performed by my Attorney exceed the amount held in trust, I agree to replenish the advance deposit upon Attorney's request. If I fail to replenish the advance deposit each time it is exhausted within ten (10) days of Attorney's request, or if I neglect to pay Attorney's fees, costs of expenses outstanding within ten (10) days of Attorney's request, I agree that, pursuant to this agreement, Attorney shall have, in addition to other rights, the right to withdraw as my Attorney based on my failure substantially to fulfill an obligation to Attorney.

Flat Fee   ____YES   ____NO

I agree to pay a flat fee of $____

2. **COSTS AND EXPENSES.** In addition to paying Attorney's Fees, I agree to pay all costs and expenses in connection with Attorney's handling of this matter. Costs and expenses shall be billed to me as they are incurred, and I hereby agree to promptly reimburse Attorney. If a retainer is being held by Attorney, I agree to promptly reimburse attorney for any amount in excess of what is being held in retainer. These costs may include (but are not limited to) the following: long distance telephone charges, photocopying ($.25 per page), postage, facsimile costs, Federal Express charges, deposition fees, expert fees, subpoena costs, court costs, sheriff's and service fees, travel expenses, and investigation fees.

Advance required   ____YES   ____NO

I agree to advance $____ for costs and expenses, which amount shall be deposited in Attorney's trust account and shall be applied to costs and expenses as they accrue. Should this advance be exhausted, I agree to replenish the advance promptly upon Attorney's request. If I fail to replenish the advance within ten (10) days of Attorney's request, Attorney shall have, in addition to other rights, the right to withdraw as my Attorney.

3. **INTEREST: ATTORNEY'S FEE FOR ENFORCEMENT.** If any Attorney's fees or costs and expenses are not paid within ten (10) days of Attorney's mailing of statement to me, I agree to pay interest thereafter on any balance due at the rate of twelve (12%) percent per annum. I further agree to pay

the reasonable attorney's fee of any attorney employed by Attorney to seek enforcement of this agreement.

4. **NO GUARANTEE.** I acknowledge that my Attorney has made no promise or guarantee regarding the outcome of my legal matter. In fact, Attorney has advised me that litigation in general is risky, can take a long time, can be very costly and can be very frustrating. I further acknowledge that my Attorney shall have the right to cancel this agreement and withdraw from this matter if, in Attorney's professional opinion, the matter does not have merit, I do not have a reasonably good possibility of recovery, I refuse to follow the recommendations of Attorney, and/or I fail to abide by the terms of this agreement.

5. **STATUTORY ATTORNEY'S FEES.** In the event of recovery under the provisions of the Longshore and Harbor Workers Compensation Act, or under Workman's Compensation laws, or under any other laws which specify attorney's fees to be paid, then the Attorney's fees shall be paid in accordance with the maximum allowed by law.

6. **CONSENT TO SETTLEMENT.** Neither Attorney nor Client may, without the prior written consent of the other, settle, compromise release, discontinue, or otherwise dispose of this matter, claim, or lawsuit.

7. **SOCIAL SECURITY FEES.** In the event of recovery under the provisions of the Social Security Act, whether disability or SSI, then the Attorney's fees shall be paid in the amount of twenty-five (25%) percent or Four Thousand ($4,000.00) Dollars, whichever is less.

8. **PRIVILEGE.** I agree and understand that this contract is intended to and does hereby assign, transfer, set over, and deliver unto attorney as his fee for representation of me in this matter an interest in the claim(s), the proceeds, or any recovery therefrom under the terms and conditions aforesaid, in accordance with the provisions that Attorney shall have the privilege afforded by _____.

9. **ALTERNATIVE DISPUTE RESOLUTION.** In the event of any dispute or disagreement concerning this agreement, I agree to submit to arbitration by the state bar association lawyer dispute resolution program. I further agree that any award by the arbitrator shall include the costs and expenses of arbitration, including attorney's fees actually incurred (if Attorney represents himself, shall record her fees and charges as they would otherwise accrue in the representation of a third party). In the event that I do not comply with the arbitrator's decision and satisfy an award within thirty (30) days of the rendering of a decision and Attorney resorts to judicial enforcement of the award, Attorney shall be entitled to recover as well as ten (10%) percent of the whole amount awarded (plus costs, expenses, and attorney's fees) as a penalty in accordance with [specific state laws inserted].

Note: Parties may also agree to submit to mediation rather than arbitration.

10. **ADDITIONAL TERMS.** Attorney and Client agree to the following additional terms:

_____

_____.

11. **ENTIRE AGREEMENT.** I have read this agreement in its entirety and I agree to and understand the terms and conditions set forth herein. I acknowledge that there are no other terms or oral agreements existing between Attorney and Client. This agreement may not be amended or modified in any way without the prior written consent of Attorney and Client.

This agreement is executed by me, the undersigned Client, on this _____ day of_____, _____(year).

_____

CLIENT

_____

CLIENT

The foregoing agreement is hereby accepted on this _____ day of _____, _____(year).

ATTORNEY _____

Note: This is only one example of an agreement. Agreements vary from state to state and also may vary depending on the specific area of law that is at issue.

Appendix C
Sample Request for Production
of Documents and Things

28TH JUDICIAL DISTRICT COURT
PARISH OF JEFFERSON
STATE OF LOUISIANA

NO. 99-1234   DIVISION "K"

ANDREA NELSON, ET AL
V.
ELIZABETH HOSPITAL, ET AL

Filed:_____   Dy.

Clk._____

REQUEST FOR PRODUCTION OF DOCUMENTS AND THINGS

TO: Ms. Jean D. Briar
      Attorney at Law
      120 N. Telley Street
      New Orleans, LA 70129

      Ms. Diana O. Cradd, IV
      Attorney at Law
      6900 Trains Drive
      New Orleans, LA 70012

General Definition: The term "information" means the originals and any annotated copies of all writings, records, printed, typed or recorded materials, graphic and photographic media, scientific tests, studies or calculations, sound reproductions, and/or computer generated or stored media wherever located which is in your possession or under your control. "Information" includes, but is not limited to, facts, opinions, decisions, discussions, memoranda, and documents. Some nonexclusive examples of the foregoing are: records, correspondence, telegrams, diaries, notes, interoffice and intraoffice communications, memoranda, work papers, manuals, policies, protocols, procedures, guidelines, calendars, telephone records, financial data, plans, specifications, inspection and investigative reports, computer tapes, computer printouts and "hard copies," stenographers' notebooks, corporate charters or articles of incorporation, corporate bylaws, corporate resolutions, corporate minutes, partnership agreements, contracts, agreements, rough drafts, scientific, laboratory, and medical tests and data, including x-rays, and all other writings and papers whether mechanically, electronically, or pictorially recorded similar to any of the foregoing, however designated. If the "information" has been prepared and additional copies have been made that are not identical or are no longer identical by reason of subsequent additions, notations, or other modifications, each nonidentical copy is to be construed as separate "information." If you provide a copy of any information in connection with your responses, give the reason the original is not produced and the name, address, telephone, employer, and position of the person who has custody of or who possesses or controls the original information.

Andrea Nelson, et al, the plaintiffs in the above entitled and numbered cause, request, pursuant to Articles 1461, 1462, and 1463 of the Louisiana Code of Civil Procedure, that each defendant produce at the LAW OFFICES OF ALEX DANDRE, RN, JD, at 10:30 AM, on the 31th day of July, 2003, and permit the plaintiff to inspect and/or copy all information on the following:

1. Any written standards, protocol, guidelines, policies, procedures, and/or directions promulgated, issued, or supplied by Elizabeth Hospital with respect to the care of skin breakdowns for the period of 1998–2003.
2. Any written standards, protocol, guidelines, policies, procedures, and/or directions promulgated, issued, or supplied by Elizabeth Hospital with respect to the use of heel protectors for the period 1998–2003.
3. Any and all materials in the personnel file of Lynn Beam, RN, including but not limited to written reprimands, evaluations, and/or letters regarding the treatment rendered by the nurse, defendant Lynn Beam, RN, found in her personnel file or other appropriate file.

Respectfully submitted:

Alex Dandre RN, JD (98902)
Attorney at Law
902 A.B.C. Building
New Orleans, Louisiana
(981) 555-1111

Appendix D
Sample Interrogatories
and Answers

28TH JUDICIAL DISTRICT COURT
PARISH OF HENDERSON
STATE OF LOUISIANA

NO.   130–138 C/W   DIVISION "L"
      186–699 C/W 422–567
      422–567

Tim and Larry Matthew, individually and on behalf of their son, Kyle Matthew,

versus

Brett Hospital, Ragus Ali, MD, and Alexes Aiken, RN

INTERROGATORIES AND ANSWERS

TO: Ms. Alexes Aken, RN
      Through her Attorney, Elizabeth Jumonville
      1323 State Lane
      Anywhere, USA 12345

INTERROGATORY NO. 1:
Please state the current address, telephone number, current position, and employment held on June 6, 2003, of Alexes Aken, RN.

ANSWER TO INTERROGATORY NO. 1:
Alexes Aken, RN, 207 Lincoln Avenue, Maro, LA 70075;
(501) 835-2500; Brett Hospital Labor and Delivery Unit.

INTERROGATORY NO. 2:
Please provide a description of the testimony to be given by Alexes Aken, RN.

ANSWER TO INTERROGATORY NO. 2:
Factual testimony on the alleged facts of the case, medical records, specifically June 6, 2003 (3-to-11 shift) and the delivery of the Matthews' infant.

INTERROGATORY NO. 3:
If a fact witness will testify, describe what facts will be testified to and how the witness was in a position to know those facts.

ANSWER TO INTERROGATORY NO. 3:

See answer to Interrogatory No. 2. As house supervisor, Ms. Aken was familiar with the daily operation of the Brett Hospital Obstetrical Unit in 2003 and learned of the facts of the case.

INTERROGATORY NO. 4:

If an expert witness will testify at the trial of this matter, please list:

a.   The expert's field in which he or she will testify.
b.   The subject to be testified about specifically related to this lawsuit.
c.   The documents, books, treatise or other information relied upon to render an opinion or in preparation of testimony.
d.   If the expert will testify regarding any standard of care for labor and delivery room nurses or services in 2003, state all information, text, journal, treatises, procedure or documents that (1) were consulted, and (2) were relied upon to form an opinion.
e.   Please list all published writings by any expert who will testify.
f.   Please list expert's educational and work background.

ANSWER TO INTERROGATORY NO. 4:

Jon Anthony Dandre, MD, OB/GYN, Board Certified, will testify as to the alleged breaches of standard of care that occurred during the labor and delivery of the Matthews' infant. See attached resume for educational and work background and publications.

Williams Obstetrics and *Danforth's Obstetrical* texts were consulted. We reserve the right to supplement and amend the answer prior to trial.

Respectfully submitted:

_____

Elizabeth Jumonville, RN, JD (92929)
Attorney for Defendant
1323 State Lane
Anywhere, USA 12345
(981) 555-8888

Note: Forms may be different depending on the state or federal court where the lawsuit has been filed.

Appendix E
Excerpt of a Sample Deposition

CIVIL DISTRICT COURT
PARISH OF LEANDER
STATE OF LOUISIANA

JEAN JACOBS
VERSUS   NUMBER 98-3156
REHABILITATION CENTER LTD., ET AL   DIVISION "K"

DEPOSITION TAKEN AT LAW OFFICES OF BRETT DANDRE, ATTORNEY AT LAW, THREE CENTER 3838 NORTH BLVD., GORGON, LA 98310
REPRESENTING THE DEFENDANTS: LAW OFFICES OF TINA E. BURNS,
ATTORNEYS AT LAW, 3838 NORTH BLVD., GORGON, LA 98310, BY TINA BURNS, ESQ.
Reported by: Shirley Donald, C.S.R., Certified Shorthand Reporter, State of Louisiana

STIPULATION

It is stipulated and agreed by and between counsel that the deposition of
ANDREA KYLE, RN, is hereby being taken under the Louisiana Code of Civil Procedure in accordance with the Code.

The formalities of reading, signing, sealing, and certification are reserved. The party responsible for service of the discovery material shall regain the original.

All objections, except those as to the form of the questions and/or responsiveness of the answers, are reserved until the time of the trial of this case.

ANDREA KYLE, RN, 4351 General Digall, New Orleans, Louisiana, 70118, after having been first duly sworn, testified on her oath as follows:

MR. DANDRE: Ms. Call, my name is Brett Dandre. I represent Mr. Jacobs in this action that he has filed against Rehabilitation Center and Andrea Kyle, RN. I am here to ask you some questions today, and if you don't understand my questions, please tell me and I will try to rephrase it so that you do.

If you do answer my question, then I will assume that you understood it and that you intended to answer it.

Would you please answer verbally and not nod or shake your head so there will be no confusion as the court reporter records it?

THE WITNESS: Okay.

ESTABLISHING A STANDARD OF CARE

Q. You have been a registered nurse for almost 5 years?
A. That is right.

Q. Is it fair to say, Ms. Kyle, that a registered nurse has an obligation to carry out reasonable physician orders?
A. Yes.

Q. The failure to carry out reasonable physician orders would constitute a violation of nursing practice?
A. Yes.

Q. Did you have a doctor's order to take vital signs and to do neuro checks every 15 minutes for 2 hours and then every 30 minutes for 2 hours?
A. Yes.

Q. Did you take Mrs. Smith's vital signs and neuro checks every 15 minutes for 2 hours?
A. No. I took everything two times—at 8:00 AM when she arrived and at 9:00 AM because I was too busy.

Q. Did you fail to follow the doctor's orders?
A. Yes.

Q. Did you violate the Nurse Practice Act by failing to use good nursing judgment?
A. Yes.

Q. What did you discover when you checked on Mrs. Smith at 12 Noon?
A. A blown right pupil and she was having difficulty breathing and hard to arouse.

Q. What did you do?
A. I called the doctor.

Q. What is your understanding of what the doctor found?
A. At 2:00 PM when the treating physician visited the patient, he found a subarachnoid hemorrhage.

Q. If the neuro checks had been performed as ordered, isn't it possible that the signs and symptoms of hemorrhage could have been detected earlier?
A. Yes, they could have been.

Appendix F
Sample Form for Request
for Admission of Facts

28TH JUDICIAL DISTRICT COURT
PARISH OF _____
STATE OF_____

NO. 96-18469   DIVISION "K"

JULIA BINE, ET AL
V.
STATE HOSPITAL

Filed:_____   Dy.

Clk._____

REQUEST FOR ADMISSION OF FACTS

Plaintiffs request that Defendants admit the truth of each of the following facts within fifteen (15) days after receipt of this request. If any of the following is denied, explain why the denial is made.

1. Do you admit or deny that patient, Mr. John Anthony, was admitted on March 1, 2003?
2. Do you admit or deny that signs and symptoms of cerebral edema can be headache, blurred vision, and change in mental status?
3. Do you admit or deny that patient, Mr. John Anthony, had the following signs and symptoms of cerebral edema:
   a. headaches
   b. blurred vision
   c. change in mental status
4. Do you admit or deny that health care providers failed to perform neurological assessments on Mr. John Anthony from 1900 to 2400 hours on March 1, 2003?
5. Do you admit or deny that the staff failed to call or contact Dr. James to discuss the neurological status of Mr. Anthony's condition between 1900 to 2400 hours on March 1, 2003?
6. Do you admit or deny that Mr. Anthony's neurological condition deteriorated between 1900 and 2400 hours on March 1, 2003?

Respectfully submitted:

_____

ELIZABETH A. KENN, RN, JD
(Bar No. 22456)
920 Jefferson Street
Metry, LA 90832
(981) 555-9669

Note: Forms may be different depending on the state or federal court where the lawsuit has been filed.

Appendix G
Sample Subpoena

CIVIL DISTRICT COURT FOR THE PARISH OF ALEXANDRA
STATE OF LOUISIANA

SUBPOENA

No.   DIVISION   Docket No. _____

JANE DOE
VS.
MIKE SMITH

TO: _____

CLERK, CIVIL DISTRICT COURT Please issue a subpoena to the above party as directed below.

SUBPOENA REQUEST

[ ] YOU ARE COMMANDED to appear in the Civil District Court, Parish of Alexandra, in Division _____. 421 Cliff Ave., New Orleans, LA, 70112, on the _____ day of _____, 2003, at _____o'clock ___m., to testify to the truth according to your knowledge, in a controversy pending herein between the parties above named; and hereof you are not to fail under the penalty of the law. By order of the Court.

DEPOSITION SUBPOENA REQUEST

[ ] YOU ARE COMMANDED to appear at the place, date, and time specified below to testify at the taking of a deposition in the above case.

PLACE OF DEPOSITION   DATE AND TIME

REQUEST FOR WRIT OF SUBPOENA DUCES TECUM

[ ] YOU ARE COMMANDED to produce and permit inspection and copying of the following documents or objects for the _____trial, _____deposition, or _____hearing (state type) _____at the place, date, and time specified below (list documents or objects) pursuant to the provisions of article 1334 et seq. of the LA Code of Civil Procedure.

_____

PLACE   DATE AND TIME

_____

Issued at the request of, and
Fees and cost guaranteed by undersigned.

ATTORNEY   _____

                                   Attorney's signature

ATTORNEY'S

NAME & BAR NO.   _____

ADDRESS &   _____

TELEPHONE NUMBER

                                   _____

                                   _____

                                   File original and two copies with Clerk
                                   Fourth copy for Attorney's File
                                   ORIGINAL REQUEST

Note: Forms may be different depending on the state or federal court where the lawsuit has been filed.

TONIA D. AIKEN, RN, BSN, JD

Key Chapter Concepts

Expert witness

General damages

Special damages

Punitive damages

Expert witness report

Chapter Thoughts

As you grow in your professional life, you gain knowledge, experience, and expertise. You may teach or write articles in your specialty, and you may be asked to be an "expert" in a case. Serving as an expert witness in a case can entail a number of different things. For example, a nurse expert may be asked to analyze medical records, to provide an opinion on an opposing expert's opinion, to determine the extent of medical damages suffered, or to provide any number of other services. A number of ethical considerations arise in the course of serving as an expert. Before agreeing to serve as an expert, nurses should clarify the specific area of expertise needed. They should not testify in an area in which they do not feel qualified and should not offer an opinion that they do not truly hold. The expert witness also does not want to be known as a "hired gun" for either plaintiffs or defendants. This title results in an instant loss of credibility and provokes questions about the expert's ethical practices.

OBJECTIVES

Upon completing this chapter, the reader will be able to:
1. Define *expert witness.*
2. Outline the types of damages in a claim.
3. Discuss the qualifications of an expert.
4. Define the "jobs" of an expert witness.
5. Discuss the types of experts.
6. Identify the pertinent sections of an expert report.

Introduction

Nurses are involved in the legal system in numerous ways, not all of them threatening in nature. Many nurses offer their expertise and knowledge to parties from both sides of the legal fence as expert witnesses. This chapter defines the qualifications, responsibilities, and types of expert witnesses and explores the need for nurse experts in malpractice cases.

What Is an Expert Witness?

An **expert witness** is a person who possesses certain qualifications, education, experience, and background in an area such as nursing or medicine and who is usually retained by an attorney, individual, or entity to assist in proving or disproving certain aspects at issue in litigation. Both plaintiffs and defendants use experts.

In medical negligence claims, attorneys routinely retain expert witnesses. In fact, in many cases, expert witness testimony is required in order to prove the standard of care. The expert evaluates documents and products to determine if a standard of care has been breached, and, if so, what damages have been caused by the breach. Expert witnesses in a malpractice suit vary depending on the issues but can include, among others, nurses, physicians, economists, physical therapists, and hospital administrators. For a health care provider to be considered an expert, attorneys consider the following points:

1. Is the health care provider expert currently practicing?
2. If not, is the expert teaching students in the specialty area that is at issue in the lawsuit?
3. Has the expert published journal articles or textbook chapters?
4. Is the expert an officer in professional organizations or associations?
5. Has the expert testified in a deposition or trial?
6. Has the expert testified primarily for plaintiffs or defendants?
7. Has the expert reviewed cases primarily for plaintiffs or defendants?
8. Is the expert considered to be a "hired gun" (one who testifies for a living)?
9. Has the expert been qualified or disqualified as an expert in the appropriate field to testify in the court?
10. Has the expert testified in depositions only or at trial?
11. Is the expert credible?
12. Does the expert have "presence"?
13. Does the expert make a good appearance?
14. Does the expert explain the case in an easily understood manner?
15. Does the expert have an accent that makes him difficult to understand?
16. Does the expert appear comfortable before a judge or jury?
17. Is the expert likable?
18. Can the expert "teach" the judge or jury?

Why Use an Expert?

An expert witness is used to prove issues related to areas of liability, causation, and damages.

BOX 15–1

Areas in which Experts Testify

1. Liability or causation issues (e.g., the cause of patient death)
2. Damage issues
   a. Economic losses (e.g., lost wages)
   b. Future health care and medical treatment needed by the plaintiff

---

Liability and Causation Issues

If it cannot be proven that the defendant committed negligent acts or omissions and that these acts or omissions caused injuries, then it is not necessary to move on to evaluating damages, because the plaintiff has not cleared the first hurdle.

Defense counsel retains experts to prove that the defendants were not negligent and followed the appropriate standards of care. The experts may also determine that even though there was a breach of the standard of care, the patient suffered few if any injuries. For example, Mrs. Flowers receives a laxative that was supposed to be given to Mr. Rose. Although the laxative causes a little discomfort, there are no true damages to Mrs. Flowers.

Evaluating Damages

Damages can be general, special, or punitive. **General damages** are awarded for the plaintiff's pain and suffering caused by the defendant's acts. **Special damages** are based on the actual monetary losses, such as lost wages or medical expenses for the past, present, and future that were caused by the defendant's acts. **Punitive damages** are damages awarded in an amount intended to punish the defendant (or person committing the tort) for the egregious nature of the tort. The defendant's actions must be willful and wanton, and the damages are not based on the plaintiff's actual monetary loss but may be doubled or tripled. Punitive damages may be awarded in some states for malpractice actions depending on state law. Factors considered include the following:

1. Concealment of the act
2. Financial position of the defendant
3. Profitability of the actions of defendant
4. Extent of harm to plaintiff
5. Duration of harm
6. Attitude and conduct of defendant

Experts are also used to prove the extent of the specific damages or injuries sustained by the plaintiff. Damages include physical, emotional/psychological, and economical losses. To establish physical damages and determine their extent, medical specialists may be appropriate. To establish economic issues, parties may retain economists.

Keep in mind, the plaintiff alone does not only suffer losses. The plaintiff's spouse and family also may have claims for damages. For example, if a wife (and mother) dies as a result of the failure to diagnose sepsis, the husband and children can receive damages for their losses. The types of damages alleged for this type of case could include, on the family's behalf, pain and suffering; emotional distress; mental anguish; loss of nurturance; loss of consortium; loss of love and affection; loss of chance of survival; premature death; medical expenses; and past, present, and future lost wages on the decedent's behalf. For types of damages commonly alleged in lawsuits, see Box 15–2.

BOX 15–2

Examples of Types of Damages Commonly Alleged in Lawsuits

Physical Damage

Death
Loss of limb
Disfigurement/scarring
Drop foot syndrome
Blindness
Premature death
Loss of life
Loss of chance of survival

Emotional/Psychological Damages

Fear of contracting a contagious disease
Loss of love and affection
Mental anguish
Emotional distress
Fear of health care providers
Decreased enjoyment of life

Economic Losses

Past, present, and future medical expenses
Pharmacy bills
Physician fees
Facility bills
Loss of past, present, and future earnings
Funeral expenses

A CASE IN POINT

The Facts

A plaintiff was injured when she fell from her hospital bed.[1]

The defendant denied the allegations of the complaint, which included that (1) both rails of the bed were improperly positioned at the time of the fall and (2) the defendants were negligent in the care and supervision of the plaintiff.

The defense was based on the ground that the plaintiff failed to file an expert affidavit supporting a claim of nursing negligence. The defendant filed a motion to dismiss and a motion for summary judgment challenging any claims of negligence and nursing malpractice.

The Court Decides

Based on the facts of the case, there was no evidence regarding specific circumstances of the plaintiff's fall. The court found that issues of material fact remained regarding whether the defendant's employees/agents exercised ordinary care in monitoring the plaintiff at the time of the alleged fall.

The Appellate Court Decides

The Court of Appeals found that the trial court erred in granting the motion to dismiss and motion for summary judgment. The allegation of negligence called into question the proper exercise of the nurse's professional judgment on the placement of the side rails. This calls into play a claim for professional negligence requiring proof by expert testimony rather than the claim for ordinary negligence alleged by the plaintiff.

Because the plaintiff failed to file an expert's affidavit outlining the acts and omissions of professional negligence together with the original complaint, the complaint was dismissed for failure to state a claim.

The Court of Appeals also held that the trial court did not err in refusing to sustain the claim of professional malpractice based on the untimely affidavit included with the amended complaint.

Qualifications of an Expert

The qualifications of an expert vary according to the type of case, the type of expert needed, and the area of the country where the case will be tried. The expert's clinical experience, educational background, professional accomplishments, and presentation (appearance and presence) are all taken into consideration by an attorney when retaining the "right" expert for the case. To establish in court that an expert is qualified to be an expert on a given matter, the attorneys must elicit testimony regarding the expert's relevant education, work experience, clinical experience, professional affiliations, and so on.

Sources of Experts

The best source for experts is in the local health care community. However, it is often difficult to find local experts to testify against local health care providers. Attorneys find experts in the following areas throughout the country:

- Universities
- Teaching facilities
- Authors and editors of textbooks and journal articles
- Expert witness locating companies
- Referrals from other attorneys
- Referrals from other experts
- Malpractice reporters, which list malpractice cases and experts used in the cases
- Professional attorney associations, which have files on experts who have testified in cases
- Internet Web sites and legal research tools

Experts: Tasks and Types

What "Jobs" Will an Expert Be Asked to Do?

Experts may be asked to do a variety of things depending on the needs of the attorney to defend or proceed with a claim or lawsuit. An expert can be asked to do any of the following:

- Determine which records are needed to properly review the case
- Review records
- Render an oral report
- Render a written report
- Determine what other experts are needed for the case
- Define the breaches of the standard of care
- Define the damages
- Outline the elements of negligence: duty, breach of duty, proximate cause, and damages
- Define the economic losses
- Assist in preparing the case for trial or a medical review panel
- Assist in preparing the case for mediation or arbitration
- Assist the attorney in preparing for depositions
- Assist the attorney in preparing discovery (e.g., interrogatories, requests for production of documents, etc.)
- Work with other experts in preparing the case for trial
- Assist in developing and selecting the appropriate visual aids and demonstrative evidence to be used at trial (e.g., medical illustrations)

- Assist the attorney in developing the theme of the case to the jury
- Determine if the claim is defensible
- Determine if the plaintiff has a claim for damages and liability

Materials to Review

Opposing counsel may ask the following questions involving the materials the expert considered in rendering an opinion:

- What materials were reviewed in forming your opinion?
- Did you know there were other materials?
- Did you ask to see them? Why? Why not?
- If yes, what were you told?
- Did you make notes?
- Did you make "good" and "bad" notes?
- Why were your notes perceived to be important by you?
- Do the notes include instructions from counsel regarding pitfalls to be avoided in expressing your opinions?
- Were you not able to form your opinion without counsel's aid?

The attorney may also ask you to read your notes and to attach your resume and any articles used in formulating your opinion.

Materials to Produce: Expert Reports

The **expert witness report** is a written opinion by the expert after review and evaluation of the documents pertinent to the issues in the case. The length of the report varies depending on what the attorney has asked the expert to review and the issues on which he or she should render an opinion for litigation purposes. The following is a suggested outline for expert reports. The report will vary according to what the attorney asks the expert to do.

? | What Would You Do?

You have been retained by defense counsel to review documents and render an expert opinion report in a nursing negligence case. Your evaluation of the documents leads you to believe that certain medical records are missing or have been lost. You contact the defense counsel to discuss the missing records, and he reveals that the nurse administrator destroyed the records at the time of the incident.

What should you do?

1. What are the potential legal implications?
2. What are the potential disciplinary implications?

1. *Start with a concise introductory paragraph.*

"I have been asked to render an opinion regarding the care and treatment received by Todd Waggnor. I reviewed the following records: St. John's Hospital records, Dr. Lucy Weir's office records, autopsy report, and death certificate."

2. *Outline of the facts of the case.*

This section should summarize the contents of all the medical and office records and pertinent documents, such as operating room logs, depositions, statements, interviews, and so on.

3. *Outline and discuss breaches of the standard of care if they exist.*

Reference authoritative texts, national standards, facility policies, and procedures.

4. *Outline and discuss damages caused by the breaches of the standard of care.*

5. *Summarize important points.*

AUTHOR TIP: *Deposition questions about your report may include the following:*

1. *What changes were made in your draft?*
2. *Did the lawyer or anyone suggest changes in your report?*
3. *Did you present the positives and negatives of the case or only one side?*

Remember to remove all "sticky" (Post-it) notes or tabs on medical records. Opposing counsel may ask you to discuss why you found each note of particular significance to mark it.

Types of Experts

Expert needs vary depending on the type of case. The following are some examples of the various types of experts that may be retained by attorneys in litigation:

- Obstetric nurse expert—reports, after reviewing the chart and fetal monitor strip, that the nurse failed to detect signs of fetal distress (e.g., bradycardia, meconium staining) or failed to notify the physician in a timely manner, which caused a delay in delivery, as well as anoxia and brain damage of the infant.
- Emergency medicine physician—testifies that the failure to perform an electrocardiogram (ECG) and laboratory work on a patient with crushing chest pains caused a delay in diagnosis and treatment, resulting in an untimely death of a 44 year old. Such a failure was a breach of the standard of care and a breach of the defendant's duty to the 44 year old.
- Long-term care nurse—testifies that the failure to perform proper skin care, use heel protectors, and rotate the patient from side to side caused decubitus ulcers, which resulted in gangrene of the leg, sepsis, and death.
- Emergency nurse—testifies that the nurse defendants did not breach the standard of care and properly monitored the cardiac patient.
- Economist—determines how much Mrs. Mays would have earned as a financial consultant if she had lived to age 65 instead of age 35 due to her premature death caused by medical negligence at Nunno Hospital.

- Metallurgist—testifies regarding whether the Luque rods and wires placed in Mr. D'Andrea's back were the correct type based on strength, length, metal composition, and use.
- Life planning expert—meets with the patient with a brain injury, her family, and her doctors and develops a plan regarding what types of services will be needed in the future, how much the services will cost, and where can services be obtained.
- Oncologist—reviews the claim and finds that the physician failed to refer the patient in a timely manner to a surgeon for consultation on a lump found, but there are no damages because cancer did not metastasize.

Health Care Specialists

Experts such as rehabilitation experts may be used to show the types of equipment, products, and treatment that the patient will need in the future. For example, if a patient suffers a stroke as a result of medical negligence, the rehabilitation expert visits the patient, family, and patient's home if it is anticipated that the patient will be discharged to the home. The rehabilitation nurse may be a vocational, physical, or occupational expert. Through interviewing and reviewing the medical records, the rehabilitation expert will determine what type of equipment, accommodations, and modifications must be done and the cost for properly caring for the patient.

The list of potential expenses may include the following:

1. Personal care attendant
   a. Home health agency
   b. Family member
2. Nurse—registered nurse (RN) or licensed practical nurse (LPN)
3. Routine medical examinations
4. Probable hospitalizations
5. Medication/supply needs
6. Durable equipment needs
7. Transportation needs
8. Home modifications/barrier removal

Expert Charges

The fees for experts vary depending on qualifications and location. See Box 15–3 for factors affecting charges.

Some experts require a retainer or a certain fee before reviewing the case and then the remainder upon completion of the report. Other experts complete what is requested by the attorney and then bill the attorney. Some experts are retained through a company and are paid by the company, which is then paid by the attorney.

BOX 15–3

Factors Influencing Expert Witness Charges

- Type of expert (e.g., physician, nurse, economist, or physical therapist)
- Level of experience (e.g., education level, status professionally)
- Years of experience
- What the expert is asked to do (e.g., review documents, assist in trial preparation)
- Location

The fees for depositions are usually higher than fees for review of records. Some experts will charge for blocking out a half or full day. Some experts require a guaranteed fee for a blocked out period, although the entire amount of time may not be used. Fees are routinely defined in a contract, retainer offer, or letter of agreement confirming the terms and what is expected of the expert. Experts may also have a contract with the attorney, the expert witness firm, or the consulting firm that located the expert for the attorney.

KEEP IN MIND

▶ An expert witness can be retained to evaluate liability, causation, and damages issues in a malpractice case.

▶ Three types of damages can be alleged in a claim—general, special, and punitive.

▶ Experts qualify to serve as experts based on their education, clinical and work experience, publications, and professional affiliations.

▶ Attorneys retain experts for a variety of tasks, among them record review and analysis, deposition or trial testimony or preparation, and damage evaluation.

▶ A variety of experts can be located from many different sources, including universities, the Internet, local hospitals, and expert services.

IN A NUTSHELL

Nurses, as well as other professionals, have numerous opportunities to be involved in the legal industry in roles other than defendant. They can earn money serving as expert witnesses for both plaintiffs and defendants in malpractice or other health-related cases. As experts, nurses can testify not only regarding the standard of care of a given practice area but also the extent and existence of damages.

AFTERTHOUGHTS

1. Define *expert witness.*
2. Discuss five services or jobs you may be asked to do as an expert.

3. Discuss the fees of an expert. Contact others who are currently retained as experts and do a survey.

4. Pull reported cases and discuss the role of the expert.

5. Create a medical malpractice scenario or use a reported case and write an expert report.

ETHICS IN PRACTICE

In a North Carolina case, a hospital was held negligent for failure of its staff to restock the code cart. The court of appeals held that the breach may have proximately caused the patient's injuries and death. The patient's condition deteriorated, and she was placed in the intensive care unit (ICU), where she coded. She was intubated and placed on a respirator. She stabilized and was extubated. The respiratory therapist could not locate an oxygen mask in ICU and went to the critical care unit (CCU) to obtain one. When he returned to the patient's room, he saw that the patient was not breathing and would have to be reintubated. The patient's heart stopped while being prepped for reintubation, and a second code was called. The respiratory therapist could not intubate the patient because he said he had too short of a blade and needed a number 4 MacIntosh medium, which was not on the cart. The 3-minute delay, during which the patient was deprived of oxygen, caused serious brain injury and ultimately death.

What theories of liability could be alleged? What types of experts would be appropriate in this case? What type of analysis would they perform?[2]

References

1. Smith et al v. North Fulton Medical Center, 408 S.E. 2d 468, 200 Ga. App. 464, June 28, 1991.
2. Dixon v. Taylor, 421 S.E. 2d 778 (NCC 1993).

Resources

Bemis, P: Power Start Your Business with Free Publicity. Cocoa Beach Learning Systems, Cocoa Beach, 2002.

Iyer, P (ed): Nursing Malpractice. Lawyers and Judges Publishing, Tucson, AZ, 2001.

Lindell, C, and Hersh, W: Internet Medical and Health Searching and Sources Guidebook and CD, ed 4. KC Press, Osceola, KS, 2001.

The American Association of Nurse Attorneys
7794 Grow Drive
Pensacola, FL 32514-7072
(850) 474-3636
(850) 484-8762 (Fax)

The American Association of Legal Nurse Consultants
401 N. Michigan Avenue
Chicago, IL 60611
(877) 402-2562
(312) 321-5177
(312) 673-6655 (Fax)

Appendix A
Sample Expert Report

June 6, 2003
Alexes Aikn, RN, JD
Attorney at Law
1200 Brett Drive
New Orleans, LA 98201

Re: Reda, Ruth
File No. 1179

Dear Ms. Aikn

At your request, I have reviewed the following documents:

Complaint, pages 1–6
Deposition of Frank Ain, RN
Incident Report, 10/4/02
Discharge Summary, 10/4/02
Interagency Referral Forms, 10/4/02
Admission History and Physical, 10/2/01
Physician's Standing Order, no date
Initial Evaluation—Problem/Goal Addendum, Nursing, 10/2/02
Daily Activity Record, 2 pages, 10/2/02
Daily Activity Record, 2 pages, 10/2/02
Daily Activity Record, 2 pages, 10/2/02
Neuropsychology Progress Notes, 10/1/02 and 10/2/02
Initial/Re-evaluation, Physical Therapy, 5 pages
Discharge Summary, Physical Therapy
Occupational Therapy General Rehabilitation Evaluation
Initial/Discharge, 4 pages, 10/4/02
Occupational Therapy Daily Attendance Records, 10/2–10/4/02
Speech/Language Pathology Initial/Discharge, 2 pages, 10/4/02
Speech Therapy Daily Attendance Record, page 202, 10/3–10/4/02
Social Service Assessment, 1 page
Rehabilitation Facility's Policy and Procedure: Use of Side Rails

I have been asked to review these records and to determine whether violations of applicable standards of nursing care caused and/or contributed to Mrs. Reda's fall and injuries.

Review and Evaluation of Medical Records

Nursing interventions must be based on assessment and knowledge of the individual patient, as well as the current standards for specific diagnoses and problems. Frank Ain, RN, indicated in his deposition that he had 5 years' experience in rehabilitation at a variety of facilities and that he did receive specialized training in rehabilitation. Mrs. Reda had Parkinson's disease, which is a common enough problem that it would be reasonable to expect that the nurse had knowledge of potential safety risks. Changes in mental status and impaired mobility can both present safety risks in Parkinson's disease.

There is the risk of injury to a patient with a known unsteady gait. The nurse must take all reasonable safety precautions. Side rails are a reasonable safety precaution. Assessment of mental status includes specific questions and testing to determine higher level cognitive functions including reasoning, judgment, and problem solving. The ability to be alert, oriented, and carry on a conversation does not in itself indicate that the person is able to make safe decisions.

Frank Ain, RN, relied on his routine conversations with the patient in making the decision to leave a side rail down. Although it is not documented, Mr. Ain stated in his deposition that he believed it posed less risk to leave the rail down due to the agitation resulting from raised side rails and that the patient was attempting to crawl out of bed. This type of patient behavior should have indicated the presence of safety/judgment issues that were not reasonably assessed prior to removing the safety device of the side rail.

The rehabilitation facility records dated 10/2/02 and 10/3/02 indicate that evaluations by the physical therapist (PT), occupational therapist (OT), and neuropsychologist were in progress. The nurse indicated in the deposition that he was aware that the patient was admitted for strengthening and improving her gait. The presence of these pending evaluations should have indicated to him that further information about mobility and appropriate intervention was forthcoming. Therefore, he should recognize that he did not have a complete assessment independently. Also, the neuropsychology consultation would have provided information about the patient's cognitive status. Again, the nurse should have recognized that the information needed on which to base nursing interventions was not complete for this patient. In his deposition he stated he had no awareness that Parkinson's could also be associated with cognitive deficits. (See Deposition Page 10.)

Rehabilitation facility policy existed regarding use of side rails. Accepted standards of practice require the nurse to be aware of, and comply with, agency policies and procedures. As a supervisor, which Mr. Ain was, this would be especially important, because the supervisory role requires that a nurse facilitate compliance with policies and procedures among those under his supervision. Accredited facilities must be sure that policies and procedures are available and that staff have been oriented to them. The nurse has admitted that he did not follow facility policy in that he did not have the patient sign a release for leaving side rails down, nor did he notify the physician of the patient's request. There is a clear breach of following facility's policy.

He did not perform a mental status exam, nor seek information about the physical or cognitive status from the other disciplines. It is not clear that he was even aware that cognitive problems could be an issue with a patient with Parkinson's. In the absence of complete information about a particular patient, the nurse must rely on general knowledge of a disease/diagnosis, including potential problem areas and safety issues. It would be safest to protect a patient from potential problems, rather than act as if undiscovered problems do not exist, until such time that complete, patient specific information is available and an individualized plan is developed.

The records dated 10/2/02 indicate that other disciplines had evaluations in progress. However, the complete assessments by the PT, OT, and neuropsychologist were not written until 10/4/02 after the fall occurred. The notes of the previous 2 days only indicate that the evaluations were being performed and that the complete report would follow. There is no indication in any of the therapists' notes that they communicated any special concerns or recommended precautions to the nursing staff. Due to the time lag of getting their written reports into the medical record, the therapists should have communicated concerns regarding safety issues to all disciplines. Furthermore, none of the therapy assessments thoroughly addressed mental status.

Damages: As a result of the fall, Mrs. Reda suffered a fractured hip and wrist, subdural hematoma, and death.

Conclusions, Summary of Important Points

Frank Ain, RN, violated applicable standards of nursing practice, which contributed to Mrs. Reda's fall and injuries.

First, Frank Ain, RN, failed to follow reasonable physicians' orders to keep the side rails elevated.

Second, Frank Ain, RN, failed to follow hospital policy concerning the use of side rails.

Third, Frank Ain, RN, made unreasonable errors in nursing judgment that demonstrated the failure to assess both the physical and mental status of the patient.

Finally, the rehabilitation facility failed to have adequate communication procedures in effect, which would require safety concerns of other disciplines from being communicated to the nursing staff.

Respectfully submitted,

Julia Green, RN, CRRN

Enclosures: Excerpt from *Textbook of Neurological Nursing*

Appendix B

SAMPLE EXPERT WITNESS CONTRACT

Professional Services and Fee Schedule Agreement

Charges:
Charges are made in $1/4$-hour increments and include time spent for clients during office consultation, review of medical records and other material research, preparation of reports, telephone consultations, testifying at depositions, hearings and trials, and travel time to and from the office. The expert cannot predict or guarantee total fees. Billing will depend on the amount of time spent on the case and other expenses.

Fees:
• The expert's time to review case materials, preparation for deposition, hearings, arbitration and/or trial, office consultation, travel time.. $175/hr.

• The expert's time for testifying at deposition.................... $175/hr.

• The expert's fee for testifying at hearing, arbitrations, or trial (minimum 6 hours, plus preparation and travel time)............ $175/hr.

• PowerPoint presentation layout.................... $100/hr.

Rates are subject to change. Charges are based upon the prevailing fee schedule when the work is performed.

Payment of Testifying Fees:
Payment of the court appearance fee is due in full seven days prior to the trial appearance date. Any balance owed will be billed following the trial. Payment of any remaining unpaid invoices and expenses, plus the court appearance fee, is to be received in full seven days prior to the expert's court appearance. An invoice for court appearance expenses (such as mileage, parking, and meals) will be sent following the appearance at the trial. In the event that the case settles before the expert leaves for court, the testifying fee will be refunded.

Invoices:
Invoices will be sent periodically to clients, and are due immediately upon receipt. Failure to make payment of invoices shall constitute a default of our agreement. Any questions pertaining to the billing must be put in writing and postmarked no more than ten business days after the date of such billing, after which time the billing will be considered correct and payable as filled. Outstanding balances over thirty (30) days are subject to an interest charge of 1.5% per month each month until paid. The expert, without liability, may withhold delivery of reports, and may suspend performance of his/her obligation to a client pending full payment of all charges.

Retainers:
For all matters, a $1050 retainer fee and a signed fee schedule and/or a retaining letter if required. Our receipt of medical records and retainer signifies acceptance by the client of this agreement. Billing will be charged against the retainer. It should be noted that _____ _____ reserves the right at his/her discretion, to require a retainer from its clients for any anticipated or requested work beyond the work covered by the initial $1050 retainer fee. Please make check payable to _____. My tax identification number is _____.

Responsibility for Payment:
Billing is not contingent upon the findings and/or conclusions reached. Responsibility for payment is that of the client (law firm/insurance company) engaging the expert's services and is not contingent upon client's contractual agreement(s) with plaintiff/defendant and/or case status. The client is responsible for paying the fees even if the outcome of the case is not favorable. As a convenience, we may agree to prepare separate invoices for testifying at a deposition. Responsibility for payment of any fees associated with the deposition remains that of the client. Responsibility for the notification of settlement of a matter is that of the engaging client. All charges incurred to the time of notification of settlement of a matter is that of the engaging client. All charges incurred to the time of notification will be billed. Lack of notification will not obviate charges incurred even when disbursement related to this matter have been made. Failure to include a billable item in an invoice shall not constitute a waiver of the right to add the charge to a subsequent billing.
In the event that it becomes necessary for _____ to retain an attorney or collection agency for collecting outstanding fees or any other breach of this agreement, the client agrees to pay _____'s reasonable attorney fees and costs incurred in enforcing her rights under this agreement. A 30% surcharge will be added to the outstanding balance if a collection agency becomes involved in the collection process.

Expenses: Including, but not limited to:
• Travel: Automobile expenses are billed at $0.40 per mile, plus tolls and parking charges. Airfare, train fare, lodging, etc. are to be paid in full seven days in advance. Meals are billed as incurred, when time away from office exceeds our hours.
• Telephone, Document Reproduction, Supplies and Delivery Costs (Federal Express, courier and other expenses): as incurred.

Modifications to the Agreement:
All modifications must be agreed to and confirmed in writing.

I have read the Expert Witness Professional Services and Fee Schedule Agreement. I understand and agree to the terms contained therein.

Case Name: _____

Date: _____   Signed: _____

Law Firm: _____

Please sign this page and return the original agreement to _____

after copying for your files.

(Reprinted with the permission of Patrica Iyer, Med League Support Services, Inc.)

Professional Liability Insurance   16

Key Chapter Concepts

Insurance policy
Occurrence basis policy
Claims-made policy
Tail insuring agreement
Liability policy
Insuring agreement
Specific performance lawsuit

Injunctive relief action
Exclusions
Reservation of rights
Named insured
Policy's limit of liability
Indemnification
Disciplinary defense insurance

Chapter Thoughts

From a historical viewpoint, litigation against health care providers is a very recent development. During the 1940s and World War II, in particular, health care made major strides in the use of antibiotics, psychotropic medications, surgery, and life-support equipment. Since then, health care has become technically sophisticated with ever-increasing success in the cure of serious diseases, treatment of critical injuries, and prolonging of life by medical and nursing interventions. With the advances in medical technology, nursing has become a skill-oriented practice working to enhance the life-saving efforts of medicine.

Unfortunately, as nursing and health care have become more dependent on technology, the treatment of patients has become less personalized. The public has begun to perceive the health sciences as infallible and health care as a person-to-institution relationship. These patients no longer feel the traditional close personal relationship between them and the health care providers. They expect successful treatment without adverse effects in all encounters. They have become more inclined to use litigation as a means of retribution for harm resulting from health care treatments, medications, or surgery.

During the 1970s the malpractice crisis exploded, and health care providers at all levels began to recognize the vast scope of potential lawsuits that could be filed against them. A medical malpractice lawsuit could be filed by any patient at almost any time. During the crisis, liability insurance rates skyrocketed, carriers stopped insuring, and many physicians couldn't afford insurance. As a result of the crisis, states passed tort reform legislation. Limits on noneconomic or total damages were imposed. Occurrence basis insurance policies were replaced by claims-made coverage.[1] On the other hand, attorneys became more aggressive in pursuing medical malpractice cases against health care providers because the attorney's fees could be very large. Because physicians were the most common early targets of malpractice lawsuits, they quickly recognized the need to increase their liability coverage under their existing malpractice insurance. Nurses, however, were much slower to acquire malpractice coverage, perhaps because lawsuits against them were much less common and it was difficult to find insurance companies that would issue malpractice policies to nurses. Even today, nurses vacillate between acquiring and not acquiring individual malpractice coverage. Most nurses are covered to some degree by their employer's insurance policy (when working as an employee), but these policies have as the primary goal protection of the employer, not the nurse.

In a perfect world, where no mistakes are ever made, where every treatment is successful, where medications have no side effects, and where every patient is physiologically the same, there would be no need for malpractice insurance. In the real world, nurses deal with increasingly complicated technology, as well as patients who are older and more critically ill, and things sometimes go wrong. The ethical principle of accountability is one of the key elements in the establishment of a profession. Nurses must be responsible for their actions as professionals, including actions that are sometimes in error. In accepting responsibility for their actions, nurses acknowledge the fact that they do make mistakes. In the litigious atmosphere of today's society, it would seem logical for malpractice insurance to be as much a requirement of nursing practice as uniforms, an automobile, a telephone, and a nursing license. If for no other reason, malpractice insurance covers the cost of defending a malpractice claim. Often the cost of the defense alone, regardless of the outcome of the case, is sufficient to destroy a nurse financially.

OBJECTIVES

Upon completing this chapter, the reader will be able to:
1. Discuss the types of insurance policies available to professional nurses.
2. Discuss whether a specific policy matches an individual nurse's practice needs.
3. Define the issues that should be considered when deciding between employer-sponsored coverage and individual policy coverage.
4. Discuss reasons for having individual malpractice coverage.
5. Discuss the sections of an insurance policy.
6. Define *disciplinary defense insurance.*

Introduction

Nurses can no longer afford to be without liability insurance. However, the kinds of decisions that must be made—whether to purchase an individual or an institutional policy, an occurrence basis or a claims-made policy—can make the selection process confusing. This chapter looks at the issues nurses should consider when choosing a policy, to ensure they have the type of coverage that will best protect them if they should be sued. From a more practical perspective, the chapter offers guidance on how to read and understand the insurance policies nurses may purchase. Box 16–1 provides an overview of the contents of an insurance agreement.

Should Nurses Have Insurance?

Opinions on whether or not to purchase personal malpractice insurance vary, some attorneys recommend that nurses have their own insurance, whereas others believe the nurse is protected under the facility's policy. The nurse will be covered under the facility's policy *if* the nurse is working for the facility at the time of the alleged act of malpractice as an employee.

However, there are circumstances when a nurse will not be covered by the facility's insurance policy. For example:

1. Volunteer Work: If the nurse volunteers to do services outside the course and scope of employment and commits malpractice, the facility will not cover the nurse.

BOX 16–1

Professional Liability Policy Sections

1. TYPE OF POLICY: Claims-made or occurrence basis.
2. PRIOR ACTS COVERAGE: Generally, prior acts are not covered by claims-made policies, but coverage can be purchased for an additional premium.
3. DECLARATIONS PAGE OR "DEC PAGE": Lists the name of the individuals or the institution, along with the total, or "aggregate," amount paid during the policy period. For example, if you see on an application "$1M/$3M," this means per incident up to $1 million will be paid and per policy period up to $3 million.
4. POLICY PROVISIONS: Insuring agreement between the insurer and insured describes the type of claims (e.g., damages due to injury) the insurer must pay and under what conditions (e.g., due to negligence in the form of acts or omissions of the insured, the nurse).
5. EXCLUSIONS: Discusses in detail circumstances not covered by the policy.
6. DUTIES OF THE INSURED: Outlines the duties of the insured (nurse), such as cooperation and notification (possibly in writing) if a claim is filed. Cooperation includes assisting in the defense of the trial in the form of securing witnesses and evidence.

(continued)

BOX 16-1

Professional Liability Policy Sections *(continued)*

7. DEFINITIONS: Insurance terms are defined and words that must be interpreted by the court (e.g., "medical incidents" or "injury") are specified.
8. NONRENEWAL OR CANCELLATION: Describes conditions or circumstances under which the insurer can cancel or decline to renew the policy.
9. RIGHT TO DEFEND OR SETTLE: States it is the duty of the insurer to defend even if it is a frivolous claim. This section may also discuss the right of the insurer to settle a claim without the approval or consent of the insured.
10. OTHER INSURANCE: Discusses how the judgment of a claim is affected and how payment priorities stand if more than one insurance company is involved.
11. PREMIUM PAYMENTS: States that premiums are payable when due. The cost of the policy varies depending on the nursing specialty. Most policies are under $100.
12. EXPENSES OF DEFENDING CLAIMS: Discusses whether or not expenses for the defense of the claim are included in the limits of liability or paid above whatever the plaintiff receives.
13. ENDORSEMENTS: Discusses added provisions or "riders" that are not part of the standard provisions (policy jacket) of the policy.

Some insurance policy applications ask the applicant to contact the company for more information on the states who have Patient Compensation Funds and the "surcharge" for the secondary layer of insurance.

---

2. At Home: If the nurse administers treatment (e.g., an injection) to a friend or neighbor and causes damage (e.g., sciatic nerve injury), the facility's policy will not cover the nurse.
3. Good Samaritan Acts: In most states where there is a statute that covers individuals under Good Samaritan situations, if the nurse is, for example, grossly or willfully and wantonly negligent, the nurse may not have the protection of the act and also will not be covered under the facility's policy.
4. Indemnification: If a nurse is sued for malpractice and the facility must pay for damages caused by the nurse's actions or inaction, the facility may sue to be indemnified or paid back.
5. Acts Not Covered: Certain acts by any employee may not be covered under the employer's policy (e.g., a patient hears a defamatory statement made about him by a nurse in the facility).

6. Merger of Facility: If a merger occurs, the new employer's policy may not cover incidents prior to the merger.

7. Policy Limits Exceeded: If the employer's policy limits are exceeded because of the severity of the damages or multiple acts of negligence, the employee may have to pay for all or part of his or her malpractice defense.

8. Acting Outside the Scope of Employment or Nurse Practice Act: If it is determined that the nurse acted outside the scope of employment or the nurse practice act, the employer could refuse coverage of the nurse. Also, conflicts can arise in defense strategy and settlement where the nurse's defense and wishes are not priority in comparison with those of the physician and facility.

9. Cost: The cost of the policy is relatively inexpensive compared with the services you receive, and it is a tax-deductible business expense.

10. Peace of Mind: You get an attorney assigned to your case who is looking out for you. Also, you prevent the loss of your personal assets by having insurance that can pay for damages if you are found negligent.

AUTHOR TIP: *Nurses must check the laws to see if their state has a prelitigation panel requirement in medical malpractice claims and a statutory cap on damages. In some states, the institution or the nurse must pay a second premium to be covered under this secondary layer of insurance afforded in their state under what is called in some states the Patient's Compensation Fund. (Check your state laws.)*

In some states, only a capped amount can be paid by your insurance company, an amount that is determined by law, and the remainder of the damage award or settlement is paid by the state's Patient's Compensation Fund. However, in some states, in order to have the right to the cap on plaintiff's damages, the insured must pay an insurance premium to the company and then a secondary premium or "surcharge" for the Patient's Compensation Fund. Also, most facilities, their employees, and their physicians pay the surcharge for the coverage or may be covered by the facility's surcharge payment.

Types of Insurance Policies

The **insurance policy** is an agreement between the insured and the insurance company stating that, in exchange for a premium, the company will pay money in the form of a settlement or award when certain injuries are caused by the person insured by the policy. There are two types of policies to consider when researching professional liability insurance.

The two types of liability insurance policies are occurrence basis policies and claims-made policies. An **occurrence basis policy** covers injuries that occur during the period in which the policy is in effect, which is known as the policy period. Occurrence policies are recommended because once the coverage is in place, the nurse is insured regardless of when a lawsuit is brought or whether or not the policy has been renewed.

BOX 16–2

What to Look for in an Insurance Policy

1. Type of insurance policy
   a. Claims-made
   b. Occurrence basis
2. The insuring agreement
   a. Types of injuries covered
   b. Exclusions
   c. Who is covered
   d. Limits of policy and deductibles
   e. Financial strength of the insurance company
   f. Legal dispute coverage
3. Right to select counsel
4. Right to consent to settlement or trial of suit
5. Cost of policy
6. Disciplinary action coverage as part of the policy or as a rider

---

On the other hand, a **claims-made policy** is in effect only if the injury occurs within the policy period and the claim is reported to the insurance company either during that policy period or during an uninterrupted extension of that policy period (the tail). A **tail insuring agreement** provides coverage for periods when the nurse is exposed to certain professional liabilities but no longer has a claims-made policy in force. For example, if a nurse leaves the practice of nursing in 2003 and has a claims-made policy, a tail should be purchased to cover the possible lawsuits that could be filed for acts of negligence that occurred in 2003 or before. If the nurse has a claims-made policy, continuous coverage in the form of a tail must be maintained to ensure that protection will be available if a claim is made in the future.

Claims-Made or Occurrence?

Nurses practicing in such "long-tail" specialties as labor and delivery or pediatrics (where there may be a long period between an injury and an assertion of a claim) need occurrence coverage or the continuous renewal of a claims-made policy. Influencing this long tail period may be the length of the statute of limitations in the state. For example, if a nurse practices in a state in which the statute of limitations is tolled (suspended) for minors, then lawsuits may be filed on behalf of a child until the child reaches the age of majority.[2]

Occurrence coverage is rarely made available to facilities, so facilities typically carry claims-made policies as their institutional coverage. This practice can present difficulties for the nurse who relies solely on an employer-sponsored institutional liability policy. The institution can cancel the claims-made policy without buying the tail. That leaves no coverage for claims asserted after the policy is canceled, even for incidents that occur while the policy is in force. If the nurse is involved in one of those incidents, the institution's responsibility or even financial ability to defend him or her and pay for the injury can become a serious issue. The nurse being sued could have to pay for the defense of the suit or for the money judgment awarded to the plaintiff.

Occurrence basis policies are available to individual professionals. Group policies that cover partnerships and professional corporations may also be available on an occurrence basis.

The Insuring Agreement

A **liability policy** is a written agreement between the health care provider and the insurance company. The insurance company agrees to pay compensation to a person for injuries caused either by an act of omission or commission by the insured health care provider. The insurance company's promise to pay in exchange for premiums is called an **insuring agreement.**

In nursing liability policies, the insuring agreement takes one of two forms:

1. Form A:

   The Company will pay on behalf of the Insured all sums which the Insured shall become legally obligated to pay as damages because of injury to a patient or client to which this insurance applies, caused by a medical incident which occurs during the policy period.[3]

2. Form B:

   The Company will pay on behalf of the Individual Insured all sums which the Insured shall become legally obligated to pay as damages because of injury arising out of the rendering of or failure to render professional services during the policy period by the Insured, or by any person for whose acts or omissions such Insured is legally responsible.[4]

Form A is limited because it covers only injuries to identifiable patients and only those injuries resulting from identifiable medical incidents. The coverage is limited to a narrow set of nursing activities: hands-on clinical care. Form B broadly covers injury to anyone in the scope of professional services.

When choosing a policy, several factors need to be considered, such as the types of injuries covered, exclusions, policy coverage, limits of liability, financial strength of the insurance company, legal dispute coverage, right to settlement on trial, cost of policy, and inclusion of disciplinary defense costs.

Types of Injuries Covered

In addition to covering specified acts, both insuring agreements refer to certain injuries. The language is both broad and limiting. In both instances, compensable injury is not defined and is broad enough to include all types of injury: bodily injury, mental anguish, property damage, and economic injury. However, the insurance company will pay only if the insured nurse is sued for damages, which means money.

The "damages-only" limitation becomes critical if the sole objective of the lawsuit is to force the nurse to do or avoid doing a certain act. This type of suit is called a **specific performance lawsuit** or **injunctive relief action.** An example would be a doctor suing a nurse to stop the "unlawful practice of medicine." The nurse's insurance policy with either of the insuring agreements (form A or B) would not kick in until a claim for monetary damages is also asserted.

Professional nursing associations, which support the expansion of nursing practice and sponsor insurance policies to ensure that their members are protected, should be aware of the limitations. They should also consider how to ensure that defense funds are available for the insured if an injunctive relief action that is excluded by an association-sponsored damages-only policy is brought against a member.

Exclusions

Items not covered by a policy are called **exclusions.** If an alleged activity or circumstance is excluded, then the insurance company may take the position that the nurse's defense costs will not be paid if it is determined that the excluded activity occurred. This insurance company's position is called a **reservation of rights,** because the company reserves the right to deny coverage once the facts are determined.

If it is ultimately determined that there is an excluded activity, then the insured must reimburse the insurance company for the defense costs. Other companies will expect the nurse to pay the bills and costs of litigation until the alleged activity is proved not to be excluded.

There are some professional liability policies that have added an exclusion for the transmission of acquired immunodeficiency syndrome (AIDS) from provider to patient. Of equal concern are exclusions for claims arising out of the following:

1. Sexual abuse of a patient
2. Injury caused while under the influence of drugs or alcohol
3. Criminal activity
4. Punitive damages (damages awarded to punish the defendant for egregious acts or omissions)

More subtle are exclusions resulting from the very nature of the insurance policy: Is it written to cover institutional or individual nursing liability?

AUTHOR TIP: *The broadest coverage available is provided by an individual liability policy in which only acts beyond the scope of nursing practice are excluded. Resolution of a dispute over the definition of the scope of nursing practice may require testimony to determine whether the acts alleged are taught as part of a nursing curriculum and therefore nursing practice. As long as the allegations are found to be within the scope of nursing practice, and not otherwise excluded, the individual nursing professional liability policy covers the nurse. Naturally, all practices taught as part of a nursing curriculum should be considered within the scope of nursing practice. Institutional liability policies offer less protection for the nurse; they exclude acts beyond the nurse's scope of employment.*

It is possible for an act to fall within the definition of nursing practice yet still be prohibited by an institution. For example, an institution could prohibit nurses from administering certain medications intravenously.

For an institutional policy to cover an alleged act, it must meet the following two criteria:

1. The act is not excluded as beyond the scope of nursing practice.
2. The act is not excluded as beyond the scope of employment as defined in a specific institution.

Policy Coverage

The party who purchases a professional liability policy is always covered by it. The purchaser is the **named insured,** who can be an individual, an institution, or a group.

In addition to the purchaser, who else is covered by the policy?

1. On an individual policy, the individual nurse's employees or agents may be covered.
2. On an institutional liability policy, usually employees and volunteers, perhaps even consultants to the organization, are covered.
3. On a group policy, a group of similarly licensed professionals and the business corporation that that group of professionals commonly owns are covered. Whether other types of professionals can be added, even as employees of the master policy owners, is a case-by-case inquiry.[5] These policies require the most scrutiny by a nurse employed by a group to ensure that coverage is extended to the nurse as an employee. The nurse employee who is evaluating coverage under an employer-sponsored program (group or institution) can request that the employer show a certificate of insurance that explicitly states that employees are covered as "insureds."

   Note that all three types of policies can be endorsed to cover not only "insureds" but "former insureds for acts committed while insureds." This can be verified with the institution so that the employee who leaves the facility's employment can continue to be covered by the former employer's in-force insurance program.

Limits of Liability

In exchange for premiums, the insurance company agrees to pay up to a certain amount on behalf of an insured. This amount is called the **policy's limit of liability.** The policy limit is always expressed in two ways:

1. The amount that can be paid for one incident (the per incident or per occurrence limit)
2. The amount that can be paid in any one policy year (the aggregate limit)

The better policy is one that provides defense costs in addition to its limit of liability because then more funds are available to pay for a plaintiff's loss and damages.

Financial Strength of the Insurance Company

Beyond the specific terms of the insurance policy, it is important to evaluate the financial ability of the designated insurance company to pay claims when they are due. This is important for any long-tail type of exposure, because there are usually a number of years between the time of the occurrence and the time the claim is paid—and a thinly capitalized carrier could go under in the meantime. Just as creditworthiness of business corporations is evaluated by firms such as Moody's and Standard and Poor's, the insurance industry relies on a firm named A. M. Best to evaluate both the financial size and the financial strength of insurance companies in the United States. An A. M. Best rating of A– or better should be a prerequisite for purchase of any insurance policy. This rating is even more important for a nursing liability policy where claims may not be made for many years. Annual editions of A. M. Best can be found in public and business libraries.

Legal Dispute Coverage

Right to Select Counsel

Some insurance companies allow nurses to select their own counsel to represent them in a medical negligence claim. Otherwise their case is referred to a law firm or attorney previously retained by the insurance company. If this is important to nurses, they should ask specifically who determines the law firm or attorney that will represent them.

Right to Consent to Settlement or Trial

Some policies allow the nurse to refuse to settle a claim, whereas other policies do not permit this decision to be made by the nurse. Therefore nurses should ask who has the right to decide if the case is settled or goes to trial.

Cost of Policy

The cost of a policy varies according to the company selling the policy and the specialty of the nurse. Many policies are less than $100.00.

Determining the Type of Professional Liability Insurance to Have

A nurse may be covered by a policy as an individual, as an employee under an institution-owned policy, or as a member of a group (e.g., CRNA and Associates, a nurse-owned corporation; Box 16–3). Determining which policy to use requires consideration of several factors. Even if coverage does indeed exist under an employer-sponsored insurance program, it is important to determine whether to rely on the employer-sponsored insurance as the sole source of protection.

In a brochure titled "Demonstrating Financial Responsibility for Nursing Practice,"[6] The American Association of Nurse Attorneys, Inc. (TAANA), states:

A. All professional nurses engaged in the practice of nursing should be insured against liabilities to third parties arising out of their professional practice.
B. The means by which a nursing professional elects to insure professional practice should be based on an informed decision.

When making a decision on the type of insurance coverage, consider individual exposure and type of clinical practice (Box 16–4).

Evaluating Individual Exposure

TAANA, along with others,[7] point to a number of important issues that should be considered when making a decision on purchasing insurance:

1. *Will the employer seek* **indemnification** *(a monetary contribution) from a nurse employee whose professional services cause losses beyond the employer's insurance policy limits or within the employer's deductible?*

BOX 16–3

The Three Types of Insurance Policies Ownership That Cover a Nurse's Professional Exposure

1. Individual liability policy
2. Institutional liability policy
3. Group liability policy

Keep in mind that individual policies offer nurses the broadest coverage. These policies offer 24-hour coverage so long as the nurse's acts fall within the scope of nursing practice.

BOX 16–4

Is an Individual Policy Best?

1. There is a belief that the availability of individual insurance converts a nurse into another "deep pocket" and makes the nurse more vulnerable to a lawsuit. However, there is no national central data bank that has information regarding the insurance status of nurses, so potential plaintiffs have no way of knowing what type of coverage a nurse has.
2. A separate insurance policy means separate legal representation for the nurse. Some argue that this may make a joint defense with the employer more difficult and perhaps more costly. Others argue it may be in the nurse's best interest because one attorney representing the hospital, physician, and nurse may be a conflict of interest.
3. There is the question of how multiple insurance policies respond to the same nursing incident. When both the employer and the nurse purchase commercial policies, which policy pays first depends on each policy's "other insurance" language.

The policy should specify how that insurance coordinates with other collectible insurance for the same loss. The most likely result is a pro-rata (even split) contribution by the available policies; however, there can be situations where the nurse's individual policy is required to pay first.[8]

When the employer is self-insured, the results differ because self-insurance is not considered "other insurance" for purposes of payment priority. The nurse's policy pays first, to the extent of the employer's self-insured deductible.[9]

The optimistic answer to this question is that the employer who faces a nursing shortage, or even one who is interested in maintaining good employee relations, will not seek indemnification from the nurse as long as the nurse acted within his or her scope of employment. There is little reported case law on this subject, which may be a good sign. Also, the unstable economic environment facing all facilities today may lead a board of trustees to conclude that the best business decision is to seek indemnification from a nurse employee (or, more likely, a former employee) rather than face financial catastrophe. It is up to the individual nurse to assess both the economic climate and the quality of the employer-employee relationship in evaluating this issue. However, this issue alone should not determine the nurse's choice of coverage.

2. *Does the nurse practice outside the primary employment setting?*

At best the institutional liability policy covers the nurse only for activities conducted while employed at that institution. If the nurse engages in private duty nursing, independent consulting, or voluntary service or determines that his or her nursing activity is controlled by more than one "master," or employer, the nurse should consider an individual liability policy. An individual policy provides the nurse with 24-hour protection regardless of job description and setting.

In an attempt at tort reform, some states have sought to limit the economic liability of any one defendant. The result, ironically, could be more nurses being named as individual defendants in lawsuits, because the more defendants in the suit, the more money to potentially tap. As the individual nurse's exposure increases, so does the need for individual liability protection.

Area of Clinical Practice

Professional liability has long-tail exposure—it may be a long time between when an incident occurs and a claim is made. The purchase of individual liability policies is particularly advisable for obstetric and pediatric nurses, who, depending on state statutes, may be at risk for lawsuits until a child reaches 21 years old. These policies are also recommended for nurses who practice in what the insurance industry views as areas with a high risk of severe injury. These high-risk areas include the operating room, emergency room, critical care areas, and home health care.

Professional Reasons to Choose an Individual Policy

When evaluating individual benefits, consider the fact that the purchase of an individual nursing liability policy acknowledges the nurse's responsibility for individual actions as a professional. Purchasing individual coverage reinforces the concept of individual responsibility. Physicians purchase individual policies because they expect to take responsibility for their professional services. Nurses must also demonstrate individual responsibility for their professional services, both financially and otherwise.

Moreover, the purchase of an individual nursing liability policy contributes to the establishment of nurse-specific claim data, which ultimately can be pooled for the development of credible nursing liability loss information. Some nurses rely on employer-sponsored insurance policies that do not identify nursing losses separately. The result can be higher premiums for nursing liability insurance. The reason for the higher premiums is that premiums are set by insurance carriers based on their perceptions of risk. The absence of credible nursing lawsuit information contributes to carriers' unacceptable conclusion that specialty nurses should pay the same rates as groups with worse, but documented, loss experience. If nurses cannot document their lawsuit experience, it is not possible to demonstrate that nursing is less risky as a profession or as a practice specialty within the profession. Questions such as "Are nurse practitioners safer than physician assistants or family practice physicians?" and "Are nurse midwives suffering because of the loss experience of obstetricians?" cannot be answered.

An informed decision whether to rely solely on an employer-sponsored policy should weigh the cost of the individual policy against the benefits that a separate liability policy confers on the nurse individually and on the nursing profession generally.

Individual policies may allow nurses more opportunity to select their attorneys and offer nurses more control in their own defense. Professional liability insurance policies are usually written so that the named insured has the right to a defense attorney. The attorney is hired by the insurance company but represents the named insured. When the nurse is not the purchaser and not the named insured of the policy, there may be reluctance on the part of the insurance company to supply the nurse defendant with counsel of his or her own. There can be situations in which the employee and the employer conflict in their defense. By not having his or her own lawyer, a nurse's interests can become secondary to the named insured who purchased the insurance policy.

Another benefit of purchasing an individual liability policy is ensuring that the state-by-state battles to broaden nurse practice acts are not in vain. Written broadly to protect the nurse for any professional service deemed to be within the scope of nursing practice, the individual liability policy best enables nursing professionals to reap the benefits of what they sow from lobbying efforts to broaden state nurse practice acts. Simply put, these policies cover more nursing activities and define nursing practice more broadly to provide greater coverage.

Before purchasing a policy, see Box 16–5 for items to consider.

Disciplinary Defense Insurance

Many facilities provide professional liability insurance policies for legal fees and expenses that you can incur if you are found to be negligent in a malpractice case. If you must defend your nursing license in an administrative proceeding, **disciplinary defense insurance** can provide for such things as the following:

1. Legal fee reimbursement or payment to the attorney
2. Wage loss reimbursement
3. Travel, food, and lodging reimbursement
4. Qualified nurse attorneys or attorneys to represent you

Check with your insurance company to see if disciplinary defense insurance is offered. The cost may be included in your premium for your professional liability policy or may be an additional rider or separate policy cost.

KEEP IN MIND

▶ An insurance policy is an agreement by the insurance company that states that, in exchange for a premium, the company will pay money when the person insured by the policy causes certain injuries.

▶ Occurrence basis policies are preferable to claims-made policies and are available to individual professionals.

▶ Individual professional liability policies are broader than employer-sponsored policies.

▶ Not all individual professional liability policies are equally broad. Look for

---

BOX 16–5

Nursing Liability Policy Checklist

Before purchasing an individual nursing liability policy, answer the following questions:

1. Named insured?
2. Coverage provided for others in addition to the named insured?
   a. Employees or agents?
   b. Volunteers?
   c. Consultants?
   d. Former insureds?
3. Occurrence basis or claims-made?
4. Scope of professional activities covered?
5. Policy limits?
   a. Per incident?
   b. Per policy year?
   c. Defense costs paid in addition to policy limits?
6. Deductible?
7. Exclusions?
   a. Sexual abuse?
   b. Under influence of drugs or alcohol?
   c. Criminal acts?
   d. Claims not seeking money?
   e. Punitive damages?
8. Authority to settle?
   a. With consent of insured?
   b. Without consent of insured?
9. If claims-made,
   a. Number of years tail continues?
   b. Cost of tail?
10. Financial strength of insurance carrier according to A. M. Best?

---

policies that cover injuries resulting from your "professional services," not from a "medical incident."

▶ An informed decision on whether to rely solely on an employer-sponsored policy should weigh the cost of the individual policy against the benefits that a separate liability policy confers on the nurse individually and on the nursing profession generally.

IN A NUTSHELL

Nurses should take the time to become familiar with their various insurance options and with the provisions in their chosen insurance policies. Decisions on whether to purchase claims-made or occurrence basis and individual or group coverage ultimately may decide the financial fate of a nurse involved as a defendant in a lawsuit. When examining and choosing an insurance policy, pay close attention to the exclusions in the policy, as well as the limits and deductibles, because these items impact coverage in critical ways.

AFTERTHOUGHTS

1. Does the purchase of an individual liability policy make the nurse more likely to be sued?
2. An employed nurse is named individually in a lawsuit, along with the employer. Is the nurse automatically entitled to an attorney separate from the employer's attorney?
3. Discuss whether tort reform measures in your state have increased or decreased the nurse's exposure to tort liability.
4. A nurse works at only one job and the employer's policy indicates that the nurse is insured under it. Should the nurse purchase an individual policy as well?
5. Discuss the various sources, nursing associations, and companies that provide professional liability insurance for nurses. How are they similar and different?
6. Discuss the types of insurance policies available to professional nurses.
7. Discuss what specific items you should look for in an insurance policy.
8. Discuss "exclusions" as seen in insurance policies.
9. Explain the differences and similarities between individual, institutional, and group policies.
10. Name and describe five sections of a policy.
11. List five reasons for having insurance and two reasons for not purchasing an individual policy.
12. Does your state have a Patient's Compensation Fund and cap on statutory damages?
13. What is disciplinary defense insurance?

ETHICS IN PRACTICE

David B., 56 years old, was admitted to the intensive care unit (ICU) with severe chest pain and a diagnosis of an acute anterior myocardial infarction (MI). After several hours in the unit, he began to have short runs (5 to 10 beats) of ventricular tachycardia (VT) that ended without treatment. The physician was called, and she ordered lidocaine.

Karen M., who was Mr. B.'s nurse, took the phone order for the medication. In writing down the order, she mistakenly wrote "1000 mg IV bolus, followed by drip at 2 mg per minute," rather than "100 mg IV bolus, followed by drip at 2 mg per minute."

Amanda K., another RN who had been pulled to the ICU from the pediatric unit, offered to give the medication because Karen was so busy. Amanda gave the medication as the order was written, and Mr. B. promptly went into cardiac arrest. Resuscitative measures, including a pacemaker, proved futile in reviving him.

It was only after the code was over and Karen was completing her chart that she realized her error in writing down a dose that was 10 times more than the usual dose. If she had been giving the medication herself, she would have discovered the error immediately, but the pediatric nurse was unfamiliar with the ICU medications and had given the full dose. The patient had arrested so quickly after the medication was given that Amanda did not have time to chart it. Because Karen was the only one who had seen the chart and the order, it would be very easy for her to change it. Amanda had already gone back to the pediatric unit and did not even realize she had given a wrong dosage of this lethal medication. It is also likely that no one else would ever discover what really happened to Mr. B.

About that time, Mr. B.'s wife arrived to collect his personal belongings. She stopped at the desk where Karen was completing her chart to thank Karen for her care of her husband. Karen feels very guilty about the incident and wonders if she should tell Mr. B.'s wife what really happened.

What should Karen do? What would be the consequences of the possible choices of action? What insurance implications would admitting her mistake have? What ethical principles should underlie Karen's decision?

References

1. Corlin, RF: American Medical News. http://www.Amedneuis.com, February 18, 2002. Tort Reform: An Idea Whose Time Has Come Again. Accessed September 3, 2002.
2. For example, effective June 30, 1984, 42 Pa. C. S. 5533 (b) tolls the statute of limitations for minors in personal injury actions in Pennsylvania. Preceding June 30, 1984, there was no tolling.
3. Chicago Insurance Co., Nursing Professional Liability Policy, Form CHIC-44-36, Chicago, June 1987.
4. Transamerica Insurance Group, Professional/Personal Liability Policy, Form 518255.
5. See Legler v. Meriwether, 391 S.W.2d 599 (Mo. 1965) and National Union Fire Insurance Company of Pittsburgh v. Medical Liability Mutual Insurance Co., 446 N.Y.S. 2d 480 (Sup. Ct. A.D., 3rd Dept. 1981). In both cases, the nurse employee was held not to be covered by the group liability policy of the employer. In the second case, National, the nurse also carried her own policy, which did respond.
6. Copies of the TAANA pamphlet are available at a nominal charge; see Resources.
7. See Northrop, C: Buy liability insurance? Some factors to consider. The American Nurse 29, October 1987; also Feutz, S: Professional liability insurance. In Northrop, C, and Kelly, M (eds): Legal Issues in Nursing. CV Mosby, St Louis, 1987, p 441.
8. See Jones v. Medox, 430 A.2d 488 (D.C. App. 1981). Court stated that in harmonizing "other insurance" provisions, nurse's individual policy must pay first, because employer's policy stated explicitly that its limits applied "excess" of other valid and collectible insurance.
9. American Nurses Association v. Passaic General Hospital, 471 A2d 66 (NJ Super. A.D. 1984). Hospital's self-insured deductible deemed not to be insurance for purpose of harmonizing "other insurance" provisions in the nurse's individual policy and the hospital's policy.

Resources _____

The American Association of Nurse Attorneys
7794 Grow Drive
Pensacola, FL 32514
1-877-538-2262
850-474-3646
850-484-8762 (Fax)

"Demonstrating Financial Responsibility for Nurse Practice" Brochure
American Nurses Association
600 Maryland Avenue, Suite 100 West
Washington, DC 20024
1-800-274-4262
292-651-7001 (Fax)

? | What Would You Do?

At Shady Rest Long-Term Care Facility, Nurse Green has cared for patient Kyle
Wayne for 2 weeks. During that period, the 80-year-old patient with diabetes,
who has peripheral neuropathy, developed decubitus ulcers on his heels and
buttocks. No documentation of skin integrity or breakdown is noted at all for 2
weeks prior to a physician's progress note describing the decubitus and treatment
ordered. Because the patient is debilitated and has diabetes, the decubitus ulcers
worsened and he became septic and died. The treating physician claims that he
was not notified of the decubitus ulcers until the day he charted in the record (2
weeks after admission).

1. Who will probably be sued by the patient's wife?
2. What theories of liability will be alleged?
3. What were the breaches of the standard of care?
4. Whose insurance may pay for damages?

Part 5

Professional

Issues

The Nurse and the Contract 17

Key Chapter Concepts

Contract

Offeror

Offeree

Acceptance

Consideration

Breach of contract

Statute of frauds

Written agreement

Merger clause

Monetary damages

Duty to mitigate

Restitution

Alternative Dispute Resolution (ADR)

Mediation

Mediator

Arbitration

Arbitrator

Facilitation

Facilitator

Summary jury trial

Independent contractor

Consultant

Chapter Thoughts

To many nurses, the term *contract* evokes visions of the murkier side of the legal system. Indeed, contract law can be complicated, confusing, and fear evoking to those not familiar with the terminology. But the reality is that nurses enter into contracts all the time. The most common contract is the nurse-employer contract, but other contracts exist between nurses and their patients, physicians, vendors, attorneys, facilities,and schools of nursing.

Although many facilities require the nurses they hire to sign written contracts, there are many other facilities that have oral employment contracts. Whether written or oral, elements such as exact work hours, job description, salary, raises, sick leave, vacation time, overtime compensation, and job expectations should be expressed clearly. In some settings, the employee's handbook serves as the written list of expectations and duties and may even have the legal force of a contract in a court of law. Whether written or oral, once agreed on, all contracts have the same weight before the law.

Once the contract is accepted and agreed on by both parties, it is in force until it is broken, or until one or the other party terminates it. It is generally accepted that the contract lasts as long as the pay period and at that time is automatically renewed or terminated. The employee may terminate the contract by presenting the employer with a formal letter of resignation at least 2 weeks or more before the effective date based on the contractual agreement. It is often more difficult for an employer to terminate an employee's contract for misbehavior, such as unsafe or negligent care, than it is for the employee to terminate the contract. However, in cases where the decision has been made to terminate an employee, employees are to be given the same 2- to 4-week termination notice as the employer is given. If there is no written contract, some states use a fire-at-will policy, which does not require notice or a reason.

Both written and oral contracts should be based on the two ethical principles of justice and fidelity. Under the principle of justice, the employer owes the nurse a safe, comfortable place to work plus a "just salary" that is equal to the work being performed. Often included under the umbrella of the term *just salary* are benefits such as health insurance, sick leave, vacation time, and so on.

The principle of justice also demands certain requirements on the part of the nurse employee. In general, the nurse owes the employer a provision of patient care that is in line with the reasonable standards and qualities of the profession. More specifically, the nurse employee should meet or exceed the standards set by the nurse practice act, continue to upgrade his or her skills through education and practice, seek the highest possible standards and quality of care for patients, and be a patient advocate seeking to follow the patient's wishes as closely as possible. Often included in these requirements for the nurse employee is the obligation to "float," or work in areas of patient care to which the nurse is not usually assigned.

The ethical principle of fidelity is one of the key building blocks of accountability, and without accountability, there can be no claim to professionalism. Although the definition of *fidelity* seems simple, "fidelity conflicts" often arise in the work setting due to opposing demands from various forces. For example, the employer hospital or institution may experience a fidelity conflict between fidelity to its employees to provide modest raises and job security and fidelity to a board of directors that is seeking reductions in overall institutional expenses by salary cuts and reduction in positions.

Nurses often experience fidelity conflicts in their day-to-day provision of care. It is usually agreed that fidelity to patients and their needs is the highest priority, yet nurses have fidelity obligations to the hospital, to the profession of nursing, to other nurses, to the government, and to society as a whole. For example, government regulations and accrediting organizations such as the Joint Commission on Accreditation of Healthcare Organizations (JCAHO) require certain types of documentation on the part of nurses. This documentation adds to the overall load of paperwork that the nurse is required to do. Many times nurses are placed in a situation where they must use valuable bedside care time to fill out forms and write lengthy notes. This conflict is really a fidelity conflict.

Awareness of the underlying ethical principles, as well as the legal intricacies, will aid the nurse in fulfilling his or her obligations in a professional manner, as well as seeing that the facility also meets its contractual obligations.

OBJECTIVES

Upon completing this chapter, the reader will be able to:

1. Discuss the principles of basic contract law.
2. Define the technical language used in contracts.

3. Explain the value of using alternatives to the court system.
4. Describe when contracts should be used.
5. List contract requirements.
6. Explain the basis for enforcement of contractual rights.
7. Discuss the different types of contracts.
8. Discuss how alternative dispute resolution, mediation, arbitration, and facilitation are used in the health care and legal arenas.

Introduction

As an alternative to the traditional employer-employee relationship, nurses are increasingly striking out on their own, opening the doors of their own businesses, entering into partnerships with other health care providers, establishing corporations, and offering their expertise to the public independent of the health care facility employer. Particularly at the executive level, nurses are entering into contractual arrangements similar to those of executives in other industries. This chapter includes an overview of contract law and focuses on the contractual needs of the nurse as an independent contractor, a consultant, an executive, and a legal nurse consultant.

Anatomy of a Contract

A **contract** is an agreement consisting of one or more legally enforceable promises between two or more parties—people, corporations, or partnerships. There are four elements in a contractual relationship: offer, acceptance, consideration, and breach (Box 17–1).

Elements

The person or entity making an offer to keep a promise is called the **offeror.** The person or entity accepting the offer is the **offeree.** An example of a contractual relationship, then, would be a hospital that contracts with a nurse so that she will perform certain nursing services. The offeree has the "power of **acceptance.**" If the offeree accepts the offer, a contract is created.

BOX 17-1

Elements in a Contractual Relationship

Offer
Acceptance
Consideration
Breach

Consideration is the economic cost of an agreement, what the offeror bargains and exchanges for the promises. For example, a legal nurse consultant (LNC) who owns a consulting business offers to analyze medical records for a lawyer for a fee. When the lawyer accepts the LNC's offer and "promises" to pay a fee, a contract is made.

If, after the LNC analyzes the records, the lawyer refuses to pay, the LNC can file a lawsuit against the lawyer and ask the court to enforce the contract between the two parties or request mediation or arbitration. Refusal to pay constitutes a **breach of contract.**

Statute of Frauds

The **statute of frauds** is a principle of common law that states that a contract does not have to be in writing to be enforced. However, there are exceptions, which include agreements involving suretyship, marriage, the sale of land or interests in land, the sale of goods, and those agreements that cannot be performed within 1 year. These exceptions do have to be in writing to be enforceable. Because they vary among the states, be sure to check your state laws.

In lawsuits involving contractual rights, the parties may need to prove to the court the express terms of the contract. A **written agreement,** expressing all the parties' intentions, is the most concrete evidence. However, subsequent communications about a written agreement can be oral, written, or behavioral and can serve as evidence of terms agreed to that are different from the original written agreement.

Merger Clause

The **merger clause** is a statement in a contract indicating that the document is the complete and final agreement between the parties. This clause indicates that the terms cannot be modified unless reduced to writing, signed by all parties, dated, and made a part of the original contract.

Remedies in Contract Disputes

Monetary Damages

The principal remedy for breach of contract is **monetary damages.** As a general rule, the goal of the courts is to make the plaintiff "whole again" and place the damaged or injured party in the same economic position he or she would have been in if the promise had been kept. For example, the legal nurse consultant would be made whole again by receiving the fee for services rendered.

If a nurse is working under an employment contract as an executive and the employer breaches the contract by wrongfully terminating her before the expiration of the contract, the nurse may enforce the contract by bringing a lawsuit to recover salary and other economic benefits agreed to for the remainder of the contract.

Duty to Mitigate

The **duty to mitigate** is the obligation to decrease or reduce the damages or award by the injured party. The wrongfully terminated nurse may be expected to reduce his or her injury by looking for and securing a new job. Any earnings made in the new job during the defunct contract period decrease the damages under the contract. The nurse has an obligation to make a reasonable effort to lessen or mitigate the damages under the contract. What the nurse is unable to recover, the court may award.

AUTHOR TIP: *The duty on the part of the injured party to a contract to mitigate his or her damages is an important one to keep in mind. Courts do not allow injured parties to a contract to sit by and wait for a court to order the breaching party to pay. Rather, courts require that reasonable efforts be made on the part of the injured party to recoup his or her losses. Then, under the "no harm, no foul" theory of law, courts will award only the remaining damages to the injured party to ensure that he or she is put in the same place that he or she would have been in had the other party not breached in the first place.*

Other Remedies

Only in certain circumstances does a court enforce a contract by requiring that a promise that cannot be measured financially be kept. For example, to prevent someone from either unjustly benefiting from or suffering a loss, a court may require restitution to the aggrieved party by canceling a contract. **Restitution** is the act of returning property or the monetary value of a loss to the property owner or party. Restitution places the plaintiff in as good a position as if the contract had been made or upheld.[1]

Alternative Dispute Resolution

For a nurse, a lawsuit can mean considerable demands on his or her professional and personal life. Today there are several alternative legal options that may be less imposing than full-blown litigation. Referred to as **alternative dispute resolution (ADR),** techniques include, among others, mediation, binding and nonbinding arbitration, facilitation, and summary jury trial.[2] Third-party impartial "neutrals" are mediators, arbitrators, or facilitators.[3] Box 17–2 outlines several advantages of alternate dispute resolution.

Mediation

Mediation is an excellent technique when parties want to maintain a positive working relationship. It involves the use of **mediators**—neutral third parties who facilitate agreements by helping both sides to identify their needs and underlying interests and work toward agreeable solutions. The nurse who wants to continue reviewing records

A CASE IN POINT

Breach of Contract

The Facts

Plaintiff nurse worked for 14 years in the critical care unit at a California hospital. She was fired for allegedly falsifying her time sheets.

The plaintiff sued the hospital for breach of an oral contract not to discharge her without good cause and for a breach of the implied covenant of good faith and fair dealing.

At the time of her termination she was 56 years old, 6 years away from retirement, and alleged that the termination was done to deprive her of accrued retirement and pension.

The Jury Decides

Jurors found that there was an oral contract; that the hospital terminated her without just cause; and that the hospital breached the implied covenant of good faith and fair dealing. The plaintiff was awarded $75,000 in damages.

The Appeal

The defendant hospital moved for a new trial based on declarations from three dissenting jurors showing the damages were inflated by one-third to cover plaintiff's attorney's fees.

Plaintiff opposed the new trial motion with declarations from several majority jurors denying any agreement to increase damages to include attorney's fees.

The Judge Decides

A substitute judge heard the new trial motion and expressed an opinion that the award was excessive and should be reduced to $56,000. Plaintiff accepted this amount to avoid a new trial.

The minute order directed counsel to prepare appropriate notices and defendant produced a notice of ruling exploring why the conditional new trial order was granted. The court failed to draft or file a specification of reasons for the decision.

Another Appeal

The defendant hospital argued that the court lacked authority to reduce the award for any reason other than excessive damages and that the court failed to prepare a list of reasons for the decision. The defendant sought an order for a new trial. However, the proper course was to reinstate the original judgment of $75,000.

The Court Decided

The defendant hospital "succeeded" in its appeal but obtained a $19,000 increase in liability.

The $75,000 awarded was the amount requested by plaintiff in her closing argument to cover lost pension plan benefits and missed overtime opportunities. The California Court of Appeals conceded that a new trial was not required as a matter of law.

Interesting Points

- The hospital's handbook stated the hospital was an "at-will" employer. The handbook also listed specific grounds for discipline, along with a three-step discipline procedure that could support the existence of an implied-in-fact contract, meaning that there was a promise not to fire except for cause.
- The plaintiff presented evidence that as an emergency supervisor she could change her own records.
- The plaintiff was terminated without a review of her evaluation reports or examination of her personnel file.
- The plaintiff was not allowed to rebut any of the charges regarding falsification of time records. (Therefore the question of whether the hospital acted in good faith was for the jury, which rendered a decision in the plaintiff's favor.)[4]

for a lawyer is much more likely to achieve that goal by mediating the dispute than by suing the lawyer. The parties can share costs for the mediator and the associated scheduling and paperwork. Mediation is the wave of the future. This process can resolve litigation (e.g., medical malpractice claims), work-related disputes, bioethical dilemmas, and patient and family conflicts in the hospital setting. Mediation not only preserves relationships between the parties, it is a much more cost-effective solution than litigation. It provides a quicker resolution, allows more creative solutions than trial, and is confidential and avoids publicity.

Nurses trained in mediation, arbitration, and facilitation techniques have a valuable skill and provide a much-needed service to the health care industry.

Arbitration

The **arbitration** process is also used for technical cases such as medical malpractice and certain employer-employee contracts. Both sides select a neutral third-party **arbitrator** with technical knowledge in the area of contention who hears the case and renders a decision and award.

Depending on what the parties agreed to before the arbitration began, the decision can be binding or nonbinding.

Facilitation

The **facilitation** process is often used to get parties to the table and to assist in difficult issues faced by the parties. A **facilitator** is an outside or impartial party neutral to the negotiations or disputes. The facilitator assists in such things as clarifying issues, overcoming obstacles, breaking impasses, and identifying needs, interests, motives, and goals of the parties. The role of a facilitator is to provide structure and advance discussions among the participants.[5]

Summary Jury Trial

A **summary jury trial** is an abbreviated, privately held trial. It is often used to give the parties an indication of the strengths and weaknesses of the case and possible outcome if the case goes to trial.

Nurses' contracts should contain a statement that provides for the use of one or more alternative dispute resolution processes. Consult legal counsel for the appropriate wording for each situation.

Types of Nursing Contracts

Independent Contractor

A nurse who is an **independent contractor** undertakes a specific job, for a person, a facility, or a corporation, using his or her own means and methods. The person, facil-

---

BOX 17–2

Advantages of Alternative Dispute Resolution

Cost savings: Court costs, lawsuit expenses, and lawyers' fees can be greatly reduced.

Time savings: Parties meet on their own schedules and do not have to wait for a court calendar date. The process often does not get drawn out and delayed with motions and discovery.

Private: The process and the result are private.

Less traumatic: Money can be saved; the process is speedier; sensitive materials are not shared with the press and general public.

More creative: Courts do not have the flexibility to create resolutions tailored to meet the needs of all parties. In mediation, for example, the parties do have the leisure to craft remedies that are more creative and benefit all parties involved.

ity, or corporation for whom the work is performed has no authority over the nurse. Many **consultants** are considered independent contractors because the consultant is his or her own boss and controls time schedules and job duties. Unlike the employer or employee, neither party has the right to terminate the contract at will. The key to independent contractor status is: How much control does the person, facility, or corporation have over the nurse?

When to Use an Independent Contractor's Contract

The traditional private-duty nurse is perhaps the nursing profession's oldest example of an independent contractor. Today nurse attorneys, legal nurse consultants, nurse paralegals, midwives, nurse-anesthetists, and nurse practitioners are among the nurse specialists who are taking advantage of the financial and professional rewards available to the independent contractor, as are nurse brokerage firms and quality review specialists. The Internal Revenue Service (IRS) has also issued private letter rulings permitting several nurses who work for nurse brokerage firms to be classified as independent contractors. However, this is a rapidly changing area of tax law, and nurses should seek legal counsel before deciding about their own classification. See Box 17–3 for the requirements to qualify as an independent contractor.

Requirements of an Independent Contractor's Contract

A contract must contain certain elements to be thorough, valid, and binding. See Box 17–4 for the list of what must be included. The following sections are recommendations of what should be in a contract. Always check with a contract attorney in your state to ensure that you are following your specific state laws.

BOX 17–3

Indications That a Worker Is an Independent Contractor: The Issue of Control

1. Employer has no right to give instructions or training.
2. Worker does not have to render services personally; may work for others.
3. Worker may hire assistants, use his or her own tools.
4. Worker does not have to keep set hours.
5. Worker does not have to work on employer's premises.
6. Worker may perform work in any sequence but has no right to quit and cannot be fired.
7. Worker is paid by the job, on commission, or by the hour, week, month, or year.
8. Worker assumes his or her own expenses and can bill for them.

BOX 17–4

Elements of Independent Contractor's Contract

Identification of parties
Recitals
Description of work
Contract price and payment schedule
Liability insurance statement
Duration of contract
Independent status
Signatures and date
Alternate dispute resolution clause

First Section: The first section of a contract should contain the full names and addresses of parties to the contract and their role in the contract, such as owner, corporation, or family and nurse.

Second Section: Recitals should address the type of business the owner or corporation is engaged in or the needs of the family or individual requiring care. They should also state that the nurse will provide nursing services for the specified persons under the terms and conditions in the contract in consideration for the promises listed in the contract.

Third Section: The contract should list a reasonably complete description of all the work the nurse will provide. For example, a private-duty nurse's description of work might be "all nursing care essential to Baby Doe's health between 7:00 AM and 3:30 PM, each Monday through Friday, until, in my judgment, in collaboration with the Doe family, all Baby Doe's health care providers, and all other professionals interested in Baby Doe's welfare, Baby Doe no longer needs such nursing care."

Fourth Section: The contract should also contain the total fee owed to the nurse and the fee schedule to be followed.

Fifth Section: The contract should have a statement about the nurse's liability insurance coverage in an amount acceptable to the other party. In some instances, a corporation may want the nurse to have a clause inserted that would hold it harmless and indemnify it from all costs arising out of the nurse's negligence or other actions. These clauses are varied and complex and have numerous and significant effects on the nurse's business. The nurse should seek legal counsel for advice and assistance in the contract negotiation process to ensure that all areas are properly covered in the contract.

Sixth Section: The duration of the contract should be clearly spelled out, the day it starts and the day it ends. In the case of Baby Doe, described earlier, a specific

BOX 17–5

Sample Contract for the Nurse Working as an Independent Contractor

This contract is made on _____ , 20 _____ ,
between _____ , whose address is _____ ,
City of _____ , County of _____ ,
State of _____ , hereinafter referred to
as Corporation, and _____ of _____ ,
City of _____ , County of _____ [address],
State of _____ , hereinafter referred to as Nurse.
Corporation owns and operates a _____ [type of business] business
at the address above, and Corporation wants to have certain nursing services
performed for Corporation's business.

Nurse agrees to perform these services for Corporation under the terms
and conditions included in this contract.

In consideration of the mutual promises contained herein, it is agreed by
and between Corporation and Nurse:

Relationship of Parties

The parties to this contract agree that Nurse is a professional person, and that
the relation created by this contract is that of employer-independent contractor. Nurse is not an employee of employer and is not entitled to any benefits
provided by employer to its employees, including, but not limited to, pension
plan, withholding of federal and state income taxes, FICA, Workers'
Compensation, Unemployment Compensation, and other insurance. Nurse
may practice nursing for others during those periods when Nurse is not
performing work under this contract for Corporation. Corporation may,
during the length of this contract, engage other nurses to perform the same
work that Nurse performs under this contract.

Duties and Responsibilities

The work to be performed by Nurse includes all services that are usually
performed by [insert type of practice] nurses, including, but not limited to, the
following: [insert type of nursing services to be rendered]

Payment Schedule

Corporation will pay Nurse the total sum of _____ Dollars ($) for the ser-
vices to be provided under this contract, according to the following schedule:
[INSERT SCHEDULE]

(continued)

BOX 17–5

Sample Contract for the Nurse Working as an Independent Contractor *(continued)*

Professional Liability Insurance

The nursing service to be provided under this contract will be accomplished at Nurse's risk, and Nurse assumes all responsibility for the condition of his/her own equipment used in the performance of this contract. Nurse will carry, for the length of this contract, liability insurance in an amount [insert limits of professional liability insurance coverage you carry].

Length of Contract

Either party may cancel this contract on _____ month(s)' written notice; otherwise, the contract remains in force for a period of _____ , from date of execution of this contract by both parties.

Dispute Resolution

For all disputes arising under or in connection with this contract that cannot first be resolved through good faith negotiations, the parties shall mediate those disputes with the assistance of a third party neutral. Costs for such mediation shall be borne equally, unless otherwise agreed to during such mediation. If the parties cannot resolve any such disputes in mediation, they shall submit such disputes to binding arbitration.

[SIGNATURES]

[DATES]

Contracts vary from state to state. This is only a sample contract. If you are creating or signing a contract, seek legal counsel.

end date should be inserted, perhaps the day the health insurance coverage ends, plus the clause that "services, in the nurse's judgment in collaboration with those mentioned above, may terminate sooner." A clause allowing either party to terminate before the end date should be included, provided written notice is given by one party to the other.

Seventh Section: A provision asserting the relationship between the professional nurse as an independent contractor and the employing party should be included, emphasizing that the nurse is not an employee. This type of paragraph is especially helpful in dealing with certain governmental agencies, such as the IRS, for the validity of certain business deductions. In fact, all the inclusions described previously are good evidence that the parties intend to pursue an independent contractor relationship, should any such agency inquire. If the employer breaches the contract by not paying according to schedule, the nurse has documented evidence of the employer's promise.

Eighth Section: The contract must have a section for signatures and dates signed. Technically, a contract does not have to be signed for a court to enforce it, but the nurse's case is stronger if such formalities are performed. Although none of the promises made by the nurse and the other party to the contract has to be written for the court to enforce them, the specific terms of the contract need to be proven, and a written contract can be clear evidence of what was promised.

Ninth Section: This section should discuss mediation or arbitration as an alternative to settling contractual disputes. See Box 17–5 for a sample of an independent contractor contract.

Consulting Contract

The traditional role of the consultant has been principally that of advice giver. This role has expanded so that it often includes performing work on or off site for an employer.

When to Use a Consulting Contract

A nurse may be hired as a consultant, for example, to advise a law firm on setting up a system to review and analyze medical records. Subsequently, the firm may want to contract with the nurse to implement that system. A nurse's consulting contract is really a variation of the independent contractor's agreement. Some of the provisions in the consulting contract, such as identifying the parties and the recitals, can be virtually identical. Other provisions are tailored for the consultants, an option that many

---

BOX 17–6

Required Elements in a Consultant Contract

Include in the contract:

1. Nurse's duties and correct title
2. Location of nurse's workplace
3. Amount of time to do the work
4. Noncompete clause (optional)
5. Payment schedule clause

Recommended:
6. Mediation/arbitration clause

nurses are choosing by taking consulting assignments for federal, state, and local governments; multinational corporations; insurance companies; law firms; and national health care providers, to mention just a few.

Requirements in the Nurse Consultant's Contract

As in any contract, certain elements must be contained in a consultant contract. See Box 17–6 for a list of these elements.

DUTIES AND RESPONSIBILITIES

In the duties and responsibilities clause, the correct title, or titles, should be included. The nurse's duties and responsibilities should be negotiated carefully and inserted in this section, with as much specificity as possible.

The description of the nurse's duties and responsibilities in the body of the contract should focus on the consulting role. The contract may include a statement about making suggestions to employees and management concerning a particular aspect of the corporation's business.

LOCATION OF NURSE'S WORKPLACE

The location of the nurse's workplace should be mentioned. Consultants often work out of their own offices, libraries and research facilities, or corporate offices or places where the corporation has contracts.

AMOUNT OF TIME TO DO THE WORK

Include the amount of time needed by the consultant to do the work. Usually consultants are paid a flat fee for a job to be finished by a certain date, but the speed at which it is accomplished is the consultant's prerogative.

NONCOMPETE CLAUSE

Some corporations may request that a nurse consultant obtain the corporation's written approval before working with competitors. A noncompete clause is a clause prohibiting a nurse from doing business that competes with the business of a client or an employer. Noncompete clauses vary regarding the type of restrictions, length of time required when the nurse cannot compete, and geographic areas restricted. If a noncompete clause is requested, the nurse should consider the full implications of this restriction on practice. Similarly, a related clause restricting the nurse from providing similar consulting services to certain types of corporations may also require the services of counsel to negotiate.

Negotiating a Contract

You are negotiating a contract as an independent contractor with a large facility in town. You have known the vice president for years as a member of the business community.

Although the negotiations have taken several weeks, you are comfortable with what has transpired thus far. You receive the final contract and note that the facility has added different language regarding termination and a noncompete clause. The vice president claims you agreed to the terms.

What would you do?

1. Were all the conditions negotiated verbally only?
2. Was anything confirmed in writing?
3. Do you have any documentation concerning the negotiation terms, such as e-mails?

PAYMENT SCHEDULE CLAUSE

The payment schedule clause should address the issue of reimbursement for all travel expenses incurred away from home or office. Seeking reimbursement and complying with IRS audit demands require scrupulous documentation of such expenses.

MEDIATION/ARBITRATION CLAUSE

The mediation/arbitration clause can be inserted to deal with any contractual disputes. Such a clause is often used to decrease legal expenses and to resolve disputes in a timely manner. See Box 17–7 for a sample consultant contract.

KEEP IN MIND

▶ A contract is an agreement that consists of offer, acceptance, and consideration.
▶ Once the offer is accepted, the contract is created, assuming the parties have exchanged consideration.
▶ Consideration is the amount paid by the offeror in exchange for a promise or agreement.
▶ To be enforced, most contracts do not have to be in writing. However, to prove what the terms of the contract are, it is helpful to have them documented.
▶ Monetary damages are the usual remedy for a breach of contract. However, enforcement of the contract may also be a remedy.

BOX 17–7

Sample Contract for the Nurse Working as a Consultant

This contract is made _____ _____ , 20 _____ , between a corporation organized under the laws of the State of _____ with its principal place of business at _____ [address], City of _____ , County of _____ , State of _____ , hereinafter referred to as Corporation, and _____ of _____ [address], City of _____ , County of _____ , State of _____ , hereinafter referred to as Nurse Consultant.

    Corporation is in the business of _____ [type of business] and wants to have the following services, as a consultant, accomplished by Nurse Consultant.

    Nurse Consultant agrees to accomplish these services for corporation under the terms and conditions contained in this contract.

    In consideration of the mutual promises contained in this contract, it is agreed by and between Corporation and Nurse Consultant as follows:

Duties and Responsibilities

Nurse Consultant will perform consulting services on behalf of the Corporation with respect to all matters relating to: [insert description of duties and responsibilities].

Location of Work

Nurse Consultant's services will be rendered at _____ [address], City of _____ , State of _____ , but that Nurse Consultant will, when requested, come to the Corporation's address at _____ [address], City of _____ , State of _____ , or such other locations as designated by the Corporation, to confer with representatives of the Corporation.

Amount of Time Devoted to Work

In the performance of the services, the services and the hours Nurse Consultant is to work on any particular day will be completely within Nurse Consultant's control and Corporation will rely upon Nurse Consultant to work such number of hours as is necessary to fulfill the intent and goal(s) of this contract. It is estimated that this work will take approximately _____ [days of work per month]. However, there may be some months during which Nurse Consultant may not provide any services or, in the alternative, may work the full week.

Payment Schedule

Corporation will pay Nurse Consultant the total sum of _____ Dollars ($) each year payable in equal monthly installments on or before the _____ day of each month for services rendered in the prior month. In addition, Nurse Consultant will be reimbursed for all traveling and living expenses while away from the City of _____ , State of _____ .

(continued)

BOX 17–7

Sample Contract for the Nurse Working as a Consultant *(continued)*

Length of Contract

The parties to this contract agree that this contract is intended to be for five (5) years from date hereof, but the contract shall be considered as a firm commitment on the part of the parties hereto for a period of _____ one (1) year commencing _____ , 20 _____ . At any time before _____ [month and day] of any year, either party hereto can notify the other in writing that the arrangement is not to continue beyond the _____ [month and day]. In the absence of any such written notification, this contract will run from year to year up to the maximum period of five (5) years.

Status of Consultant

This contract contains the performance of the services of the Nurse Consultant as an independent contractor and Nurse Consultant will not be considered an employee of the Corporation for any reason, including, but not limited to, payment of taxes and insurance.

Services for Others

Because Nurse Consultant will acquire or have access to information that is of a confidential and privileged nature, Nurse Consultant shall not perform any services for any other person or firm without Corporation's prior written consent.

Services after Contract Ends

Nurse Consultant agrees that, for a period of one (1) year following the termination of this contract, Nurse Consultant shall not perform any similar services for any person or firm engaged in the business of _____[specify business] in the County of _____, State of _____ .

Dispute Resolution

For all disputes arising under or in connection with this contract that cannot first be resolved through good faith negotiations the parties shall mediate those disputes with the assistance of a neutral third party. Costs for such mediation shall be borne equally, unless otherwise agreed to during such mediation. They shall submit such disputes under this contract to binding arbitration if they cannot be resolved first through good faith negotiations and mediation.

[SIGNATURES]

[DATE]

Contracts vary from state to state. This is only a sample contract. If you are creating or signing a contract, seek legal counsel.

▶ Using alternative methods to resolve contract disputes is less expensive, faster, less traumatizing, and provides a higher level of confidentiality and privacy than pursuing a lawsuit in court.

▶ The appropriate alternative dispute resolution method should be included as a contract term. Some of the methods include mediation, arbitration, facilitation, and summary jury trial.

▶ Independent contractors and consultants must arrange to pay their own federal and state income taxes, social security, and unemployment obligations.

▶ Breach of employment executive contracts by either party is often handled through binding arbitration.

IN A NUTSHELL

The way nurses are compensated for their work has changed almost as rapidly as the health care delivery system. Nurses are no longer confined to hourly wages. They function as consultants, business owners, executives, and independent contractors. Consequently, nurses need to know when to use a contract.

The easiest contracts to enforce are those in which the terms are committed to writing, signed, and dated. After all, enforcement proceedings in a court can be expensive, time consuming, and emotionally draining. Use of the appropriate alternative dispute resolution mechanism can eliminate these problems.

Before creating, signing, or approving any contract, you should seek legal advice, because every contractual relationship is different and many require various clauses to protect you and your company. The sample contracts in this book are not intended to be used without seeking legal advice regarding your specific circumstances relating to state and federal laws.

AFTERTHOUGHTS

1. Discuss the four elements in a contractual relationship.
2. What is the purpose of a merger clause?
3. Why should an alternative dispute resolution be included in a contract?
4. Discuss contractual remedies.
5. a. Describe the types of contracts and when they should be used.
   b. Describe the employment issues that should be covered in each type of contract.
   c. Develop a sample contract using one of the types of contracts discussed.
6. Explain the advantages of using mediation and arbitration rather than the court system to resolve disputes.
7. Why should a contract be in writing?
8. Why should nurses understand basic contract law?

9. Discuss instances when legal counseling is helpful in the contract process.

10. Discuss the role of the nurse mediator or nurse facilitator in the health care setting.

11. Obtain a copy of a contract and discuss the specific sections.

12. Find a case based on an allegation of breach of contract. Discuss with the class.

13. Contact a legal nurse consultant or nurse attorney to discuss his or her experience with contracts and potential problem areas.

14. Perform a mock discussion between the employer and nurse consultant about a contract dispute.

ETHICS IN PRACTICE

Betty A., registered nurse (RN), graduated from an associate degree program 2 years ago and is now the 3 PM to 11 PM charge nurse on the medical unit of a small rural hospital. Most of her experience for the past 2 years has been in the medical unit, although she has occasionally floated to the maternity unit, emergency room (ER), and intensive care unit (ICU). The usual staffing for her unit on her shift is an RN, a licensed practical nurse (LPN), and an aide.

One Friday evening, the nursing supervisor called Betty at the beginning of her shift and stated that she needed Betty to go to the six-bed intensive care unit (ICU) to cover for 1 to 1.5 hours because the scheduled RN for the ICU had been in a minor accident on the way to work. The supervisor felt Betty was the best qualified of the nurses who were in the hospital at that time and that the medical unit was quiet enough so that the LPN could handle it while Betty was gone.

Betty quickly went to the ICU, where she received an abbreviated report on the four unit patients from the 7 AM to 3 PM nurses who were waiting to leave for the weekend. The day shift RN also mentioned that there was a patient in the ER who was experiencing some chest pain and might be admitted to the ICU.

Within minutes of receiving the report, the ER called and said they were admitting a 46-year-old male with an acute anterior myocardial infarction (MI) to the ICU. They also relayed the facts that they had begun streptokinase therapy and that the patient required very close monitoring for arrhythmia, blood pressure changes, and bleeding.

Betty had never administered or cared for a patient receiving streptokinase and felt incompetent to care for such a patient. Although the LPN working with her had worked with these types of patients, she was not permitted to administer any of the many intravenous (IV) medications this type of patient requires. Just as the patient was being brought through the ICU doors, Betty called the nursing supervisor to let her know that she would need help with this patient. The nursing supervisor said that because of call-ins, there was no help available at this time, but that Betty just needed to admit the patient. The regular ICU RN should be in at any time.

Betty assessed the patient and checked his vital signs. He was cold and diaphoretic, and he appeared pale and gray. His blood pressure was 88/42 with a pulse of 52, and he was having frequent premature ventricular contractions (PVCs). The monitor technician also informed Betty that he was in a 2:1 atrioventricular (AV) block. Betty wanted the supervisor to come to the floor and relieve her of the responsibility for the care of this patient. Betty did not know the ICU protocols for arrhythmia and did not feel competent to care for this seriously ill patient. It would be at least another 45 minutes before the regular RN arrived.

What are Betty's obligations under her contract with the hospital? What are the hospital's obligations in this situation? Where do the issues of justice and fidelity fit into this situation? Are there any fidelity conflicts in this situation? How should Betty resolve the dilemma?

References

1. Law.com Dictionary. http://dictionary.law.com, accessed November 10, 2002.
2. Aiken, T, Aiken, J, Grant, P, and Warlick, D: The basics of alternative dispute resolutions. In Legal and Ethical Issues in Health Occupations. WB Saunders, Philadelphia, 2001.
3. Marcus, L, et al: Renegotiating Health Care: Resolving Conflict to Build Collaboration. Jossey-Bass, San Francisco, 1995.
4. Thompson, V: Friendly Hills Regional Medical Center, 71 Cal. App. 4th 544, 84 Cal. Rptr. 2d 51, 99 Cal. Daily Op. Serv. 2847 (Cal. App. Dist. 4 04/20/1999).
5. Marcus, p. 434.

Resources

Association of Conflict Resolution
1527 New Hampshire, NW
Washington, DC 20036
202-667-9700
202-265-1968 (Fax)
http://www.acr@acresolution.org

American Bar Association
Section of Dispute Resolution
740 Fifteenth Street
Washington, DC 20005
202-662-1680
202-662-1683 (Fax)
http://www.abanet.org/

American Arbitration Association
335 Madison Avenue
Floor 10
New York, NY 10017
212-716-5800
212-716-5905
800-778-7879
http://www.adr.org/

Recommended Reading

Weeks, D: The Eight Essential Steps to Conflict Resolution. Penguin Putnam, New York, 1994

Conflict Management and the Nurse 18

James B. Aiken, MD, MHA, FACEP

Tonia D. Aiken, RN, BSN, JD

Key Chapter Concepts

Conflict	Mediation
Brainstorming	Arbitration
Constructive criticism	Facilitation
Negotiation	Communication

Chapter Thoughts

Conflict is a part of life, whether we experience it at home or in the workplace, and is not necessarily a bad thing. It usually means there is a problem with communication or a need that is not being met. **Conflict** can be described as interpersonal experiences arising from fundamental diversity of needs, perceptions, attitudes, culture, and past learning that offer opportunities for growth and enduring partnerships.

There are many different signs and symptoms that might suggest a conflict, such as body language, voice, increased heart rate, increased blood pressure, decreased communication, passive-aggressive acting out, or team splitting in the form of cliques. In the workplace, conflict can be very costly because it causes the following:

1. Stress-related illnesses
2. Decreased ability to focus
3. High employee turnover
4. Disability claims
5. Increased sick time
6. Friction
7. Low morale
8. Sexual harassment claims
9. Strikes
10. Poor patient outcomes
11. Sabotage in the form of withholding information or "forgetting" to tell someone about a meeting or a report that is due
12. Inefficiencies when tasks have to be performed over again (e.g., "Fax the form again, we didn't get it.")

In the health care setting, conflict can additionally involve ethical issues, such as right to die issues; do not resuscitate orders, advance directives (living wills and medical durable power of attorney/health care proxies), resource allocation, and patient care issues.

The ethical principles of beneficence (to do good for the patient) may be at issue if conflicts between health care providers and patients and families are not timely and appropriately resolved. This chapter focuses on the anatomy of a conflict and offers suggestions on effectively resolving conflict situations.

OBJECTIVES

Upon completing this chapter, the reader will be able to:

1. Define *conflict* and its signs and symptoms.
2. Outline the causes of conflict.
3. Discuss the anatomy of conflict.
4. Discuss how needs, desires, values, and diversity affect resolution of conflicts.
5. Define the alternative dispute resolution processes—mediation, arbitration, and facilitation.
6. Define *negotiation*.
7. Discuss how communication and body language can affect conflict resolution.

Introduction

Conflict has many causes. Some of the causes of conflict include the following:

1. Unequal treatment
2. Unmet needs
3. Scarce or finite resources
4. Competition
5. Differences (which may be based on culture, ethnicity, religion, or other things)
6. Communication problems[1]

How Do You Assess Conflict?

Assessing conflict can be likened to assessing a patient and using the nursing process. You use all your senses to get an accurate picture of what is going on with the conflict (patient).

- Look
- Listen
- Perform a "physical" (e.g., "Is the person perspiring, breathing rapidly, etc.?")
- Perform a history

- Review written documents
- Study behaviors
- Use intuition

As we said in the beginning of this chapter, conflict is a symptom that something in a relationship is amiss. Conflict should make you curious about what is causing this conflict. For example, if someone complains "I am tired of her taking such long breaks," think about why the person is taking long breaks and why this is causing a problem.

Common types of conflict faced on the units include the following:

- Staff requests for time off
- Time commitment problems with the staff
- Traveling/pool nurses refusing to take assignments or the fact that the hospital uses them at all
- Refusal of assignments by individual staff members
- Staff refusal to float to another unit
- Individual staff member not pulling his or her weight
- Competent staff covering for incompetent staff or doing more than what is outlined in the job description
- End-of-life issues
- Drug/alcohol abuse by nurses
- Staff absences or call-outs
- Turf wars
- Interdepartmental/intradepartmental disputes
- Patient/family complaints about perceived lack of caring and poor attitude

Before you can resolve such conflicts, you must know what your needs are. For example, as a unit manager you are faced with staff refusing assignments. As a manager your needs may be to:

- Cover your unit.
- Provide quality care.
- Be liked or respected.
- Avoid escalation.
- Maintain unit harmony.
- Be equitable and fair.
- Hold staff accountable for their actions.
- Ensure staff knowledge of liability issues.
- Maintain predictability.

Once you understand your motivation, you must discover the needs or motivations causing the conflict.

For example, in the situation mentioned earlier, you may ask the staff member, "What would be necessary for you to take shorter breaks and be back on time?" "What would it take for you to accept this assignment?" or "Why do you feel this way?"

To avoid escalating the conflict or creating a new one, use the "me *and* you approach," not the "me *versus* you" approach.

Many times the real conflict is at the bottom of the iceberg, related to values acquired from school, background, or work or diversity issues based on ethnic or cultural backgrounds or religion.

The conflict may also be related to desires of the parties. For example, due to hospital staffing shortage, a nurse may be asked to perform duties, such as changing bed linens, that other employees normally do. Although most nurses will do what has to be done in trying times for their patients, they certainly would prefer to concentrate on the duties they were trained to perform.

Steps in Conflict Resolution

There is no one solution that will resolve every conflict. Like choosing a nursing intervention, deciding what will work will take analysis of the situation and exploration of your options. It may also be trial and error. However, here are some points that may help set the stage for resolution or actually help resolve the conflict.

- Select a discussion site away from the "war zone." For example, if the unit has numerous conflicts that have not been resolved, move the meeting to a neutral environment, such as a restaurant, home, or coffee shop, to create a more relaxed atmosphere.
- Listen, listen, listen…to everyone's side without interrupting. Clarify perceptions and your understanding of the issues on the table. Focus on needs—your needs and the needs of others.
- Share the discussion and the power. Do not dominate the conversation. Have a positive attitude—you must learn from the past but look to the future for new and creative options and resolutions.
- Use openings to a conversation such as "How can I help you?" or "How can we work this out together?"
- After listening to everyone's side of the story, distinguish needs from desires or expectations.

Brainstorming

One of the most creative parts of the conflict resolution is **brainstorming,** the process of freely and nonjudgmentally exploring all possible issues and solutions. For a successful brainstorming process, keep the following rules in mind:

- Define your purpose for the meeting and select a facilitator to keep the meeting on track and to stimulate ideas, options, and discussions.[2]
- Keep a nonjudgmental atmosphere. Remember that no answer is bad, no answer is wrong, and no answer is ridiculous.

- Use techniques such as mind mapping (a building block technique used to flush out a problem, concept, or option).
- Group and emphasize the areas of commonalities together to build momentum.
- Encourage people to work "outside the box" and to be creative.
- Position parties who have a conflict side by side because it reinforces the idea of working together to tackle and solve the problem. Sitting across a table or using a rectangular or square table reinforces turf and opponent attitudes and positions of power. A round table puts everyone on equal footing.
- After you have examined all options and possibilities from every angle, write them down as evidence of collective achievement by the group. This also helps to stimulate more ideas and reinforces the idea that all suggested options are wanted to use in solving the problem.
- Always use **constructive criticism**—for example, "What I like best about your idea is _____."

Alternative Dispute Resolution

When the conflict cannot be resolved within the group, trial and litigation can be one method of resolving the conflict. However, litigation is often not the best choice because it:

- Blames and points fingers.
- Is very costly.
- Produces lengthy court delays.
- Causes ill will.
- Is a win-lose situation rather than a win-win situation.
- Does not value underlying relationships, interests, desires, or needs.
- Does not foster ongoing or enduring relationships.
- May cause unwanted publicity.

Less threatening and less costly methods of dealing with disputes and avoiding trial or litigation include negotiation, mediation, arbitration, and facilitation and are referred to as alternative dispute resolutions (ADR). The ADR processes can be used to get parties to the table without having an emotionally draining and costly litigation. These processes also allow for the application of more creative and mutually beneficial solutions for parties.

Methods of ADR

Negotiation is a process of communications with exchanges (not always overtly) of needs and priorities to achieve consensus on critical issues and hopefully to gain advantages that otherwise would not be achievable without negotiation. Ultimately the process, if conducted in good faith and respect, will provide a foundation for a subsequent mutually satisfactory relationship. Negotiation differs somewhat from conflict resolution in that the negotiation process is more issues oriented. But the principles of conflict resolution (e.g., separating people from certain issues and differentiating absolute needs from desires) will quite often be called into use as negotiations proceed.

Mediation is a process in which a neutral third party facilitates and assists the parties in resolving a dispute. The mediator can be a nurse attorney, attorney, nurse, legal nurse consultant, social worker, judge, layperson, or other professional who has been trained in mediation techniques.[3]

Arbitration is a process of resolving issues in a more structured setting. The decision may be binding or nonbinding, and discovery and witnesses are allowed.[4]

Facilitation is a process in which a third party assists in the resolution of a conflict by meeting with parties to learn about the individual and shared needs of the parties. The facilitator then aids the parties in discussing options that benefit all parties. During facilitation, the facilitator uses language at the beginning of the meeting to get initial agreements, focusing on getting the parties to agree on the positive points, such as the following:

- "Can we agree to let the other party tell his side of the story without interrupting?"
- "Can we look at both positive and negative ideas of both parties' positions?"
- "Can you clarify for me what you just heard the other party say?"

Communication and Conflict

Good **communication** skills are key to resolving or preventing conflicts. Using listening skills and knowing your personality type and conflict style will also aid you in resolving conflict more efficiently and effectively. There are many personality indicator tests that can be taken to learn your type. By studying your type and knowing the traits of others, you gain added insight into the process to help you better manage conflicts and resolve them.

Analyze body language. Noticing eye movement; posture; position of the legs, hands, head; and even the tone and pitch of a voice can aid you in determining how your "opponent" is feeling about what is being said or done.

1. For example, folding your arms across your chest can be seen as a sign of defense or "blocking out" the other side.
2. Leaning toward a person can signify that you are interested in what they are saying.
3. Looking away and failing to focus on the person's face when they are speaking, can be interpreted as being "uninterested."

Learning how to use active listening and positive body language are extremely useful in the conflict resolution process.

? | What Would You Do?

Conflict Resolution

You have recently moved from out of state and are the new nursing manager on 2 East. You have noticed a problem in morale and bickering among the staff, particularly when one nurse is working. It seems to you that whenever this nurse works, the staff changes their body language to the "defensive mode" and avoids any contact with this nurse.

When you ask what the problem is, they respond, "She is a troublemaker." "She is different." "She is out for herself and not a team player."

You decide to use some conflict management techniques to get to the real issues.

1. What techniques can you use?
2. What kinds of questions can you use?
3. What must you determine with regard to the "players" and their styles?

KEEP IN MIND

▶ Conflict is a part of life and has many signs and symptoms.
▶ Causes of conflict can involve needs, resources, competition, differences, and communication problems among other things.
▶ Assessment of conflict involves the same skills used in the nursing process such as assessment, planning, monitoring, and evaluation of the situation and participants.
▶ Know the needs and desires of the participants and yourself before attempting to solve a conflict.
▶ Use brainstorming and effective communication techniques to find creative solutions.
▶ Know what alternative dispute resolutions are available to you such as mediation, arbitration, and facilitation.
▶ The negotiation process is more issues oriented than conflict resolution.

IN A NUTSHELL

Conflict is a part of our life, but there are methods of dealing with conflict that allow the participants to maintain a future relationship. Conflict manifests itself differently in different people and situations. Although workplace and ethical issues provide a breeding ground for conflict, if the nurse is trained and possesses the tools to effectively deal with the needs and causes of conflict, resolution can be obtained. During conflict, negotiation may also be required and techniques must be learned to be a skilled negotiator in today's cutthroat environment. With the use of active listening, good conflict management, and communication tools, alternative dispute resolution processes such as mediation, arbitration, or facilitation may not be necessary to resolve disputes.

AFTERTHOUGHTS

1. Define *conflict*.
2. Discuss how conflict can manifest itself.
3. Discuss how conflict can affect the health care industry.
4. Define common workplace and ethical issues that can cause conflict.
5. Outline how you would assess conflict.
6. Discuss three conflicts that you are currently experiencing in school or the workplace.
   a. What are the signs and symptoms?
   b. How are they affecting you and your environment (school or workplace)?
   c. What are your needs and the needs of those involved in the conflict?
7. Discuss the steps in conflict resolution.
8. Define *brainstorming* and list several of the ground rules.
9. Discuss why litigation is not always the best alternative for conflict.
10. Define the following:
    Mediation
    Arbitration
    Facilitation
    Negotiation
11. Discuss how communication can affect conflict management and resolution.

ETHICS IN PRACTICE

A nurse has complained to administration about being harassed by a coworker. A nurse facilitator is called in to facilitate a meeting among the nurse, the alleged harasser, witnesses, and the director of nursing (DON).

When the nurse arrives, she sees the nurse facilitator laughing and joking in the hallway with the alleged harasser and the DON.

The meeting did not go well, and the nurse later learns that the nurse facilitator dated the brother of the alleged harasser. The alleged harasser also worked with the DON at a previous facility.

What are the ethical implications for all in this situation? What are the options for the nurse?

References

1. Aiken, JA, Aiken, TD, Gerardi, D, and Morrison, G: Stanford University Hospital Center Course of Healthcare Mediation. Stanford, CA, 2002.
2. Ibid.

3. Aiken, JA, Aiken, TD, Grant, P, and Warlick, D: The basics of alternative dispute resolution. In Legal and Ethical Issues in Health Occupations. WB Saunders, Philadelphia, 2002.
4. Ibid.

Resources

http://www.Mediate.com
Reference articles on the mediation process.

Associations:

Association for Conflict Resolution
1527 New Hampshire Avenue, NW
Washington, DC 20036
(202) 667-9700
(202) 265-265-1908
http://www.acresolution.org

International Association of Facilitators
7630 West 145th Street, Suite 202
St. Paul, MN 55124
(952) 891-3541
(952) 891-1800 (Fax)

Recommended Reading

Ahronheim, J, Morem, J, Zucherman, C: Ethics in Clinical Practice. Aspen, Gaithersburg, MD, 2000.
Fisher R, Ury W: Getting to Yes, ed. 2. Penguin, New York, 1991.
Madonik, B: I Hear What You Say but What Are You Telling Me? The Strategic Use of Nonverbal Communication in Mediation. San Francisco, Jossey-Bass, 2001.
Marcus, L, Dorn, B, Kritek, P, et al: Renegotiating Health Care—Resolving Conflict to Build Collaboration. Jossey-Bass, San Francisco, 1995.
Ury, W, Brett, J, and Goldberg, S: Getting Disputes Resolved. Designing Systems to Cut the Cost of Conflict. Program on Negotiation at Harvard Law School, Cambridge, MA, 1993.
Weeks, D: The Eight Essential Steps to Conflict Resolution. Penguin Putnam, New York, 1994.

Index

A "t" following a page number indicates a table, "f" indicates a figure, and "b" indicates a box.